Innovative Approaches to Researching Landscape and Health

Innovative Approaches to researching Landscape and Health

Open Space:
People Space 2

Edited by
Catharine Ward Thompson,
Peter Aspinall and Simon Bell

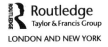

Routledge
Taylor & Francis Group

LONDON AND NEW YORK

First published 2010

This paperback edition published in 2014
by Routledge
2 Park Square, Milton Park, Abingdon, Oxon OX14 4RN

and by Routledge
711 Third Avenue, New York NY 10017

Routledge is an imprint of the Taylor & Francis Group, an informa business

British Library Cataloguing in Publication Data
A catalogue record for this book is available from the British Library

Library of Congress Cataloging-in-Publication Data
Ward Thompson, Catharine.
Innovative approaches to researching landscape and health : open space: people space 2 / Catharine Ward Thompson, Peter Aspinall and Simon Bell.
p. cm.
Includes bibliographical references.
1. Environmental health. 2. Landscape–Health aspects. 3. Medical geography. 4. Landscape–Psychological aspects. 5. Open spaces. 6. Public spaces. 7. Spatial behavior. I. Aspinall, Peter. II. Bell, Simon, 1957 May 24- III. Title.
RA566.7.W37 2010
362.196'98–dc22
2009043120

978-0-415-54911-0 (hbk)
978-1-138-78793-3 (pbk)
978-0-203-85325-2 (ebk)

Typeset by Saxon Graphics Ltd, Derby

Contents

Contents

Acknowledgements

We are very grateful to all our authors for their generous and patient cooperation in preparing their contributions and throughout the many stages to final production of the book. We are fortunate in having had two excellent editorial assistants, Anne Boyle and Nessa Johnston, whose commitment, dedication and tact have helped immeasurably in getting this book to publication; we thank you especially for your care and good humour throughout it all. We are also grateful to Anna Orme who, as OPENspace administrator, has managed the whole process from the original conception and development of the conference ideas, assisted by Lucy Ribchester in liaising with our many conference contributors. We thank the designers and photographers who allowed us to use copyrighted visual material in this book. Finally, we are grateful to our publisher, Alex Hollingsworth, who supported the book in its development, Catherine Lynn and Louise Fox our editorial assistants, and Nick Ascroft, our production editor at Routledge, Taylor and Francis books.

Catharine Ward Thompson, Peter Aspinall and Simon Bell
September 2009

List of contributors

Peter Aspinall is associate director of OPENspace Research Centre and holds a Masters degree in Psychology and a Ph.D. from the Faculty of Medicine at the University of Edinburgh. He has undertaken teaching and research in architecture and landscape architecture at the University of Edinburgh. He was appointed research director of Environmental Studies and research director of the college before moving to the School of the Built Environment at Heriot-Watt University. In addition to being an associate director of OPENspace, he is co-founder of VisionCentre3, a new collaborative research centre for visually impaired people, and has introduced new courses for disabled people on inclusive access and environmental design. He is currently an honorary fellow of the University of Edinburgh and emeritus professor of vision and environment at Heriot-Watt University.

Simon Bell is associate director of OPENspace at the University of Edinburgh and professor of landscape architecture in the Institute of Agriculture and Environment at the Estonian University of Life Sciences, Tartu, Estonia. He is a forester and landscape architect, educated at University of Wales, Bangor, the University of Edinburgh, and recently gained his Ph.D. at the Estonian University of Life Sciences. He is an international expert on forest and park landscapes, outdoor recreation and large-scale landscape evaluation and design. His research interests include landscape and recreation planning and design, and he is author or editor of several books published by Taylor & Francis. He has undertaken many projects in Britain, Canada, the United States, Ireland, Latvia and Russia, and is involved in several European-level research projects.

Inga-Lena Bengtsson is a medical doctor: general practitioner and psychiatrist, licentiate in medicine, and registered psychotherapist. She is working part-time in the therapeutic garden in Alnarp.

William Bird trained as a GP and still practises part time in Reading. He set up the Green Gym and Health Walks from his practice, and is developing the Blue Gym and NHS Forest, which link people with the natural environment. He is strategic health advisor for Natural England and a senior lecturer at the Peninsular

Medical School, Plymouth. He chairs the Outdoor Health Forum and the new Physical Activity Alliance set up with the Department of Health. He is on the expert group to deliver the government report on National Ecosystem Services.

Fiona Bull holds faculty appointments in the School of Population Health at the University of Western Australia and School of Exercise and Sport Science at Loughborough University (UK), and co-directs the British Heart Foundation's National Centre on Physical Activity and Health in the United Kingdom. Professor Bull's work includes a focus on measurement methods, patterns of participation in physical activity in developed and developing countries, environment and health, international physical activity policy analysis and intervention research.

Ruth Conroy Dalton is the Bartlett's Lecturer in Architectural Morphology and Theory. Her research interests include spatial navigation and cognition, visibility field analyses/measures and environment complexity measures. Additionally she is a chartered architect with many years of practice experience.

Nilda G. Cosco is education specialist, the Natural Learning Initiative; research associate professor in the College of Design, and former director of the Center for Universal Design, at North Carolina State University. Dr Cosco holds a degree in educational psychology, Universidad del Salvador, Buenos Aires, Argentina and a Ph.D. in landscape architecture, School of Landscape Architecture, Heriot-Watt University/Edinburgh College of Art, Scotland. Her primary research interest is the impact of outdoor environments on child and family health outcomes such as healthy nutrition, active lifestyles, attention functioning and overall well-being, particularly as they relate to natural components of the built environment. She is also involved in direct intervention and pre/post-evaluation of outdoor improvement programs in childcare centres.

Billie Giles-Corti is director of the Centre for the Built Environment and Health, School of Population Health, University of Western Australia, and a National Health and Medical Research Council senior research fellow. Professor Giles-Corti is recognized internationally for her research on the built form, and in 2006 won an NHMRC Capacity Building Grant to establish the Centre for the Built Environment and Health focusing on the impact of the built environment across the life course. She serves on numerous international, national and state committees, and was awarded a Fulbright Senior Scholar Award in 2007.

Patrik Grahn is a professor in landscape architecture with aim and direction in environmental psychology. He is the head of Research and Development as regards evidence-based health design in landscape architecture and in nature-assisted therapy in the Swedish University of Agricultural Sciences, Alnarp.

Julienne Hanson is professor of house form and culture at University College London. Her research interests include profiling the housing stock for older people, investigating the design of care homes in relation to residents' quality of life, studying the housing needs of older and working-age adults with impaired vision, mainstreaming telecare services, remodelling sheltered housing to extra care housing and designing open spaces in residential areas so as to minimise opportunities for antisocial behaviour.

Harry Heft holds the Henry Chisholm Chair in the Natural Sciences, Department of Psychology, Denison University, Granville, Ohio, USA. He is the author of *Ecological Psychology in Context: James Gibson, Roger Barker, and the Legacy of William James' Radical Empiricism* (Erlbaum, 2001). His research interests include the study of affordances, children's environments, and way-finding. He also publishes in the area of the theory and philosophy of psychology.

Carina Tenngart Ivarsson is a landscape architect and a doctoral candidate concerning evidence-based health design, the Swedish University of Agricultural Sciences, Alnarp.

Brian R. Little received his Ph.D. in psychology from the University of California at Berkeley. He has taught at Oxford, Carleton, Harvard and McGill universities and is currently Distinguished Research Professor in psychology at Carleton University. Dr Little pioneered the study of personal projects analysis as an approach to the study of human personality in context, and his edited book *Personal Project Pursuit: Goals, Action and Human Flourishing* applies this framework to a wide range of theoretical and applied fields. For 2010–11 Professor Little will be Visiting Fellow in the Faculty of Politics, Sociology, Psychology and International Relations at Cambridge University.

Robin C. Moore is professor of landscape architecture and director of the Natural Learning Initiative, North Carolina State University. Professor Moore is an urban designer and design researcher, specialising in child and family urban environments. He previously taught at the University of California, Berkeley and Stanford University. He is a member of the UNESCO Growing Up in Cities international research team. He holds degrees in architecture (London University) and city and regional planning (Massachusetts Institute of Technology). His publications include *Natural Learning* (1997), *Plants For Play* (1993), *The Play For All Guidelines* (1987, 1992) and *Childhood's Domain* (1986).

Ulrika K. Stigsdotter is an associate professor in landscape architecture at the University of Copenhagen. Her research focus is on the connection between people's health and the design of the outdoor environment. The research has an applied perspective and is aimed at both scientists and practitioners and students.

Sjerp de Vries is senior social scientist at Alterra. Wageningen University and Research Centre (WUR), the Netherlands. He has pioneered the use of GIS to research the relationship between green space and health. His research interests focus on the interaction between people and their physical environment, especially landscape appreciation, outdoor recreation behaviour as well as the relationship between nature and green space on the one hand and health, well-being and liveability on the other. Recent work includes a national survey on landscape appreciation, modelling landscape appreciation using GIS data, modelling the need for recreation opportunities (normative) and visits to forests and nature areas (descriptive/predictive), as well as an epidemiological study on the relationship between the amount of green space in residential environments and self-reported health indicators (secondary analysis).

Catharine Ward Thompson is research professor of landscape architecture at the University of Edinburgh. She is Director of OPENspace – the research centre for inclusive access to outdoor environments – based at the University of Edinburgh and Heriot-Watt University, and directs the University Landscape Architecture Ph.D. programme. She is a qualified landscape architect and a fellow of the Landscape Institute. She has led several multidisciplinary research collaborations investigating relationships between environment and health, including I'DGO (Inclusive Design for Getting Outdoors) and Mobility, Mood and Place, which focused on access outdoors and quality of life for older people. She has also led teams in developing innovative research techniques and programmes to elucidate causal links between landscape and health, including the use of biomarkers to investigate environment–body interactions and development of longitudinal studies based on natural experiments to investigate the effects of environmental interventions on wellbeing. She was a member of the Scottish Government's Good Place, Better Health Evaluation Group.

Lisa Wood is a postdoctoral fellow on a National Health and Medical Research Council funded capacity building grant based at the Centre for the Built Environment and Health, School of Population Health, University of Western Australia. Dr Wood has worked with both government and nongovernment organizations, and her research interests include social capital and sense of community, urban design/built environment and health, social determinants of health, life-course approaches to health, Aboriginal health, and the translation of research into policy and practice.

List of figures

List of tables

Foreword

William Bird,
Strategic Health Advisor, Natural England

About half of all GP consultations are related to stress. Stress causes illness. Some of the time the illness is self-limiting but the majority of patients now treated are those with long-term conditions such as depression, heart disease, cancer or asthma that account for 80 per cent of the UK's National Health Service (NHS) budget and a similar amount of GP workload. These long-term conditions can both be caused and exacerbated by constant stress. The stress can be due to poverty, insecurity, bereavement, isolation, poor relationships or bad health itself. But it can also be due to an unhealthy environment, not just from toxins or pollution but because it is barren, deprived of life and isolated from the order of the natural world.

Medicine has little to offer chronic stress. But creating a healthy environment and engaging the person with this environment may have a greater rôle than previously thought. The concept of a healing environment is not new. For people recovering from illness, the healing garden has long been seen as part of convalescence. 1000 yrs ago, St Bernard said of the healing garden in Clairvaux, France: 'The sick man sits upon the green lawn ... he is secure, hidden, shaded from the heat of the day. For the comfort of his pain all kinds of grass are fragrant to his nostrils. The lovely green of herb and tree nourishes his eyes ... the choir of painted birds caresses his ears ... the earth breathes with fruitfulness' (Cooper Marcus and Barnes, p. 10).

Humans have not changed in that 1000 years but attitudes have. The desire for expensive drugs and technology has made medicine the powerful force in healthcare. Life expectancy is the prime metric, with quality of life its poorer relation. There is a noble effort to fight disease and prevent death but this often occurs at the expense of prevention. The natural world is where we belong, where humans evolved and where our genetic memory may still be active. Our balance with the natural world may have a significant rôle in preventing illnesses such as diabetes and depression by buffering the stress from other sources. Finally, society is realising its importance. Getting more people physically active in the natural world is now part of a key government target to tackle the obesity epidemic. The value of the local, natural environment is being recognised by the

Dr William Bird

UK's NHS for its contribution to health with hospitals and clinics, and once again there is interest in incorporating the building into landscaped gardens and parks. The National Institute for Health and Clinical Excellence (NICE) is recommending health walks that take older people to green space specifically for the benefit of their mental health.

This book is timely in that only now are some health professionals trying to understand how we can tap into the resources of the natural environment. But of equal importance is that the UK Government is looking for other ways to reduce health inequalities and improve the mental health problems that costs this country £75 billion a year. Landscape designers, architects and planners may have as much effect on the health of a community as conventional public health measures. *Innovative Approaches to Researching Landscape and Health* is about public health since, if we create a healthy environment, a healthy population will follow.

However, we still do not understand the specific ingredients of the landscape that reduces stress and how the context of this interaction can create different responses in different people at different times. To create a truly Natural Health Service will require harder evidence and a disentangling of these complex relationships, requiring researchers from many different disciplines working together. *Innovative Approaches to Researching Landscape and Health* goes beyond any other text to further our understanding. By every measure, our understanding of what components constitute a healthy environment is of great importance and the researchers who have contributed to this comprehensive book are already the pioneers to help make the world a better and healthier place in which to live.

Reference

Cooper Marcus, C. and Barnes, M. (1999) *Healing Gardens, Therapeutic Benefits and design Recommendations,* New York: Wiley

Preface

Catharine Ward Thompson, Peter Aspinall and Simon Bell

The development of this book builds on the OPENspace research centre's growing expertise in researching access to and experience of green and open space for different groups in society. Since its establishment in 2001, OPENspace has explored the potential offered by urban and green open space at all scales to provide opportunities for outdoor activity, positive engagement with the natural environment, and to build social capital and social inclusion while contributing more generally to people's health and well-being. The first book, published by the centre in 2007 on the theme of 'Open Space: People Space', focused on issues relating to inclusive access outdoors and on how research could inform policy and practice in this field. This current volume takes a more challenging view of where gaps and opportunities lie in researching landscape and health, drawing on a number of recent reviews and mapping of research literature undertaken by OPENspace, as well as its own, innovative research projects. The book arose from contributions made to the second Open Space: People Space conference on the theme of 'Innovative Approaches to Research Excellence in Landscape and Health', organised and hosted by the OPENspace research centre in 2007. In planning the conference, OPENspace researchers were enthusiastic about inviting some of the key researchers whose methods and theories we admired and whose contribution, past and future, was likely to be significant. For three days in late September, researchers and professionals from landscape architecture, urban design, public health and psychology were brought together in Edinburgh to debate the links between landscape and health. We were delighted that so many agreed not only to present at our conference but also to contribute to this book. The authors have since had the opportunity to reflect on the issues and their contribution, so that what is presented here goes beyond that debate and is in many ways a distillation of the key messages emerging. We hope the book will move the debate forward and contribute to an expanding research agenda recognised as important internationally as well as core to the focus of work in OPENspace.

Introduction

*Catharine Ward Thompson, Peter Aspinall
and Simon Bell*

It is a characteristic of developed countries that life expectancy continues to increase yet, at the same time, their populations are experiencing a serious range of health problems, especially associated with diet, lack of exercise and poor mental health. Obesity levels are increasing and, with them, cardiovascular diseases and diabetes, while depression, especially among young people, is being diagnosed more than ever before. This is in part a consequence of our more sedentary but also more stressful lifestyles, as a result of changing family structures, travel demands and work–life balances, and partly a result of increased access to, and promotion of, calorie-rich foods. In a recent advertising campaign by the British Heart Foundation, a poster shows young boys reclining on a sofa surrounded by soft drink bottles and confectionery wrappers, with each one either talking on their mobile phone, watching television or playing with a computer game. The caption beneath reads: 'The early signs of heart disease'. This image is both hard-hitting and accurate and shows how the risks associated with this modern lifestyle are not just affecting adults or older people but often start with habits established early in life.

If we compare this lifestyle with that of 60 or so years ago, we can see that people spend less time outdoors doing activities that help to keep them fit and in good health. In the nineteenth and early twentieth centuries, the public health issues were infectious and communicable diseases or pollution, dangerous working conditions and poor housing, which combined to kill many thousands of people each year. Now that we have largely conquered these (at least in the developed world) through clean water supply, better drainage, pollution control, health and safety regulations, planning of building works and public parks, as well as mass vaccination programmes and better and more effective medical treatment, a new set of challenges faces the public health arena. In the same way that the environment had a major effect on the public health issues of bygone days, so it has an effect on the modern range of concerns, due to the way we have retreated indoors and placed greater reliance on motorised transport.

While many of the issues can be treated by medical interventions and health campaigns – diet advice and treatment to reduce obesity, drugs to reduce stress and alleviate depression, promotion of gyms to increase levels of exercise,

1

for example – there seems to be something missing in the equation. This, we suggest, is the experience of being engaged in activities outdoors - in an environment which can potentially provide multiple benefits.

Many people would agree with the notion that access to fresh air and green space or nature can contribute not only to a healthy body but also to a general sense of well-being and a richer engagement with place. However, there is much that we don't understand about how outdoor environments can make a difference to health. What exactly is it about the landscape that brings benefits, and in what ways? What are the characteristics or qualities of green space necessary to make a difference in terms of people's health for different ages or social groups? Indeed, whether we can adequately identify, describe and quantify these characteristics, and translate an understanding of them into practical policies, which can be implemented by landscape architects and health professionals, is also a matter of contention and debate.

This book arose out of the growing interest in salutogenic environments – environments that support healthy lifestyles and promote well-being – and the need in particular for appropriate methods to research the links between outdoor environments and health (taking the broad, World Health Organization (WHO) definition of health to include physical, mental and social well-being). In this context, the editors set out to explore the challenges that are thrown up by research into the relationship between landscape and health or quality of life. This highlighted the difficulties in understanding the mechanisms and patterns behind any such relationship. We were particularly interested in going beyond the conventional theoretical and methodological approaches that have been used to date, to explore what new approaches might offer both to theory and to practice.. For this reason, we invited international experts who have led the way with new conceptualisations and approaches to contribute their insights from diverse perspectives. The book thus brings together views from a range of disciplines to show how research on people's engagement with the environment can illuminate links between landscape and health in different ways.

Since the book's theme is about salutogenic environments, it has a focus on positive relationships between the outdoor environment and health, rather than on pollutants and environmental risk factors, although inevitably the latter are also implicated to some extent in understanding what benefits the landscape may confer on quality of life. We have taken a broad definition of the landscape, recognising that, in the words of the European Landscape Convention (Council of Europe, 2000), it is "an area of land as perceived by people", so we are interested in more than environment alone. Our conception of landscape embraces the way we experience, engage with and respond to it. The perceptual aspect is important as it encompasses our multiple senses and mental processes, including issues of aesthetics and preference, which may play a significant part of the salutogenic possibilities of certain landscapes. In terms of the categories of landscape used here, it includes urban and rural contexts, public open space and private gardens, urban streets, parks and squares, as well as woodlands and countryside green and natural spaces, including rivers and coastal landscapes. It also focuses on the multidisciplinary nature of research into salutogenic land-scapes, where research and its associated practice must take into account both the person (as an individual and as part of a larger population) and the envi-ronment (as the neighbourhood where an individual or community lives as part of a larger city or region), using a range of approaches coming from the world of public health, environmental psychology, urban design, landscape architecture and horticulture, to name just some of the disciplines represented here.

The choice of authors for the book and the range of approaches and themes – theoretical, methodological and practical – reflect several factors of relevance. The first is the nature of the evidence acceptable to the different arenas of planning, public health and medicine and the robustness of the method-ologies being used. The quality hurdle for health research has a high bar, and one with which researchers from a non-medical background may be unfamiliar, so that developing and supporting research excellence is vital. The second factor is the need to be able not only to demonstrate the links between nature or land-scape and health, but also to begin to identify the causal factors so as to maximise the benefits. The third factor is the need for a better theoretical underpinning to the developing empirical evidence base.

The book is organised into four parts, plus an overview, although there are many themes that span several parts and chapters. One of the key theories that runs through the book is that of 'affordance', as initially developed by James Gibson in the 1970s, linking environment and human behaviour, or opportunities for action. In Part I, Harry Heft's opening chapter sets out the basis for this theory in the psychology of environmental perception and goes on to articulate the value of such a conceptualisation for researchers today. He empha-sises the relational importance of the concept, arguing for an understanding of environmental perception that links the properties of the environment to their functional significance for an individual. He highlights the value of affordance in offering a dynamic understanding of how environments are experienced by users in the course of action - a key issue of relevance to investigating healthy activity in the landscape. In Chapter 2, Robin Moore and Nilda Cosco take up the theme of affordance and apply it to children's environments, reflecting Eleanor Gibson's contribution to the concept through her work on infant and child development. They also draw on Roger Barker's theoretical framework of 'behaviour settings' as the basis for their detailed exposition of behaviour mapping as a practical research tool. They show how such tools can be used to identify specific environ-mental features associated with higher levels of physical activity or imaginative engagement, through children's play. Together, these first two chapters illustrate the value of a strong theoretical basis to inform practical tools for undertaking research on the links between landscape and healthy behaviour.

Part II of the book presents evidence on the relationship between landscape and health, moving from an overview of evidence for the different ways that landscape, especially green space, might benefit health at a population level, to a detailed exposition of one landscape and the evidence of its therapeutic effects on a very particular group of people. In Chapter 3, Sjerp de Vries examines four categories of potential mechanisms linking 'nearby nature' and health. 'Nearby nature' encompasses green space and natural or semi-natural environments near to people's everyday living and work places. He looks at the evidence for such environments offering health benefits through mitigating air pollution, reducing stress, stimulating physical activity and facilitating social contact, and considers what the implications might be for landscape design. In Chapter 4, Fiona Bull, Billie Giles-Corti and Lisa Wood take the theme of landscape and physical activity further, outlining the many methodological issues and challenges in undertaking and interpreting research on this theme. They argue that an understanding of environments that support and encourage physical activity provides a strong basis for a population-level approach to health and this, in turn, should inform landscape and urban design. By contrast, in Chapter 5, Patrik Grahn, Carina Tenngart Ivarsson and Inga-Lena Bengtsson explore links between landscape and health through stress reduction, and take a particular therapeutic garden and individual responses as the focus of their research. The value of action research is highlighted in this chapter, showing how a longitudinal programme of therapy within a landscape setting can contribute to knowledge and theory building, informing both our understanding of links between natural environments and well-being, and practical considerations for environmental design.

Part III explores different perspectives on methodology, highlighting approaches whose potential for researching landscape and health may not have been fully realised to date. In Chapter 6, Brian Little's work on personal projects provides a valuable framework for understanding, at the individual level, how the environment may support or thwart plans and opportunities for action. He underlines the importance of understanding differences in the 'fit' between environment and each person's needs and desires, their personal projects, and offers a method to help illuminate the motivations behind affordances for certain individuals or groups. This offers insights into the diversity of landscape experience that may be necessary in salutogenic environments and underlines the need for choice in the environments of daily life. Peter Aspinall, in Chapter 7, takes the theme of choice and examines the difficulties in researching people's preferences and choice in meaningful ways. He then illustrates the value of conjoint analysis as a method to address some of these challenges through examples relating to choice in housing and in local park planning and design, showing how different subgroups' preferences can also be elicited.

Part IV looks at applications of research methods in practice, with contributions from architecture and landscape architecture on themes of spatial structure, landscape design and landscape use. Bill Hillier and Julienne Hanson were responsible for one of the great innovations in analytical tools for understanding spatial patterns of human use in the built environment – space syntax – developed at University College London in the 1970s. Ruth Conroy Dalton and Julienne Hanson, in Chapter 8, take the concepts and applications of space syntax, as they have been developed and refined in the intervening years, and explore their use in a more natural landscape context. They identify the challenges involved and argue for interdisciplinary collaboration to resolve ways of using space syntax to quantify the experience of being in and moving through the landscape. In Chapter 9, Catharine Ward Thompson brings a landscape architect's perspective to such challenges, pointing to the particular qualities of the landscape and people's engagement with it that must be taken into account. She illustrates how George Kelly's personal construct theory and Brian Little's personal projects approach can illuminate understanding of relationships between neighbourhood environments and older people's well-being. She highlights the challenges in assessing the 'walkability' of built or natural environments and illustrates new approaches and tools developed at OPENspace research centre to assess how aspects of the landscape may support or inhibit use.

In the Conclusion, Simon Bell takes an overview of the book's content and summarises the debates, challenges and opportunities identified. He makes a personal assessment of the key issues and possible ways forward for researching the relationships between landscape and health in the future. He highlights the need for a strengthening of the theoretical ground on which such research is based and for more work to understand the mechanisms behind any observed relationships. He also points to the opportunities that computer-based technologies such as GIS and virtual environment modelling offer in taking the research forward.

This book offers a basis for beginning to address the challenges of innovative research in landscape and health. The theories presented offer new insights across disciplines and fields of action with real opportunities for synergistic aligning of methodologies and, just as important, illuminating interpretation of results. Heft's development of affordance theory has already inspired a number of researchers working in environment–behaviour landscape studies, as chapters by Moore and Cosco, Grahn and colleagues and Bell illustrate, since the transactional relationship between person and environment is at the core of the theory of affordance. Brian Little's work helps us understand the motivations behind affordances and *why* the relationships between individuals, their projects and their environment may lead to stress or to restoration. Both Heft and Little remind us that these relationships are idiosyncratic and therefore the same place can have multiple meanings and, indeed, be experienced as a different place by different people.

5

Heft, de Vries and Grahn and colleagues discuss theories about the evolutionary basis for perception of and engagement with the landscape, which may have an increasing role to play in our understanding of the therapeutic benefits of the landscape. This is especially important for a world population increasingly characterised by poor mental health and stress as well as physical inactivity.

Moore and Cosco underline how we need to understand and value a real, embodied experience of the physical environment for children today, since the omnipresent virtual world of computers and television increasingly offers the disengaged 'looking at' experience of life that Heft decries. Ecological models of engagement with the world are part of their approach and are, indeed, a common theme discussed by many authors in this book. Ward Thompson discusses the range of scales with which landscape researchers need to engage, and Bull and colleagues show how socio-ecological models have reinvigorated research approaches to environment and health relationships, with multilevel modelling increasing the sophistication of such approaches. These techniques highlight the importance of examining a range of scales and socio-spatial contexts if environmental design is to be effective in supporting human well-being.

Addressing the need to deliver evidence or guidance that planners and designers will use, Aspinall offers practical approaches to understanding how changes in the environment will impact on people's choice, with particular emphasis on choice relating to action, rather than simply attitudinal change. The links with affordance and with personal projects are evident here, as in the work of Grahn and colleagues and Ward Thompson's research. Conroy Dalton and Hanson's research builds on the theories of space syntax towards developing better predictive tools for understanding patterns of landscape use and here, too, they emphasise the contribution from environmental psychology (including affordance theory) as well as practical methods from landscape architecture (including new information technologies highlighted by Bell) to record and characterise the landscape.

Since this book first appeared, interest in research on links between landscape and health has grown, as has policy-makers' demand for evidence on what characterises salutogenic environments. For example, the UK's National Institute for Health and Clinical Excellence (NICE) has an ongoing review of evidence to support its public health guidance on physical activity and the environment (NICE, 2008). The volume and quality of evidence is increasing, although it can take many years to complete a well-founded study as recommended, in their different ways, by our authors here. New methodologies have also been developed, partly in response to the refinement of technologies such as GPS recorders and accelerometers, that make it easier and more affordable to collect data on individuals' locations and behaviours, but also in response to interest in psychophysiological evidence of environment-body interactions when people are in built or natural environments. Our own research centre (OPENspace) has recently contributed to development of methodologies that open up new possibilities for understanding environment-body interactions. Firstly we have been able to obtain evidence using a physiological biomarker (cortisol levels in saliva samples) that suggests neighbourhood green space is associated not only with a reduction in feelings of stress but also with healthier diurnal patterns of stress hormones in the body (Ward Thompson et al., 2012; Roe et al, 2013). This supports the work of others (e.g. Park et al, 2007; Van den Berg & Custer, 2010; Lee et al, 2011) in pointing to a pathway through which the environment may impact on health. Secondly, by use of a neural cap originally developed for video gaming, we have been able to monitor brain activity (EEG signals) while people are walking through an urban environment. Results show changes in brain activity as people move from a busy shopping area into green space that are in keeping with restoration theory, i.e. the move into green space was associated with a reduction in arousal and increase in meditative activity (Aspinall et al., 2013). Such developments enhance the techniques available for future research while the innovative methods, theories and approaches outlined in this book remain equally valuable and pertinent. They offer a guide to future, robust research and point to what is still needed in terms of evidence.

Ultimately, we are interested in how researchers can provide and present good evidence that is useful for policy makers and practitioners. This reflective examination of the field should help the research, policy and practice community in framing, commissioning, undertaking and applying the results of research in a more organised and focused way. In particular we hope that researchers working in the field will find the discussion within these pages of help in framing research questions and developing appropriate methods. We suggest there is much that landscape design, planning and management can offer for well-being, not only to support health and avoid illness but, further, to provide choice and options for human flourishing through support for individual fulfilment and meaningful engagement with the world. We hope that this book will inspire and encourage new research towards this end.

References

Aspinall, P., Mavros, P., Coyne, R. & Roe, J. (2013) 'The urban brain: analysing outdoor physical activity with mobile EEG.' *British Journal of Sports Medicine*, bjsports-2012-091877 Published Online First: 6 March 2013.

Council of Europe (2000) *European Landscape Convention*, Strasbourg: Council of Europe.

Lee, J., Park, B.J., Tsunetsugu, Y., Ohira, T., Kagawa, T. & Miyazaki, Y. (2011) 'Effect of forest bathing on physiological and psychological responses in young Japanese male subjects.' *Public Health 125*, 93–100.

NICE (2008) *Physical Activity and the Environment, Public Health Guidance 8*, Manchester: National Institute for Health and Clinical Excellence. Available online at: www.nice.org.uk

Catharine Ward Thompson, Simon Bell and Peter Aspinall

Park, B.J., Tsunetsugu, Y., Kasetani, T., Hirano, H., Kagawa, T., Sato, M. & Miyazaki, Y. (2007) 'Physiological effects of Shinrin-yoku (taking in the atmosphere of the forest)—Using salivary cortisol and cerebral activity as indicators.' *Journal of Physiological Anthropology, 26*, 123–128.
Roe, J.J., Ward Thompson, C., Aspinall, P., Brewer, M.J., Duff, E.I., Miller, D., Mitchell, R. & Clow, A. (2013) 'Green space and stress: Evidence from cortisol measures in deprived urban communities.' *International Journal of Environmental Research and Public Health, 10*, 4086–4103.
Ward Thompson, C., Roe, J., Aspinall, P., Mitchell, R., Clow, A. & Miller, D. (2012) 'More green space is linked to less stress in deprived communities: Evidence from salivary cortisol patterns.' *Landscape and Urban Planning* 105, 221–229.
Van den Berg, A.E. & Custer, M.H.G. (2010) 'Gardening promotes neuroendocrine and affective restoration from stress.' *Journal of Health Psychology, 16*, 3–11.

Part I

Affordances in the landscape: a theoretical approach

Chapter 1

Affordances and the perception of landscape:
an inquiry into environmental perception and aesthetics

Harry Heft

What is the nature of our experience in environments? Travel diaries and nature writing are filled with first-hand descriptions of environments. These accounts range from the pedestrian and mundane to the artful and even inspirational. However, for the purposes of systematic analysis expected of scientific inquiry and for the practical concerns of environmental design, we must also delve deeper than mere description. A more analytical path creating possibilities for experimental investigation is essential. This path, though, is not without its hazards.

Sometimes *analyses* of perceiving – which after all are intellectual exercises – can overshadow some of the essential, immediate qualities of perceptual experience. This is because what researchers and designers assume is *experienced* often becomes entangled with their suppositions about *how* perceiving occurs. If uncertainties surrounding perceptual processes were well settled, then this might not seem too problematic. But such is not the case. Even after centuries of inquiry, accounts of perception continue to be contested, and our understanding is murky at best.

The overarching thesis of this chapter is as follows: *the way that environmental psychologists and designers think about processes of perceiving has a direct bearing on how they think about the visual experience of landscape, and in turn how they approach landscape perception research and aesthetics.*

Research within environmental psychology concerning environmental perception and aesthetics over the past three decades has been dominated by a specific approach to perception, and to visual perception in particular. This approach, which can be traced at least as far back as Renaissance and Enlightenment science, has shaped the specific way that twentieth-century research in environmental aesthetics has proceeded both methodologically and conceptually. By the same token, it has led researchers to construe narrowly the nature of aesthetic experience in environments.

We begin by examining the dominant approach to environmental perception and aesthetics and its theoretical assumptions. Some of its limitations are best identified in contrast to an alternative perspective, the ecological approach, which will be taken up in due course.

Thinking about perceiving

The modern study of visual perception in psychology has its origins in sixteenth and seventeenth-century philosophical inquiries concerning the nature of knowing (epistemology). It is essential to emphasize two related points about this historical period of inquiry at the outset:

- These efforts *precede* any serious scientific consideration of *biological evolution*. This historical fact partially explains why the *functional role* that perceiving plays in the activities of organisms receives little attention in this early work.
- The central concerns of these inquiries were *epistemological*, with questions such as 'what are the origins of knowledge?' and 'what role does vision play in knowledge acquisition?' at the forefront. Clearly, these are *not* central concerns for visual scientists today, much less for those studying environmental perception. But it is important to recognize that the impetus for most early theories of vision was such epistemological concerns.

Taken jointly, these two points highlight that the dominant, contemporary approaches to visual perception, and perception more generally, arose in a pre-Darwinian age in order to address a set of epistemological rather than functional questions.

A third feature of these inquiries, in this case specific to the analysis of vision, also needs to be pointed out. Vision is conceptualized as primarily an image-capturing process. From otherwise divergent philosophers such as Descartes and Berkeley, the assumption is maintained that the starting point for an analysis of vision is the pattern of light projected on the retinas of the eyes.

The reasons for this way of thinking about vision are tied up, in part, with the discovery that light from environmental features can pass through a narrow aperture and project an image of these features on the rear surface of a hollow chamber, such as a mammalian eye. This finding led to the invention of the camera obscura, a device which had a profound impact on creating techniques for representational painting (Pastore, 1971; Steadman, 1995). Importantly, these developments converged with the proposal based on anatomical investigations that the mammalian eye operates in this manner. By the early nineteenth century, experiments with pinhole camera devices in conjunction with methods to capture traces of light chemically resulted in the development of the photographic camera (Benson, 2008). From the perspective of theories of vision, this way of thinking set the major problems that an explanation of vision must address, namely, how three-dimensional qualities of visual experience are recovered from a static, two-dimensional retinal image (Gregory, 1990).

A watershed event occurred in the mid-nineteenth century which altered the type of questions being asked about vision. This event, of course, was the Darwinian revolution. And with it the questions concerning vision began to shift from solely epistemological ones to more functional ones – namely, what role does perceiving play in the life processes of organisms? It is critical to note, however, that *while the nature of the question shifted, the approach to vision did not*. That is, while there was a shift from an epistemological to a functional orientation in the study of vision, *the original sixteenth/seventeenth-century explanatory frameworks were adopted without much reassessment*. They were, and remain today, adjusted slightly to make allowances for functional questions, but fundamentally they have not changed.

The continuity of these earlier approaches to those of the present day can be seen in several ways:

- Although vision researchers no longer talk of stimulus input as if it produced a picture or image in the visual system, but instead refer to patterns of neural firings in the visual pathway, *the image-like properties of stimulation* (for example, forms, patterns, elements) continue to dominate the discourse (Marr, 1983). This proclivity clearly marks writings in environmental aesthetics.
- Directly related to this point is the assumption that the perceiver is stationary, temporarily positioned like a camera at a fixed observation point. From this perspective, the perceiver is 'at a remove' from the perceived, adopting the stance of a detached spectator rather than that of an engaged agent (Dewey, 1948).
- Psychological processes tend to be conceptualized as distinct and compartmentalized. Hence, perception is considered to be one process, touching another process, moving yet another process, and so on – a tradition long called 'faculty psychology' which still holds psychology in its grip (Uttal, 2001).

One final, and admittedly rather philosophical, stance needs to be mentioned, which marks most theories of vision from Descartes to the present day.

Because of the three factors (among others) just mentioned – that perceiving involves image-like input to a stationary perceiver, with the sensory systems operating as separate channels – there would appear to be an enormous disparity between the environment as it is conveyed in stimulus input and the environment as it is experienced. Directly stated, the way we experience the environment would seem to be much *underdetermined* by stimulus input. Take the case of continuity of visual experience. Whereas we experience the environment in a continuous, ongoing manner, the stimulus input is typically assumed to be temporally discrete, providing information about what can be seen with a succession of eye fixations. Hence, it would seem that temporally continuous experience is underdetermined by stimulus input. The continuity that is experienced must then be attributable to constructive processes 'in the head' which assemble the discrete inputs into a dynamic, ongoing stream. From a theoretical standpoint, this move (and others like it) preserves a dualism that was initiated by sixteenth-century Cartesian thought between physical stimulation issuing from a world 'out there' and a wholly subjective, inner, mental realm. In contemporary cognitive psychology, this subjective realm of mental phenomena is underwritten by mental representations, schema, mental images, cognitive maps, plans, scripts and the like. The result is that our experience of environments is considered to be necessarily subjective.

Apart from the unresolvable philosophical challenges that such a view creates (Edelman, 1993; McGinn, 2000), this position would seem to present insurmountable obstacles for designers who are at work in the public, socially shared realm. To wit, *if the environment is experienced privately by countless separate individuals, how do we even begin to think about a common, public domain?*

More broadly, we can locate this theoretical perspective within a taxonomy of meta-theories ('world hypotheses') developed by Pepper (1942), and later applied to theories relevant to environmental psychology by Altman and Rogoff (1987). Specifically, the dualistic, image-capturing approach to visual perception is an instance of an *interactionist* worldview. This worldview is characterized by taking the environment and the person as two distinguishable, separate realms. On the one hand, there is the physical world that can be described rigorously using measures of light, sound, chemical composition and so on, or geometrically in terms of patterns and forms. In marked contrast, there is the subjective realm of mental phenomena. A hallmark of interactionist theories is that occurrences in the environmental domain are viewed as having linear (unidirectional) causal effects, producing mental states in the organism. Accordingly, much of perception research since the 1950s has involved trying to unravel the causal chain from optical stimulation to brain processes resulting in our mental experience of the world.

Environmental perception and aesthetics

When environmental psychologists turned their attention to the perception of landscape in the late 1960s and early 1970s, this interactionist approach to perception was adopted without much critical scrutiny. Most of this research attempted to answer questions such as 'why are some environments preferred more so than others?' and 'what makes for a pleasing environment?'

Wohlwill (1968, 1976, 1983) initiated some of the earliest of these investigations, which were formulated as an effort to identify the environmental bases for curiosity and exploratory behaviour, and ultimately preference (Berlyne, 1971). This research programme rested on the assumption that environments could be characterized as possessing varying degrees of arousal-producing stimulus properties, such as the degree of complexity and harmony/disharmony among its features. It was assumed that individuals tended to prefer intermediate levels of arousal, and so environments that produced these levels (that is, that were intermediate in degree of complexity and so on) would generally be preferred (Heft, 1998). This approach can be seen as a partial extension of Hullian drive-reduction thinking to the domain of environmental perception. From such a perspective, the motivational bases for behaviour are attributed to efforts that, in most cases, lower arousal from some elevated levels. Whereas in a Hullian model, elevated arousal is ultimately tied to essential tissue needs (for example, hunger), Berlyne's extension looked to environmental conditions as precipitating factors.

A second line of research developed initially as a critique of this prior effort (Kaplan, Kaplan and Wendt, 1972). Although less clearly grounded theoretically than the Berlyne-inspired approach just described, it was rooted in the information-processing models of 1970s cognitive psychology. Broadly, this approach, championed over the years by the Kaplans (for example, R. Kaplan and S. Kaplan, 1989; S. Kaplan and R. Kaplan, 1982) considers the relationship between, on the one hand, the composition of an environmental scene conceptualized as a two-dimensional image or picture, and on the other hand, preference. More specifically, a distinction was drawn between two types of properties: those two-dimensional properties such as complexity or coherence that are present in 'the two dimensional aspects, or picture plane before one ... that is immediately available' (R. Kaplan and S. Kaplan, 1989: 52); and those properties suggested in the picture plane, such as mystery and legibility, that lead one to infer what lies beyond that which is immediately available. Because visual perception is assumed to operate on only what is immediately available from a *fixed observation point*, rather than being a dynamic process, the implications of exploration for perceiving were not seriously considered.

This image-based (picture plane) model has led to a substantial body of research concerning the stimulus correlates of environmental preference (for example, R. Kaplan and S. Kaplan, 1989). In recent years, this line of thinking has shifted emphasis somewhat in an effort to offer an explanation for the apparently restorative psychological effects of 'green' natural settings (for example, Kaplan, 1995; Hartig and Staats, 2006; Herzog et al., 1997). This explanation rests on the notion of 'attentional fatigue', which has few counterparts in the contemporary psychological and neuroscience literature, although it may resonate with everyday observation and reprise some work on attentional load conducted in the 1970s and on vigilance in earlier decades. William James's psychological writings are often cited as an influence, but as Kaplan (1995) duly notes, James did not posit that attention was something that could be depleted. Indeed, James did not view attention as having a limited capacity (see James, 1909; Meyers, 1986; Spelke, Hirst and Neisser, 1976).

In spite of the theoretical differences between Wohlwill's research program and that of the Kaplans, both camps had far more in common than not. Both shared the outlook that landscape perception research proceeds *by identifying stimulus properties considered independently of the ongoing actions of the perceiver*. That is, critically, in both approaches, the perceiver is taken to be an observer of the environmental layout standing apart from it while surveying its qualities or possibilities. Any considerations of the perceiver's actions are minimal, or at best promissory notes that are rarely cashed.

There is much of value that has come out of these lines of research. I cannot but wonder, however, whether those gains have more to do with 'taking in a view' of landscapes, or most often their photographic surrogates, in a detached manner and at a remove from them, rather than perceiving landscapes in the course of active engagement. (I shall return to this point.) If so, such 'interactionist' formulations of perceiving uncritically applied to environmental perception might broadly constrain research in landscape perception, and in turn, overlook some essential properties of environments from the point of view of an active perceiver.

Experiencing landscape and the ecological approach

Let us now return to the question prompted by the Darwinian revolution: what role does perceiving play in the everyday functioning of an organism? One answer to this question is that perceiving is the process by which the organism stays informed about its immediate environment. That is obviously true; and yet it is a somewhat superficial answer. It does not get to the heart of the nature of perceiving. In order to appreciate perceiving more fully, it is necessary to consider it in the context of the *ongoing life processes of the organism*. For this we shall need to take a longer view of the place of perceiving in the evolution of living things.

Acting, exploring, and perceiving

Clearly, it is essential that all living things obtain the resources necessary for their survival. The problem is that often these resources are not close at hand. This challenge has been met in various ways. In the case of plant life, we find geotropic and phototropic growth responses of roots and shoots. Among animals there has been the selection of a variety of bodily structures and the functions they make possible, which permit organisms to propel themselves through water, to fly through the air, to burrow in the ground, to climb in trees, and to walk, crawl and manoeuvre on surfaces.

But animacy is not enough. Living things must be able to *detect* a resource once they reach it; and further, most animate beings require some perceptual means to *guide* their actions and to support exploration, sometimes over considerable distances. Perceiving *and* acting, then, are fundamental to nearly all complex organisms for sustaining life. Critically, these processes operate *synergistically*. That is, perceiving guides actions, and actions facilitate perceiving.

Let me illustrate this latter point by way of a very simple demonstration. If a familiar object is placed in the hand of a blindfolded individual who has been instructed to keep her hand stationary, it will be quite difficult for her to identify the object. However, as soon as she is permitted to manipulate the object, to turn it in her hand and to examine it tactually, identification is usually quite easy (see Heller and Myers, 1983). What does this simple exercise tell us? It indicates something that is commonly, and in retrospect, surprisingly overlooked in discussions of perceiving – something quite simple and yet profound. Perceiving typically involves more than the passive imposition of stimulation on receptors. Actions participate in perceiving in a fundamental way.

Perceptual systems

It cannot be overemphasized that examples such as this case of active touch represent *normative* instances of perceiving rather than exceptions. The least bit of observation of living things (when they are unconstrained by research equipment, that is) reveals that organisms are continually active, turning their head, moving around while looking, as well as feeling, sniffing, tasting, cocking an ear and so forth. Individuals employ these actions in the process of perceiving the environment.

Perceiving and acting are intertwined. Indeed, the separate terms 'perception' and 'action' can be somewhat misleading. More accurately put, *perceiving* is a perception–action process. In his groundbreaking book *The Senses Considered as Perceptual Systems*, J. J. Gibson (1966) explained in detail why consideration of stimulation imposed on receptors alone is insufficient as an account of perceiving, and he offered – as the book's title indicates – a radical reformulation of perceiving. Returning to the above example, perceiving an object by touch from a *perceptual systems* perspective involves the collaboration of movements of the hand and stimulation of the haptic sensory system. What purpose do these movements serve in perceiving? They produce a changing array of stimulation, and in so doing, allow the selective nature of perceiving to isolate or 'foreground' unchanging structure specifying the object (Gibson, 1966).

Likewise, from a perceptual systems view, *looking* includes movements of the eyes, head, and entire body of the individual. These actions in moving about produce a changing array in the reflected light that makes the identifying structure (invariant information) specific to features of the surround easier to detect (for more details, see Gibson, 1966, 1979; Heft, 2001; Reed and Jones, 1982; Michaels and Carello, 1981; Reed, 1996).

At first glance, this account of perceiving might seem to involve little more than adding movements of the body to a standard treatment of perceiving. But in fact, *it necessitates a complete transformation of the standard accounts of perception* as the receiving of stimulation to one of perception/action. This alternative approach to perceiving, which is partially rooted in William James's writings and those of John Dewey (Heft, 2001), is referred to as *the ecological approach*, in part because of its emphasis on the dynamic, reciprocal relationship between perceiver and environment (Gibson, 1979).

How does the position that visual perception is a process of detecting what is immediately in view to a stationary perceiver in the 'two-dimensional picture plane' hold up in relation to the view that organisms are fundamentally animate and that perceiving is best characterized as a perception–action process? It would seem, not very well. If animate organisms are continuously moving for the purposes of facilitating perceiving, which in turn supports all manner of activities of daily living, then visual perception considered as a process of solely detecting what is 'immediately present' would seem unworkable.

There are several problems here. First, what does 'immediately present' actually mean? If it refers to what can be perceived 'from here', introduce a moving perceiver and 'here' is an elusive place. At best, one might say that what is being detected are 'snapshot-like' images at each momentary pause in eye movements. But then one must speculate that there exists somewhere complicated brain machinery that continuously assembles these discrete 'snapshots' (Hochberg, 1971). Such a mechanism may exist, but I am unaware of any evidence for it. I suspect that it is unlikely to be found. Perceiving is more likely to be a continuous, dynamic, 'online' (immediate) process.

Second, especially significant from a functional standpoint, as the passive versus active touch demonstration indicates, a stationary animal would be considerably *disadvantaged* when it comes to perceiving environmental features. The fact is that action facilitates detection of environmental properties (Gibson, 1966; Lee, 1976; Lederman and Klatzky, 1987; Mark et al., 1990). The selection of a wide variety of action possibilities or 'action systems' (Reed, 1982) across all types of organisms, from insects to birds, fish and humans, can be viewed with respect to the essential place of animacy in perceiving.

In the end, however, what are most critical are the tangible research directions a perspective offers and the fruits of that work. It is precisely the research outcomes stemming from the ecological approach that have drawn the most attention to it. For present purposes, let us consider only one consequence of adopting an ecological perspective which raises novel possibilities about what properties of the environment are perceived.

Perceiving affordances

From an ecological perspective, what is immediately perceived is not an array of two-dimensional forms, or picture-like images, or mental constructions of the environment, much less stimuli, but rather what the environment affords – that is, its *affordances*.

Let me explain this perspective using a hypothetical, but common-place example. Imagine a trail through a wooded area leading to a pond. An indi-vidual could walk along the trail until reaching the impasse of the pond, which is an impediment to further locomotion. The reasons for these outcomes are plain. Whereas the relatively unobstructed ground surface of the trail will support the weight of the striding hiker, the water surface of the pond will not. Stated differ-ently, the trail *affords* walking-on for a person, but the pond does not. Such is not the case, however, for all organisms. For example, a fisher spider (*Dolomedes triton*), a North American pond-dweller, can walk on both surfaces.

What does this simple comparison indicate? It shows that a feature of an environment can be described in both *organism-independent* ways and *organism-dependent* ways. As to the former, one could readily describe the physical properties (for example, material composition) of the trail and of the pond apart from consideration of any specific organism. However, if our aim is to offer a description of the functional possibilities of an environment, such an account must necessarily be offered relative to some individual organism. That is, a functional description requires a *relational* stance.

Simple enough; but now consider some philosophical implications of this example. Where do the functional possibilities of these surfaces, their affordances, reside? Are they properties of the environment, or are they prop-erties of the organism? From the point of view of standard formulations of visual perception and its interactionist worldview, these two options – the environment or the organism – are the *only* ones available to choose from. But clearly, neither of these options will do. The affordance of a 'walk-on-able' surface refers to the *relationship* of an organism to an environmental property. Affordances are *rela-tional* properties of the environment taken with reference to a specific individual.

19

Defining an affordance

When Gibson (1979) introduced the concept of affordance it was fairly novel in the psychological literature (Heft, 2001). That is no longer the case. It has been appearing with growing frequency over the years, but not always with much definitional specificity among environmental psychologists. Terms that are lacking in specificity soon become vacuous, and the distinctive contribution they might make to systems of thought becomes lost. There is a voluminous literature on affordances as such, and some of the finer points of the concept are still being debated (see Jones, 2003). Still, there is a wide agreement among ecological psychologists as to the essential features of this idea.

Further, in spite of the increasing familiarity of the concept of affordances, it is necessary to take full measure of this concept. Just as the idea of a *perceptual system* does not suggest merely adding action to standard image-capturing accounts of vision, the concept of *affordance* is not just an additional way of describing environments that can supplement existing modes of description, such as physical or material accounts. It is far more radical than that.

Altman and Rogoff (1987) accurately locate affordances within a *trans-actionalist* worldview that rejects the interactionist position that environment and organism are separate, though interacting, entities. From a transactionalist perspective, *entities exist and manifest the qualities that they do by virtue of their relationships within a dynamic system of mutual influences*. The philosophical groundwork for transactionalism as it is manifested within psychology was laid by William James and John Dewey, among others (see Heft, 2001). In contemporary writing, some of the best expressions of a transactional worldview appear in the literature of developmental biology (for example, Lickliter and Honeycutt, 2003; Oyama, 1985) and motor development (Thelen and Smith, 1995).

Affordances are perceptible properties of the environment that have functional significance for an individual. Consider, for example, a ledge approximately 150 mm (6 inches) high, located in a public area. It may function as an edge marker for adults, delineating one region of the landscape from another, and it may be liable to be tripped over if an adult is not paying attention to where she is walking. Other than those two functions, it has few other apparent uses for an adult. However, for a young child such a ledge is typically a very salient functional feature: it can function as a place to sit, as a structure to climb on and to leap over, and as a challenging edge on which to walk. Casual observation as well as data from observations of children at play (Heft, 1988) attest to the allure of these affordances.

A more detailed consideration of this example will illuminate what it means to claim that affordances are relational properties of the environment. Why is it that this ledge is likely to be perceived and used as a place to sit on by young children, but not so for adults? The reason should be obvious. The ledge considered relative to a small child – its height relative to the child's leg length – is a feature that affords sitting on. In contrast, the relative scaling for a typical adult is all wrong. So if it is said that the ledge affords 'sitting-on' for a child, what is the nature of this affordance property? Is 'sit-on-able' a property of the ledge considered independently of any prospective individual? Clearly not. It is a relational property.

Can affordances be defined in a more rigorous way? After all, physical measures may seem to be preferable to affordances if for no other reason than that they can be specified in systematic and precise ways. In principle, this is also true of affordances. In a seminal study, Warren (1984) has shown that a horizontal surface is perceived as 'step-up-on-able' by an individual if the ratio of step height to perceiver's leg length is a specifiable value. This value (a pi number) captures a property of the environment scaled with reference to the body. Because leg length can vary substantially across individuals (for example, children versus adults), obviously there is not a uniform height required for all steps. However, the pi number (for example, step height/leg length ratio) that specifies a 'step-on-able surface' is constant across all individuals. This finding demonstrates that this affordance is a *specifiable property* of the environment taken relative to a person. (For other examples, see Turvey, Shockley and Carello, 1999; Lee, 1976; Mark et al., 1990.)

These seemingly simple observations, validated by experimental findings, have deep implications for psychological theory. They reveal a *domain of relational properties* which has been overlooked when environment and person are considered independently. Affordances are not mental constructs that a perceiver subjectively imposes on the world, nor are they interpretations of a physical world in the 'head' of a perceiver. Affordances are properties of the environment that are both objectively real *and* psychologically significant. In the dualistic framework invoked by standard psychological theory, objective reality is attributed to a physical domain that stands apart from the individual; and psychological significance is a subjective property residing 'in' the individual. Affordances transcend this historically problematic dichotomy.

Affordances of the landscape

To date, as we have seen, most of the research in environmental perception has attempted to identify stimulus correlates, or image-like properties, that are predictive of perceivers' positive assessments of environments. The standard methodological paradigm is to ask perceivers to evaluate landscapes as represented by photographic displays on rating scales provided by the investigator. Typically, perceivers are asked to offer relative preference judgements of these displays.

What is striking about this method is that participants in these investigations do little more than look at photographic displays and provide check marks on a rating scale. In effect, these assessments are akin to gazing at the landscape through a window. This analogy is intended to indicate that what is at issue here is not solely the two-dimensional character of these photographic displays of landscapes, nor the obvious framing and the absence of occlusion effects that reveal them to be photographs as such. Just as critical, if not more so, is the detached, passive stance of the perceiver standing apart from that which is being viewed. It is precisely for this reason that the defence that judgments of photographs and judgments in situ are highly correlated is really beside the point. *Both* circumstances assume a passive observer.

If the findings from this body of research were stated as applying primarily to conditions where perceivers 'take in a view' of the landscape from a fixed vantage point, then that would be one thing. But these findings are rarely couched in that limited way. Instead, they are presented as being characteristic of environmental perception and aesthetics in a general sense. If, however, researchers (and designers) are interested in the experience of environments in the course of action, it is not self-evident that this approach speaks to this commonplace phenomenon.

Affordances are the *functional properties* of an environmental feature for an individual. Although one can often perceive affordances from a fixed vantage point, they are all about action. They indicate what one can do in some setting, and what activities may be ruled out. How would an affordance analysis of landscape proceed? Initially, one would need to identify the potential affordance properties of environments from the standpoint of prospective users of those settings. To do this, the *activities* of individuals representative of the group (for example, school-age children) could be observed in the environment of interest (for example, a city park), or alternatively in one quite similar to it. Systematically observing activities in everyday environments will begin to illuminate some of the affordance properties of the environment.

To illustrate, some time ago I applied an affordance perspective to a pre-existing detailed record of a day in the life of a nine-year-old boy (Heft, 1988). This data source was one of a number of records produced by Roger Barker and his co-workers based on observations of elementary school children as they went about their day's activities in a small town. In my analysis, Barker's published record of 'one boy's day' was examined by noting every instance of an observed action recorded in the transcript of activities. From these behavioural criteria, the environmental features cited in the observational record that supported each of these actions were then enumerated. The total list of supportive environmental features was then categorized according to common actions. In other words, the environmental features were clustered as to their affordance properties. The result of this analysis was a catalogue of affordances available for that boy on that day. Expanding on that catalogue by drawing on other sources, a preliminary taxonomy of children's environments was offered (Table 1.1).

Table 1.1 A Preliminary Functional Taxonomy of Children's Outdoor Environments (from Heft, 1988).

---

1. Flat, relatively smooth surface:
    affords walking, running
    afford cycling, skating, skateboarding

2. Relatively smooth slope:
    affords coasting down
    affords rolling, sliding, running down
    affords rolling objects down

3. Graspable/detached object:
    affords drawing, scratching
    affords throwing
    affords hammering, batting
    affords spearing, skewering, digging, cutting
    affords tearing, crumpling, squashing
    affords building of structures

4. Attached object:
    affords sitting-on
    affords jumping-on/over/down-from

5. Non-rigid attached object:
    affords swinging-on

6. Climbable feature:
    affords exercise/mastery
    affords looking out from
    affords passage from one place to another

7. Aperture:
    affords locomoting from one place to another
    affords looking and listening into adjacent place

8. Shelter:
    affords microclimate
    affords prospect/refuge
    affords privacy

9. Moldable material (e.g., dirt, sand)
    affords construction of objects (e.g., pottery)
    affords pouring
    affords sculpting

10. Water
    affords splashing, pouring
    affords floating objects
    affords swimming, diving, boating, fishing
    affords mixing with other materials

The taxonomy based on this record has several limitations. It is not an exhaustive list of all the affordances that might have been available to the boy, but shows only those affordances that were suggested through his actions on that day. Nor is it a list of affordances for any individual who might visit those same places, but only for him and possibly for children who share some of his physical and psychological tendencies. At best, it is only a first approximation of the functional possibilities of the environment for that individual, and perhaps others similar to him.

A methodological limitation of this exercise is that it is entirely a posteriori. How adequate an approximation it is can be determined with subsequent observation of the activities of this individual or others. Further, its adequacy can be assessed in a predictive manner. To illustrate in the case of the taxonomy cited above, a sample of young children were asked to show an investigator their favourite play areas in the places adjacent to their homes. The taxonomy captured most of their choices (reported in Heft, 1997). Such data can also refine the taxonomy, or even expand it in ways appropriate to specific individuals assessed (see Kytta, 2002).

Environmental design and affordances

Designers interested in how particular environments are utilized and experienced quite reasonably might turn to the environmental psychology research literature for guidance. They are likely to be disappointed. Although there is an extensive literature addressing how individuals assess environments (or rather environmental surrogates) on rating scales, information is sorely lacking about how environments are experienced by users *in the course of action*.

One general consequence of adopting an affordance perspective – as illustrated by the affordance taxonomy study – is that it leads environmental psychology researchers and designers back to considering behaviour, that is, activity, in everyday environments. Now, nearly 40 years since the emergence of environmental psychology, it seems trite to say so, but much could be learned by considering psychological processes in situ. Social psychologists too are once again recognizing that those in their area of work rarely examine behaviour (Baumeister, Vohs and Funder, 2007).

The concept of affordances can be useful for highlighting several interrelated qualities of environments and environmental features that often fail to appear in conventional accounts of environmental perception. Two of these qualities, *function and meaning,* are conveyed by the very definition of affordances. Both function and meaning are qualities that reside in the dynamic, reciprocal relations of persons and environmental features.

In addition, in view of the emphasis in this chapter on *environmental aesthetics*, perhaps the concept of affordance can shed new light on aesthetic experience, or what I call below 'attraction'? Here we will be breaking somewhat new ground. I will propose that approaching environmental aesthetics from an affordance perspective will open up a new set of phenomena to be explored. In the present context, I can only offer some preliminary ideas in this regard.

Let us briefly consider each of these interrelated qualities, with an eye toward applying them to the matter of landscape perception.

Function

Affordances are most essentially about function. Their relational character specifically invites a consideration of the possibilities for activities in any specific environmental setting.

Applying an affordance 'lens' to a setting will not result in an exhaustive list of the possibilities for action in the setting. However, with a particular individual, or group of individuals in mind, many of a setting's affordances can be anticipated. Still, it is a mistake to think about affordances as causing an action. Affordances in no way suggest any degree of environmental determinism. Instead, affordances identify possibilities for action, as well as constraints on action.

Environmental psychologists have long been critical of neighbourhood and community designs that are not sufficiently sensitive to user needs or that constrain desirable actions. For example, over the past decade, psychologists and designers with interests in children's activities in everyday environments have called attention to the limited access children often have to environmental amenities (for example, Gill, 2007). Efforts at providing resources such as parks and playgrounds amount to little if they are not readily accessible. To this end, designs that afford access to such community resources are essential for residents of all ages.

This issue ties into a broader concern that is addressed elsewhere in this book. Evidence is accumulating that children's independent exploration and mobility contribute positively to psychological development and health (see Bull, Chapter 4, and Moore and Cosco, Chapter 2, this volume). At the same time, trends suggest that both have been in decline over recent decades (Kytta, 2004). The concept of affordance provides a framework for thinking about such functional concerns *explicitly*. If this way of thinking were commonplace in the design area, one might expect that questions of access and mobility, and more generally, of environmental design for human use, would occur early in the design process rather than as an afterthought.

Meaning

One of the benefits of working from an affordance perspective is the prospect of developing a terminology that describes environments in psychologically meaningful ways. Owing to its historical lineage, psychology's referents to the environment – most notably the catch-all 'stimulus' and similar terms – do not convey the significance of particular environmental features for individuals. Symptomatic of this state of affairs, environmental psychology researchers and designers have employed a mixed bag of terminology – from physical descriptors to geometric terms – which also tend not to be up to this task of offering a psychologically meaningful description of environments.

As we have already seen, much of the conventional terminology results in the abstraction of specific properties from environments, such as complexity and coherence. Although concepts such as these are useful for some purposes, in moving via abstraction from the level of particulars to that of general concepts such as these, the meaning of specific environments can be lost. To offer a simple example, one could imagine two different playgrounds that might be judged as being comparable in complexity or coherence while offering quite different affordance possibilities (see Moore and Cosco, Chapter 2 of this volume). In such a case, what might seem as being equivalent from the analytical stance of the researcher might be strikingly different in terms of the functional possibilities and meaningful experiences for young children.

Alternatively, sometimes we find the reverse situation where environmental psychologists employ concepts that do have psychological meaning, but otherwise are not grounded in any specifiable properties of the environment. For example, in their introduction to a collection of papers on 'place', Altman and Low (1992) noted how rarely the idea of place is tied to properties of environments. Instead, this concept, and others like it, seems to float free of any specifiable environmental properties.

In contrast, if we consider environments from a relational perspective along the lines that the affordance concept conveys, then meaning resides in the relationship between the environmental feature and the perceiver. Imagine, for example, a public square that can be entered by walking down three stairs, and that contains low concrete ledges, an arrangement of flat, smooth surfaces, and a pair of benches positioned at 90-degree angles from each other. Describing the square in this way, and even offering more physical specifics – such as the materials utilized or the physical dimensions of the structures – while being useful for some purposes, tells us little about the psychological significance of the square for individuals who might enter it. Alternatively, if we begin to consider the potential affordances of the square in relation to the activities of a potential user group, its value as a place for each should become apparent. For example, to thirteen-year-old skateboarders, this place is loaded with meanings which are directly tied to features that make certain manoeuvres possible. For elderly users of the square, its functional meanings will be quite different – perhaps the particular arrangement of benches in the plaza might afford opportunities for social encounters with friends.

It is worth mentioning, on the heels of postmodernist thought, that alternative uses for the public square are *not* a matter of different users interpreting the *same* setting differently. Rather the square has multiple use possibilities and in some respects, is not fully the same place for each user group. The alternative functional significances reside in possible environment–person relationships. This is not a relativism, but rather a *pluralism* grounded in the relationship between the setting and its potential users.

Finally, one might conclude from the preceding that affordances apply only to physical, material features of the environment, having little relevance for meanings that are more culturally laden. This conclusion is unwarranted. For one thing, it is based on the dubious distinction between the natural and the cultural domains (Gibson, 1979; Heft, 2001, 2007; Reed, 1996). The culturally saturated character of most affordances indicates that the concept of affordances goes beyond solely body-scaling parameters to encompass a wider set of sociocultural considerations (for extended discussion of these issues, see Heft, 1989, 2001, 2007).

Attraction

Meaningful things can take hold of us. Whereas the presence of an unfamiliar person might not produce for us much of a reaction, the presence of a loved one draws us to him or her. Kurt Lewin (1951) proposed decades ago that the objects of experience have a valence, that is, significance *in the context of a person's actions and history*. This viewpoint led Lewin to propose that we should think about the individual's momentary psychological field as an array of dynamic, multiple influences (vectors or lines of force), some drawing the individual toward them, and others repelling the individual.

Likewise Barker and Wright (1955), two students of Lewin, pointed out in their study of children's daily activities that environmental features possess 'physiognomic' qualities that influence actions. For example, observing the penchant for children to be drawn into open places for running and playing, they remark: 'Open spaces seduce children.' That is, open fields lure children to run, tumble, and so forth. They do more than offer the possibility for running; they entice children to do so.

I suggest that we consider affordances as having in many cases such motivating qualities. To offer another example, I have rarely observed an instance when a young child walking in the proximity of a low ledge fails to climb up on it and walk along its elevated surface. Conversely, things of the environment can appear repelling, as in the case of a child's description of a residence in the neighbourhood as 'the house with the dog that bites' (Hart, 1978). In short, affordances are not usually properties of the environment at which individuals gaze indifferently. They are meaningful, value-rich features of experience that *in the course of action and in the context of an individual's history are often alluring,* and sometimes repelling.

These comments only touch on matters of aesthetic experience, but they do point to the fact that affective experience can reside *in our relationships to* features of the environment. Considering the environment with *activity as a frame of reference* raises questions such as *how well* and *in what ways* the environment prompts or supports some ongoing activity.

Often individuals are drawn to certain locales because of the distinctive experiences those places afford. Just as the 'feel' of a utensil or tool can be a matter of considerable *value* for users, there can also be *a value in engagement* that makes some settings especially desirable. Frozen ponds for skating, snowy slopes for skiing, even suitable trees for climbing – to name only a few possibilities – have a quality that goes beyond pleasure in the narrow sense of liking how something looks. Indeed, the affective experiences arising from engaging certain features of the world can be challenging and even demanding, pleasurable being too narrow a descriptor of some positive experiences. And *skilful engagement,* often with the support of well-fashioned tools and equipment, brings a delight which, rather than being of a generalized nature (for example, 'I like this feature'), is tied to the unique 'feel' of that the specific action.

Travel and 'nature' writing abound with reports that describe 'the feel' of a locale. For example, in *The Maine Woods,* Thoreau (1864) describes a portion of a hike in the following way: 'The evergreen woods had a decidedly sweet and bracing fragrance; the air was a sort of diet-drink, and we walked on buoyantly in Indian file, stretching our legs' (Ktaadn, part 2, 1). Rather than describing the qualities of the setting in a detached manner, this is an embodied description that stems from action – from the breathing of the air to walking with buoyancy. There is no denying its aesthetic character. Similarly, consider this passage from Dewey:

> The man who poked the sticks of burning wood would say he did it to make the fire burn better; but he is none the less fascinated by the colourful drama of change enacted before his eyes and imaginatively partakes of it. He does not remain a cold spectator.
>
> (Dewey, 1934: 3)

The qualities that arise from engaging the environment are vital to the affective experience of landscape.

What I am suggesting then, is that affordance considerations can lead environmental aesthetics research beyond broad assessments of preference per se from a detached stance, to the qualities of experiencing the environment in the course of action. We do not merely like to look at forest scenes and cityscapes. We also like to engage them.

Conclusions

An examination of the treatment of perception in much of the psychological literature can readily leave one with the impression that the image-based approach to vision is an inevitable outcome of our understanding of how vision works. This claim, however, is contestable (Gibson, 1966). Moreover, I have tried to show, if only briefly, that rather than being an inevitable formulation, this approach is in large measure a product of our intellectual history. Our long-standing preoccupation with images is intimately intertwined with this history. Even after psychology took a more functional turn on the heels of evolutionary theory, the received image-based view was not reassessed for its adequacy; instead, proposals were offered to explain how animals function *in spite* of the limitations of images being presented to the visual system.

That is the state of the field today, for the most part. However, a reassessment was indeed called for. Although some initial steps in this direction were made (for example, Dewey, 1896), an alternative framework was not realized until the 1960s and 1970s, with the formulation of Gibson's ecological approach to perception.

Likewise, research of environmental perception and aesthetics to date within environmental psychology and the design fields has almost exclusively assumed the image-based approach to vision, and accordingly, the literature consists of instances of individuals, often in experimental conditions, 'looking at' landscapes from the stance of a detached spectator. In contrast, empirical investigations of environmental perception and aesthetics from the point of view of individuals as active, embodied participants engaging the environment are exceedingly rare. The ecological approach to psychology offers one theoretical framework for guiding investigations from this perspective; and in this endeavour, the concept of affordance may play a key role.

Are there grounds for claiming that 'the spectator stance' and the engaged, active perceiver stance are distinctive modes of experiencing the environment? The conceptual analyses offered in the foregoing indicate why this is a reasonable expectation, and identify some likely differences between these two modes of perceptual experience. Further, empirical support for this distinction is emerging from environmental perception research (Heft and Nasar, 2000; Heft and Poe, 2005; Hull and Stewart, 1995), and evidence compatible with it can also be found in experimental research (Anderson and Runeson, 2008; Heft, 1993).

In addition, we can find discussions of the distinctive character of 'image-based' experience of environments – as compared with first-hand experience – in writings on the perception of photographs. Photographs offer the *spectator mode* of experience par excellence. The cultural theorist Susan Sontag was among the most astute commentators on photography and its impact on cultures. She argued that the *feelings engendered* when viewing photographs are dissimilar from those accompanying first-hand experiences of the subjects of those representations. '[P]hotographic images tend to subtract feeling from something we experience firsthand and the feelings they do arouse are, largely, not those we have in real life' (Sontag, 1977: 68). Perceiving images is a special kind of visual experience. It is characterized by a distancing of oneself from the subject represented, a holding the world at arm's length. In this respect, representations of the world through photographs are a natural extension of landscape, portrait and still life paintings. This detached yet appreciative stance is 'the aesthetic attitude' as classically understood, and it establishes 'the picturesque' as the standard criterion for environmental assessment (Carlson, 2000). Arguably, the attitude of the 'picturesque' has come to dominate much of our thinking about landscape perception.

To conclude, then, let us review and summarize several of the interconnected claims offered above, highlighting their implications for environmental design:

1 There is reason to believe that experiencing landscapes as detached spectators and experiencing them in the course of actively engaging with them are qualitatively dissimilar.

2 The ecological approach prompts designers to think about landscapes as *arenas for action*. Emphasizing the experience of landscape through active engagement readily lends itself to consideration of the functional possibilities that landscapes afford individuals. Further, it opens up new possibilities for thinking about aesthetic experience in landscapes. By the same token, it might remind designers – if any such reminding is necessary – that designing 'picturesque' landscapes to gaze upon in a detached manner is only one design goal among many.

3 This action-based perspective should prompt designers to take up often-neglected approaches in the design field that emphasize the experience of landscapes over time (for example, Cullen, 1961; Thiel, 1997; also, see Heft, 1996). In doing so, qualities of environmental experience *over time* can be revealed that are otherwise masked by the dominance of static pictures on our thinking. This approach may shed new light on current inquiries concerning the relationship between environments and psychological well-being.

4 Because affordances are action-related properties of environments, they are particularly well suited for considering the implications of environmental design for health promotion and 'active living'. Landscapes vary in the degree to which they support, and even promote, action, and such environmental properties typically differ across user groups (for example, children and

elderly people). With the concept of affordance in mind, matters of access, navigability, use possibilities and so on, relative to individuals are maintained at the very forefront of design and evaluation.

5   Finally, the ecological approach sidesteps a vexing theoretical problem that environmental psychologists and designers typically sweep under the carpet. Traditionally, the environment is assumed to be subjectively experienced 'in the heads' of so many separate individuals. This conceptualization does not seem to trouble designers *as much as it should.* And why should it? In reality, designers go about their work assuming a high degree of shared environmental experience among potential users. After all, their designs are typically for a public domain. And yet, the standard account of perceiving informs the designer that *environmental experience is idiosyncratic and intra-psychic.* That view would seem to render the goal of designing shared public settings as rather hopeless. In short, theories that locate perceptual experience 'in the head' would seem to be ill suited to the goals of design.

In contrast, an action-based approach highlights the properties of environments that are engaged by users, pointing to properties that are located 'where the action is'. Environments offer an abundance of relational affordance properties, some of which might be realized by particular users at a given time. As noted earlier, this view of environments is pluralistic, grounding as it does environmental properties in the relationship between the setting and its potential users. Not only does this conceptualization better undergird what designers actually attempt to achieve, but this theoretical move has practical implications as well. One can begin to anticipate many of the environmental properties in some locale that are significant for a user group by taking into consideration the range of users' body-scaling and their action possibilities as realized in sociocultural contexts (Heft, 1989, 2001). Conceptualizing the environment as something experienced in the head offers few constraints, and hence few design guidelines.

Individuals engaged in both environmental perception research and in environmental design will be well served if they bear in mind that perceiving most fundamentally is a process that supports action and exploration. I anticipate that from this vantage point we can begin to contemplate new ways to understand the nature of aesthetic experience in environments. In this work, the following reflections will be an instructive, if general, guide:

Perceiving the environment from within, as it were, *looking not at it* but *being in it*, nature becomes something quite different. It is transformed into a realm in which *we live as participants, not as observers.*

(Berleant, 1992: 83)

Harry Heft

Acknowledgements

I would like to thank the editors of this volume for their comments on an earlier draft of this chapter.

References

Altman, I. and Low, S. (1992) 'Place attachment: a conceptual inquiry', in I. Altman and S. Low (eds), *Place Attachment: Human Behavior and the Environment*, 12: 1–12, New York: Plenum.

Altman, I. and Rogoff, B. (1987) 'World views in psychology: trait, interactional, organismic, and transactional perspectives', in D. Stokols and I. Altman, *Handbook of Environmental Psychology*, 7–40, New York: John Wiley.

Andersson, I. and Runeson, S. (2008) 'Realism of confidence, modes of apprehension, and variable-use in visual discrimination of relative mass', *Ecological Psychology*, 20: 1–31.

Barker, R. G. and Wright, H. F. (1955) *Midwest and its Children*, Evanston, Ill.: Row, Peterson.

Baumeister, R., Vohs, K. and Funder, D. C. (2007) 'Psychology as the science of self-reports and finger movements: whatever happened to actual behavior?' *Perspectives on Psychological Science*, 2: 396–403.

Benson, R. (2008) *The Printed Picture*, New York: Museum of Modern Art.

Berleant, A. (1992) 'The aesthetics of art and nature', in A. Carlson and A. Berleant (eds), *The Aesthetics of Natural Environments*, 76–88, Ontario: Broadview Press.

Berlyne, D. (1971) *Aesthetics and Psychobiology*, New York: Appleton-Century Crofts.

Carlson, A. (2000) *Aesthetics and the Environment: The Appreciation of Nature, Art, and Architecture*, London: Routledge.

Cullen, G. (1961) *Townscape*, New York: Rheinhold.

Dewey, J. (1896) 'The reflex arc concept in psychology', *Psychological Review*, 3: 357–70.

Dewey, J. (1934) *Art as Experience*, New York: Minton, Balch.

Dewey, J. (1948) *Reconstruction in Philosophy*, Boston: Beacon Press (originally published by Henry Holt, 1920).

Edelman, G. M. (1993) *Bright Air, Brilliant Fire: On the Matter of the Mind*, New York: Basic Books.

Gibson, J. J. (1966) *The Senses Considered as Perceptual Systems*, Boston: Houghton-Mifflin.

Gibson, J. J. (1979) *The Ecological Approach to Visual Perception*, Boston: Houghton-Mifflin.

Gill, T. (2007) *No Fear: Growing up in a Risk Averse Society*, London: Calouste Gulbenkian Foundation.

Gregory, R. L. (1990) *Eye and Brain: The Psychology of Seeing*, Princeton, N.J.: Princeton University Press (originally published in 1966).

Hart, R. (1978) *Children's Experience of Place: A Developmental Study*, New York: Irvington.

Hartig, T. and Staats, H. (2006) 'The need for psychological restoration as a determinant of environmental preferences', *Journal of Environmental Psychology*, 26: 215–26.

Heft, H. (1988) 'Affordances of children's environments: a functional approach to environmental description', *Children's Environments Quarterly*, 5: 29–37 (reprinted in J. Nasar and W. Preiser (eds), *Directions in Person-Environment Research and Practice*, 43–69, Aldershot, UK: Ashgate).

Heft, H. (1989) 'Affordances and the body: an intentional analysis of Gibson's ecological approach to visual perception', *Journal for the Theory of Social Behavior*, 19: 1–30.

Heft, H. (1993) 'A methodological note on overestimates of reaching distance: distinguishing between perceptual and analytical judgments', *Ecological Psychology*, 5: 255–71.

Heft, H. (1996) 'The ecological approach to navigation: a Gibsonian perspective', in J. Portugali (ed.), *The Construction of Cognitive Maps*, 105–32, Dordrecht: Kluwer Academic.

Heft, H. (1998) 'Towards a functional ecology of behavior and development: the legacy of Joachim F. Wohlwill', in D. Gorlitz, H. J. Harloff, G. Mey and J. Valsiner (eds), *Children, Cities, and Psychological Theories: Developing Relationships*, 85–110, Berlin: Walter De Gruyter.

Heft, H. (2001) *Ecological Psychology in Context: James Gibson, Roger Barker, and the legacy of William James's Radical Empiricism*, Mahwah, N.J.: Lawrence Erlbaum Associates.

Heft, H. (2007) 'The social constitution of person-environment reciprocity', *Ecological Psychology*, 19: 85–105.

Heft, H. and Nasar, J. L. (2000) 'Evaluating environmental scenes using dynamic versus static displays', *Environment and Behavior*, 32: 301–22.

Heft, H. and Poe, G. (2005) 'Pragmatism, environmental aesthetics, and the spectator approach to visual perception', paper presented at the meetings of the American Psychological Association, Washington, D.C.

Heller, M. and Myers, D. S. (1983) 'Active and passive tactual recognition of form', *Journal of General Psychology*, 108: 225–9.

Herzog, T., Black, A., Fountaine, K. and Knotts, D. J. (1997) 'Reflection and attentional recovery as distinctive benefits of restorative environments', *Journal of Environmental Psychology*, 17: 165–70.

Hochberg, J. (1971) *Perception*, Englewood Cliffs, N.J.: Prentice-Hall.

Hull, R. B. and Stewart, W. P. (1995) 'The landscape encountered and experienced while hiking', *Environment and Behavior*, 27: 404–26.

James, W. (1909) *A Pluralistic Universe*, New York: Longmans Green.

Jones, K. (ed.) (2003) 'What is an affordance? Special issue', *Ecological Psychology*, 15(2).

Kaplan, R. and Kaplan, S. (1989) *The Experience of Nature: A Psychological Perspective*, New York: Cambridge University Press.

Kaplan, S. (1995) 'The restorative benefits of nature: toward an integrative framework', *Journal of Environmental Psychology*, 15: 169–82.

Kaplan, S. and Kaplan, R. (1982) *Cognition and the Environment: Functioning in an Uncertain World*, New York: Praeger.

Kaplan, S., Kaplan, R. and Wendt, J. S. (1972) 'Rated preference and complexity for natural and urban visual materials', *Perception and Psychophysics*, 12: 354–6.

Kytta, M. (2002) 'Affordances of children's environments in the context of cities, small towns, suburbs and rural villages in Finland and Belarus', *Journal of Environmental Psychology*, 22: 109–23.

Kytta, M. (2004) 'The extent of children's independent mobility and the number of actualized affordances as criteria for child-friendly environments', *Journal of Environmental Psychology*, 24: 179-98.

Lederman, S. J. and Klatzky, R. (1987) 'Hand movements: a window into haptic object recognition', *Cognitive Psychology*, 19: 342–68.

Lee, D. (1976) 'A theory of visual control of braking based on information about time-to-collision', *Perception*, 5: 437–59.

Lewin, K. (1951) 'Defining the 'field at a given time', in D. Cartwright (ed.), *Field Theory in Social Science: Selected Theoretical Papers*, 43–59, New York: Harper Torchbooks (original work published in 1943).

Lickliter, R. and Honeycutt, H. (2003) 'Developmental dynamics: toward a biologically plausible evolutionary psychology', *Psychological Bulletin*, 129: 819–35.

McGinn, C. (2000) *The Mysterious Flame: Conscious Minds in a Material World*, New York: Basic Books.

Mark, L. S. (1987) 'Eyeheight-scaled information about affordances: a study of sitting and stair climbing', *Journal of Experimental Psychology: Human Perception and Performance*, 13: 361–70.

Mark, L. S., Balliett, J. A., Craver, K. D. and Douglas, S. D. (1990) 'What an actor must do in order to perceive the affordance for sitting', *Ecological Psychology*, 2: 325–66.

Mark, L.S., Dainoff, M. J., Moritz, R. and Vogele, D. (1991) 'An ecological framework for ergonomic research and design', in R. Hoffman and D. Palmero (eds), *Cognition and the Symbolic Processes: Applied and Ecological Perspectives*, 477–505, Hillsdale, N.J.: Lawrence Erlbaum Associates.

Marr, D. (1983) *Vision: A Computational Investigation into the Human Representation and Processing of Visual Information*, San Francisco: W.H. Freeman.

Meyers, G. E. (1986) *William James: His Life and Thought*, New Haven, Conn.: Yale University Press.

Michaels, C. and Carello, C. (1981) *Direct Perception*, Englewood Cliffs, N.J.: Prentice-Hall.

Oyama, S. (1985) *The Onotogeny of Information: Developmental Systems and Evolution*, New York: Cambridge University Press.

Pastore, N. (1971) *Selective History of Theories of Visual Perception (1650-1950)*, New York: Oxford University Press.

Pepper, S. (1942) *World Hypotheses: A Study in Evidence*, Berkeley: University of California Press.

Reed, E. S. (1982) 'An outline of a theory of action systems', *Journal of Motor Behavior*, 14: 97–134.

Reed, E. S. (1996) *Encountering the world: toward an ecological psychology*, New York: Oxford University Press.

Reed, E. S. and Jones, R. (1982) *Reasons for Realism: Selected Essays of James J. Gibson*, Hillsdale, N.J.: Lawrence Erlbaum.

Sontag, S. (1977) *On Photography*, New York: Farrar, Straus & Giroux.

Spelke, E., Hirst, W. and Neisser, U. (1976) 'Skills of divided attention', *Cognition*, 4: 215–30.

Steadman, P. (1995) 'In the studio of Vermeer', in R. Gregory, J. Harris, P. Heard, and D. Rose (eds), *The Artful Eye*, 353–72, New York: Oxford University Press.

Thelen, E. and Smith, L. (1995) *A Dynamic Systems Approach to the Development of Cognition and Action*, Cambridge, Mass.: MIT Press.

Thiel, P. (1997) *People, Paths, and Purposes*, Seattle, Wash.: University of Washington Press.

Thoreau, H. D. (1864) *The Maine Woods*, in The Thoreau Reader, available at: <http://thoreau.eserver.org> (accessed 19 August 2009).

Turvey, M. T., Shockley, K. and Carello, C. (1999) 'Affordance, proper function and the physical basis of perceived heaviness', *Cognition*, 73: 17–26.

Uttal, W. (2001) *The New Phrenology: The Limits of Localizing Cognitive Processes in the Brain*, Cambridge, Mass.: MIT Press.

Warren, W. H. (1984) 'Perceiving affordances: visual guidance of stair climbing', *Journal of Experimental Psychology: Human Perception and Performance*, 10: 683–703.

Wohlwill, J. F. (1968) 'Amount of stimulus exploration and preference as differential functions of stimulus complexity', *Perception and Psychophysics*, 4: 307–12.

Wohlwill, J. F. (1976) 'Environmental aesthetics: the environment as a source of affect', in I. Altman and J. F. Wohlwill (eds), *Human Behavior and Environment*, 1: 37–86, New York: Plenum.

Wohlwill, J. F. (1983) 'The concept of nature: a psychologist's view', in I. Altman and J. F. Wohlwill (eds), *Human Behavior and Environment*, 6: 5–37, New York: Plenum.

Ye, L., Petrovic, M., Dainoff, M. J. and Mark, L. S. (2007) 'Guerilla ergonomics: perceiving the affordances for the workplace', *Ergonomics and Health Aspects of Work with Computers*, 163–8, Berlin: Springer.

Chapter 2

Using behaviour mapping to investigate healthy outdoor environments for children and families:
conceptual framework, procedures and applications

Robin C. Moore and Nilda G. Cosco

This chapter focuses on a methodological approach to assess the health impacts of the places where children spend most of their time when not at home: childcare centres, schools, parks, residential neighbourhoods, and community institutions such as zoos, museums and botanical gardens – where families spend quality time away from the pressures of everyday life. These commonplace environments and mission-driven institutions are potential supporters of preventive health and disease prevention objectives to get children outdoors in contact with nature and engaged in physical activity. They fall within the scope of healthy community design, where this chapter is situated at the intersection with the built environment.

Environments and programmes used daily by children and families require innovative research and evaluation tools to assess their support for new health mandates. A body of knowledge is required to provide evidence-based guidance to help guarantee the success of design strategies and policy decisions.

To this end, this chapter presents three selected case examples (neighbourhood parks, a children's museum and childcare centres) to illustrate an approach based on behaviour mapping, which objectively measures the actual use of environments. The authors developed the methodology to investigate relationships between designed environments and intended behaviours, including those related to childhood public health and disease prevention.

Behaviour mapping is an unobtrusive, objective, observational method for measuring actual use of space. Compiled data disclose the pattern of behaviour in a given space, which may help design researchers and practitioners visualize children's physical activity in specific behaviour settings. The method is presented from a normative point of view, as part of a methodological approach aimed at improving the quality of relationships between people and the built environment.

Behaviour mapping can yield information about relationships between environment and behaviour and can answer questions such as, 'Which settings or components are most heavily used?' or 'Which physical components support significant amounts of physical activity, or social interaction, or interaction between children of different ethnic backgrounds?' The resulting graphical maps, accompanied by descriptive statistics, could add strength to the designer's decision-making process using an understandable visual language required for the design field. The method allows environmental components of interest to be linked with operationalized behavioural variables. For example, Moore and Cosco (2007) presented a behaviour mapping case study of community park design showing that, out of 12 identified behaviour settings, the five most heavily used (composite structures, swings, primary pathways, gathering settings, sand play settings) accounted for more than three-quarters (77 per cent) of the park use by children (p. 99). Settings such as swings within playgrounds and parks, within neighbourhoods, within cities, within climatic regions, within political jurisdictions, and so on, can be considered as nested ecosystems of the built environment, with each level structurally linked to the ones above and below. In an effort to bring the methodology to the attention of other professionals beyond landscape architects and designers, and before describing the case examples, a discussion about the broader context of application follows.

Measuring built environment variables relevant to design

According to US National Institute of Environmental Health Sciences (NIEHS):

> The built environment encompasses all buildings, spaces and products that are created, or modified, by people. It includes homes, schools, workplaces, parks/recreation areas, greenways, business areas and transportation

systems. It extends overhead in the form of electric transmission lines, underground in the form of waste disposal sites and subway trains, and across the country in the form of highways. It includes land-use planning and policies that impact our communities in urban, rural and suburban areas.

(NIEHS, 2009)[1]

Extending the NIEHS definition for the purposes of this chapter, the term 'built environment' is used to refer to all manufactured human artefacts and natural elements in children's everyday environments that might be present in streets, playgrounds, parks, greenways, nature preserves, childcare settings, schools, out-of-school programmes and community institutions. At the small scale at which children are physically engaged with the environment, this includes play equipment, trees and plants, topography, water, all other landscape features potentially influencing children's behaviours – and the pathways that connect them to children's homes (Moore and Cooper Marcus, 2008).

Health-related environmental issues have been researched and described in the field of environment and behaviour since the field emerged in the 1970s. Currently, the field needs to move beyond generalized environmental variables such as 'exposure to nature'/'not nature' to identify specific environmental components or characteristics more tightly related to health outcomes. An appropriate example is neighbourhood walkability, where sidewalk (pavement) connectivity is commonly used as a validated, reliable measure (Bull, Giles-Corti and Wood, Chapter 4, this volume). Relevance would be increased if detailed attributes that may differentiate sidewalk quality for users were included, such as the presence of shade trees and floral displays in neighbours' front gardens. Neighbourhood walkability measures for children would include detailed traffic counts and street engineering measures such as street width, intersection 'necking,' marked crossings and traffic lights, as well as the presence of adjacent parks and playgrounds. We assume that such detailed environmental design attributes and components may influence behaviour – especially of parents when deciding limits to their children's independent mobility and/or the voluntary, inner-directed decisions of the children themselves.

Built environment designers (architects, landscape architects, and urban designers) visualize environments that do not yet exist. As managers of environmental change, they (and the professional associations that accredit design education programmes) need to show how visions of new or retrofitted environments can be brought to fruition. Considered as a public health intervention, design innovation must be informed by evidence of success and developed into policy to have real impact. As partners in this task, design professionals need evidence to support development of built environment design policy to promote healthy human habitats, including places where children can engage with nature and enjoy active lifestyles as an integral part of daily life. This task requires new methodologies to investigate the design details of spaces scaled to the size and needs of children.

Healthy community design

The US Centers for Disease Control (CDC) focal policy area 'healthy community design' is based on the assumption that 'The way we design and build our communities can affect our physical and mental health' (CDC, National Center for Environmental Health, 2008). Healthy community design emphasizes two key factors at a higher level in the built environment ecosystem: density and mixed-use development. These factors are still relevant to design policy related to children and families. Increased density can decrease automobile dependence (reducing contributions to global warming) and make it easier for people, particularly children, to move around on foot and bicycle, which encourages residents to be more physically active (Frank, Engelke and Schmid, 2003).

Density may be associated with development of children's friendship networks, which can provide a protective social shield for groups of friends and siblings outdoors (Moore, 1986). Increased mixed use can encourage a more diverse mix of housing and related community and commercial facilities. In turn, this may increase community stability by making it easier for families to remain in higher-density environments to 'grow in place' (that is, not to move to the suburbs when children arrive) and 'age in place' (live on in the same community once children have left home).

Together, growing in place and ageing in place may support stability of extended families, which can provide a source of social and economic support, especially when times are hard. Combinations of higher-density and increased mixed-use development may augment social engagement and the growth of social capital (Frank, Engelke and Schmid, 2003), thus supporting improved physical, social, and mental health (CDC, National Center for Environmental Health, 2008). Hypothesized relationships such as these, between place, social life and healthy lifestyles, are under-researched, especially for children. And yet, according to the CDC website:

> Healthy community design can benefit children in many important ways. At a time when obesity and diabetes are rising among children, when asthma continues to be highly prevalent, and when conditions such as attention deficit disorder may be on the rise, it is crucial to seek, understand, and implement environmental design solutions that might help with these health challenges. Research increasingly suggests that children benefit from the opportunity to play outdoors, where they can explore and enjoy natural environments.
>
> (CDC, 2009)

A statement such as this, by an authoritative US government health agency, underscores the beneficial health implications of designing nature into spaces where children spend time in daily routines. Naturalizing such places, including childcare centres, schools, parks, and safe routes integrated with residential communities, can be seen as a potentially powerful community design strategy for the healthy nurturing of children. These ideas echo those of Frederick Law Olmsted, Jr. (1870–1957), 'arguably the intellectual leader of the American city planning movement in the early twentieth century' (Reps, undated). A century ago, about the same time the first commercial automobile appeared in the US, he proposed that:

> well-distributed public playgrounds and neighbourhood parks become one of the urgent needs if the health and vigour of the people are to be maintained. And the most important classes to provide for are the children and the women of wage-earning families. Most important because of their numbers, and of the direct influence of their health and vigour upon the efficiency of the coming generation; but most important also because they have less energy to seek out healthful recreation at a distance from their homes.
>
> (Olmsted, 1911)

The younger Olmsted's vision is supported by rapidly accumulating research, which suggests that nature can impact several health dimensions, including longevity (Mitchell and Popham, 2008). Diverse, stimulating environments offered by nature help children thrive (Maller et al., 2006); even so, today's children are growing up disconnected from nature's healthy offerings (Louv, 2005). This change coincides with, and is likely linked to, a decrease in children's physical activity (Roemmich et al., 2006). The most obvious and serious consequence is the rise in childhood levels of obesity (Andersen et al., 2006; Ogden, Carroll and Flegal, 2008). An association between children's time outdoors (where nature is) and physical activity has been established (Sallis et al., 1993), as well as the positive influence of nature on child development (Cornell et al., 2001; Wells and Evans, 2003), including key factors such as attention functioning (Berto, 2005; Faber Taylor and Kuo, 2008), healthy eyesight (Rose et al., 2008), and general health (Maller et al., 2006). The accumulated evidence suggests that childhood time outdoors may delay or prevent the onset of chronic diseases later in life.

To resolve healthy community issues related to children and families, environments need to be designed to support healthy behaviours. There is increasing recognition that shaping healthy behaviours, such as increased physical activity, will involve influencing social norms (Williams, 2007), like reintroducing the natural world as a backdrop to children's play (Staempfli, 2009) and encouraging individuals of all ages, friends, families, neighbourhoods and other identifiable social groups to be physically active (Watanabe et al., 2006).

The process, form and content of community design

Designing is 'to plan or produce with special intentional adaptation to a specific end, to devise or propose for a specific function' (Webster's Third International Dictionary, 1981: 611). Design professions are concerned with changing the conditions of community environments (buildings, open spaces and products), and their proposals for design interventions contain detailed descriptions of how environments should work, be laid out and managed (Moore and Cooper Marcus, 2008). Designers think about design problems through visual imagery, and express solutions as visual statements. Designing outdoor environments generally falls under the professional purview of landscape architecture, which, according to the American Society of Landscape Architects (ASLA), 'encompasses the analysis, planning, design, management, and stewardship of the natural and built environments' (ASLA, 2009).

Design is concerned with both built environment *form* (that is, the layout of space, its boundaries, pathway systems, and interrelationships between subspaces or behaviour settings) and built environment *content* (that is, the subspaces themselves, their physical components and supported behaviours).[2] Although these factors vary between one design and another, successful designs must knit them into compelling places, attracting users who perceive and use them as coherent wholes. To understand the success of design from this holistic point of view, methodologies are needed that link designed environments to behaviour and address both form and content. Research guided by this conceptual framework is more likely to create useful evidence required for design interventions for healthy child development. As Aboelata (2004: 1), asserts, 'The designated use, layout, and design of a community's physical structures including its housing, businesses, transportation systems, and recreational resources, affect patterns of living (behaviours) that, in turn, influence health.'

The promise of a transdisciplinary field

The American Academy of Pediatrics (2009) has recently added its considerable voice to the expanding chorus of concern about preventable childhood lifestyle diseases, for which modifications to the built environment are part of the solution. Bringing together different fields of expertise in a truly transdisciplinary[3] field to focus on built environment change holds promise for innovation and the required massive changes in both form and content. Interdisciplinary progress has been made for several years but the transdisciplinary goal of creating a new, integrated field has yet to be reached. It is no small task to create a field where differing research and practice traditions can develop a shared problem-solving strategy and language. One reason is that design still has much research ground to cover before achieving full respect and attention from potentially allied, research-driven disciplines such as public health. Equally, the potential allies of design do not yet understand the workings of the complex production processes of the built environment in a way that will inform the challenging task of changing those processes to support healthy built environment design.

Development of a shared methodology can be seen as a crucial strategy that could yield early results focusing attention on design of the built environment. As Jackson and Kochtitzky urge:

> We must integrate our concepts of 'public health issues' with 'urban planning issues.' Urban planners, engineers, and architects must begin to see that they have a critical role in public health. Similarly, public health professionals need to appreciate that the built environment influences public health as much as vaccines or water quality.
>
> (Jackson and Kochtitzky, 2001: 15)

Because it is adaptable to many types of environments, different scales and varied settings, behaviour mapping is the type of methodology that may add impetus to a strategic push towards a common ground where a wide range of disciplines can contribute.

Creating evidence-based community design policy

To be effective, community design interventions need to be evaluated to demonstrate whether the desired improvement has resulted. In this policy arena, there is a growing desire in the scientific and design practitioner communities for increased rigour, validity and reliability in measuring the impact of the built environment on human behaviour (Frank, Engelke and Schmid, 2003).

Interest is particularly strong in the burgeoning interdisciplinary field of active living research, driven by recognition that built environment factors may help to explain the variability of active lifestyles across different populations and urban contexts (Frumkin, Frank and Jackson, 2004). In order to evaluate, adjust and, if necessary, create new policy to support active living and liveability in general, reliable, empirical evidence is needed, matching the level of regulatory detail appropriate to different sectors of urban development, including building envelope and setback regulations; street engineering; zoning and building density; location of parks, playgrounds and greenways; storm water management; and design of civic spaces. Many of these regulations apply at the 'site design' level. Those responsible for designing, managing and regulating built environments need access to precise site-design-level data that relates to specific designed elements in those environments in order to make informed decisions.

In addition, built environment moderators (and potential mediators) such as zoning regulations, parking requirements and building codes need to be researched and understood if policy is to be developed to encourage built environment design in a healthy direction. Behaviour mapping can provide a research tool to measure the behavioural effects of these secondary policy variables related to the physical settings and elements of children's environments.

Environment and behaviour (E&B) research has a 40-year track record and a developed repertoire of methodologies to study healthy lifestyle issues and help build the evidence base necessary to develop design and management solutions. Kevin Lynch, a design researcher and practitioner, who conceived the city as a human artefact designed to serve human needs, was one of the first to recognize the practical utility of an environment-behaviour approach in his concept of 'fit' (Lynch, 1981: ch. 9).

Lynch also instigated the first international study of children's urban environments (*Growing Up in Cities*, Lynch, 1977), which was replicated in expanded form in the 1990s (Chawla, 2002). The research subfield of children and family settings has developed a substantial conceptual framework and effective methodology, which Lynch helped to shape by establishing a multi-method direction that has evolved over many years. Direct observation of behaviour, objective measurement of physical activity, combined with qualitative, child-friendly methods (for example, drawings, child-taken photographs with or without audio-tagging, journals, semi-structured interviews and child-led safaris, Driskell, 2002) offer data-gathering tools to measure children's behaviour and perceptions useful to inform design. These complementary methods used to explore and identify environmental discriminatory items produce data that can be linked to behaviour mapping data, thus improving interpretation of results produced by both qualitative and quantitative research designs.

Theoretical framework

The theoretical basis of the authors' ecological approach to design research and the methodology presented here (behaviour mapping) are the key concepts of *behaviour setting* (Barker, 1976; Heft, 2001) and *affordance* (E. Gibson and Pick, 2000; J. Gibson, 1979) fully described in the previous volume in this series (Moore and Cosco, 2007; Cosco, 2007) as well as by Heft in this volume. Together, affordance and behaviour setting offer a common framework for researchers and designers to both analyse the quality of environments and use findings to improve designs.

Behaviour setting

Behaviour setting has been employed as a concept by environmental design researchers in a variety of areas with variable degrees of complexity (Lynch, 1981). The present authors have applied the concept as a unit of analysis in environment–behaviour research studies over several decades, which has resulted in the development of a stable set of behaviour setting types used in the ongoing design assistance and research programs of the Natural Learning Initiative at North Carolina State University, USA. Each application provides an opportunity to retest the relevance of individual types or the whole set of types.

Behaviour setting provides an evidence-based method of subdividing an environment or area behaviourally so that environment and behaviour can be linked directly, which is essential for understanding the impact of design on children's behaviour and for guiding design interventions. As a unit of analysis, behaviour setting provides a common language for linking design to research by disaggregating designed outdoor environments or areas into their functional parts as a designer would (that is, pathway, climbing area, sand pit, water play setting, gathering place, tricycle path, vegetable garden and so on).

Behaviour setting has the potential for linking research findings to design policy to provide an analytical tool for managers of built environments in a way that can inform decision making and policy development in the professions responsible for public and institutional environments. Measurable user response could provide crucial data to inform investment or management decisions and increase confidence that specific designs would support desired behaviours.

Affordance

Affordance also has practical applications. Applied to environmental management and design, the concept of affordance can be used to identify and analyse similarities and differences among behaviour settings such as manufactured play equipment, sand play areas, pathways and vegetated settings. It can explain how design details afford variations in activity across behaviour settings of the same type. For example, why one sand play setting is more popular than another for caregivers with young children could be explained by the elevated sand enclosure that affords a sitting wall for the adult. Museum curators can use affordance concepts to understand how different exhibits' physical components or attributes may affect desired learning behaviour responses. Characteristics of plants such as fragrance or fruiting habit may influence their 'smellability' or 'pickability'. Identified affordances can provide valuable information for managers by focusing attention on detailed design of components that affect costs balanced with benefits for users.

Behaviour mapping

Behaviour mapping can be applied in a variety of built environment contexts, particularly as they relate to the behaviour of children and families, where environment–behaviour interaction is qualitatively different from interaction where only adults are engaged. Application of the method began in the 1970s with indoor environments (Ittleson, Rivlin and Proshansky, 1976). However, several early applications focused on children's outdoor behaviour, mainly settings at the level of residential neighbourhood (Björklid, 1982; van Andel, 1984–85), park and playground, and renovated schoolyards (Moore, 1974; Moore and Wong, 1997). These early examples used pencil and paper techniques to gather data, and hand graphics to spatially represent results. An exception was van Andel (1984–85), the first investigator to create a digital program to code both behaviour and attributes of the built environment linked through a relational database. The development of geographical information systems (GIS) now makes this task easier since GIS software programs in general allow the recording of not only events and activities on the ground but also their location (Longley et al., 2005). This and the availability of hand-held digital coding devices provide researchers with a choice of methods for gathering, processing, analysing and representing data.

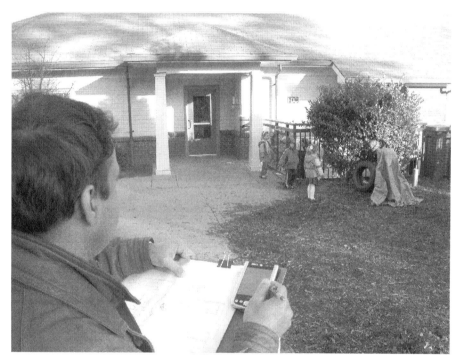

Figure 2.1
Field researcher gathering behaviour mapping data in a childcare centre preschool outdoor play and learning space. The paper base plan scaled drawing is fixed to large clipboard. Location of observed individuals are being marked with a red ink fine point 'Pilot' pen on the base plan. Behavioural and environmental data are being entered in the PDA, using the stylus taped (for convenience) to the other end of the ink pen.

Behaviour mapping procedures

A key criterion of behaviour mapping, as discussed here, is that the behaviour map is compiled from direct field observations of individuals in situ, where both environment variables and behaviour variables are observed simultaneously and coded at precisely the same site location (Figure 2.1). To develop a behaviour mapping protocol, several typical dimensions are addressed: *study site boundaries, behaviour setting boundaries, observation sessions* (or data-gathering site visits) and *session scheduling,* and the *number and duration of rounds of data gathering* to be conducted during each session.

Study site boundaries

It is not necessary for the whole site to be observed, only those areas accessible to users that can be used by them. The Bay Area Discovery Museum (BADM) outdoor exhibit areas studied by Moore et al. (2008) contained large, steep, landscaped slopes that were not used by even the most intrepid young visitors and so were excluded from the 'effective net study site'. The site boundary for Moore and Cosco's (2007) park study was clearly marked by a chain-link fence. Lacking such conditions, effective site boundaries must be defined post hoc as a result of the behaviour mapping. For large and/or heavily used sites, where observation times may be curtailed, the space can be subdivided to create a manageable protocol. For the Environmental Yard (an urban schoolground's renovation project) behaviour mapping study, the site was divided into two subareas observed by two observers during the 30-minute lunchtime recess (Moore and Wong, 1997: 239).

Behaviour setting boundaries

Behaviour setting boundaries (the subareas of a site) can often be defined by the 'lines on the ground' of physical components such as pathways or a meeting space such as a gazebo. Frequently, however, children's actual behaviour attached to settings spills over beyond boundary lines on the ground. Boundaries must then be defined post hoc by the clusters of actual behaviour.

In an unpublished study of Minnesota suburban school playgrounds conducted by the authors, play equipment was installed in subareas defined by use zone safety surface boundaries, which attracted the bulk of play activity. However, a proportion of behaviour spilled onto adjacent areas of mown grass and asphalt, extending the behaviour setting boundaries. In other cases, the behaviour defined separate behaviour settings (around a grove of trees and a free-standing cluster of rough-and-tumble play). Such settings were also mapped to show both the amount and type of behaviour compared with behaviour associated with manufactured equipment.

45

To study new or unfamiliar types of site design, two waves of data may need to be gathered; first, to define behaviour setting boundaries; and second, to code behaviour and physical attributes of each defined setting. To investigate early science learning and its relationship with the environment (a topic lacking research literature) in the Bay Area Discovery Museum (BADM) outdoor exhibit space, Moore et al. (2008) conducted a pilot project, including gathering sufficient data to define behaviour setting boundaries for later application.

Observation sessions – scheduling

To investigate moderators such as seasonal change, observations should ideally be conducted over a twelve-month period. Typically, this scope of observation is impractical because of the time commitment and cost involved. However, if suspected underuse or nonuse of the space is an issue, the only way to provide convincing evidence is to devote long hours observing what might turn out to be an unused space. The I-PARK (Investigating Parks for Active Recreation of Kids) team observed twenty inner-city parks in 2007 during eight summer weeks (the assumed high-use season). Preliminary results show that the majority of parks were relatively underused in contrast with a small minority of recently retrofitted parks that were heavily used. The finding rather convincingly illustrates the positive effect of park renovation. However, interpretation of the issue of underuse or nonuse was limited by the lack of interview data in the sparsely used parks. Were potential users frightened by the lack of upkeep, or was the old, worn-out equipment unattractive, or was the weather too hot? We don't know.

If a research objective is to measure the relative use or 'loading' across behaviour settings, observation sessions should be conducted during assumed high-use periods (which could be established through a pilot study), to yield as much data as possible. Cosco (2006) observed preschool playground use during outdoor playtimes programmed by individual childcare centres. Cooper Marcus (in Moore and Young, 1978: 117) observed behaviour in the St Francis Square residential development during a multi-session 'composite day' covering the period 8:00 am to 8:00 pm. Moore and Cosco (2007) gathered multiple rounds of park use data on all days of the week and weekends to ensure that data reflected weekly park use.

Observation rounds per session – number, duration and interval

Resources available to support observation time, including the number of observers available and the number of sites to be observed, often dictate decisions about the number of rounds per session. Climate, seasonal effects on activity, special events, often associated with public holidays, and cultural celebrations may affect the choice of both number and duration of rounds per observation session. Such external influences are also important control variables, which the researcher(s) should attempt to either exclude or hold constant during the observation period.

Because data gathering is expensive (see below), a typical objective is to gather as much data as possible in a short period of time. Pairs of observers are most commonly employed, thus yielding twice the number of rounds and double the data possible with a single observer. Pairs of observers also allow for reliability testing to be conducted as part of the protocol. For efficiency of observer deployment, rounds should be conducted sequentially, with a predetermined round duration and interval. Round duration defines the approximate time taken to conduct a round, which will vary slightly depending on the number of observations coded. Round interval defines the predetermined time between the start of each round. To ensure that round interval remains constant, allowance should be made in the schedule for slack time between rounds, typically five to ten minutes.

Round interval and duration is typically determined by the size of the site and density of users to be observed. Larger sites usually require longer round interval and duration. The more dense behaviour is, the slower the round navigation will be because of the time required to record behaviour. Round intervals of less than ten minutes are rare, first, because most moderately sized sites such as urban parks with moderate use levels, for example, require at least ten minutes to conduct a single round, and second, because round intervals of less than ten minutes indicate low-use conditions, suggesting consideration of a different session schedule. In any case, short round intervals result in higher levels of double counting, which may threaten study validity.

Large sites may require much longer round intervals. The behaviour mapping study of downtown Davis, California, conducted by Francis (1984), employed a single daily round covering twenty-two subareas with three observers, totalling thirty-three rounds in total, conducted over a period of four weeks (total number of individual observations not noted). Francis replicated the study in 2008 and observed 2,743 individuals (personal correspondence).

Control issues

To protect a behaviour study from external threats such as the climatic cycle, local variation in weather conditions, periodic changes in school schedules, public holidays and community-wide cultural events, the observation schedule should be framed as tightly as possible. For example, Moore et al. (2008) gathered BADM data during one springtime week including the weekend (when visitor population was known to be high and as a strategy to include more fathers in the sample).

Robin C. Moore and Nilda G. Cosco

Using behaviour mapping to investigate healthy outdoor environments for children and families

Three recent behaviour mapping studies illustrate the versatility of behaviour mapping applications in three different types of outdoor environments:

- *Neighbourhood parks*: key components of healthy neighbourhood design. Investigation of neighbourhood park behaviour by children and families can inform policy development to counteract sedentary lifestyles at neighbourhood level. The illustration used here is *Investigating Parks for Active Recreation of Kids (I-PARK)*, a study of park use by children and families, conducted in Durham, North Carolina.[4]
- *Children's museums*: community destinations offering active outdoor environments that afford children's play as a vehicle for informal learning. Investigation of children's play and learning in outdoor exhibit areas can improve understanding of how behaviour setting (exhibit) design can afford desired behaviours. The illustration used here is *My Place by the Bay: Prepared Environments for Early Science Learning*, a study of early science learning conducted in the outdoor exhibits at the BADM.[5]
- *Childcare centres*: community institutions where the majority of children under five in the United States spend most of their waking hours while parents work. Centre outdoor environments are particularly important because they can afford higher levels of physical activity. Investigation of relationships between setting physical attributes and preschool physical activity can influence policy developed by regulatory bodies. The illustration used here is *Measuring Physical Activity Affordances in Preschool Outdoor Environments*, a study of outdoor preschool areas in 30 childcare centres located in the Research Triangle urban region of North Carolina.[6]

Healthy neighbourhood parks

Neighbourhood parks provide a potentially important neighbourhood destination for regular healthy outdoor activity for children and families. They have therefore become an important research topic in the field of active living. The most commonly used research tools to measure physical activity behaviour include those developed by McKenzie and colleagues, beginning in 2002 with SOFIT (System for Observing Fitness Instruction Time), followed by SOPLAY (System for Observing Play and Leisure in Youth), and SOPARC (System for Observing Play and Recreation in Communities, McKenzie and Cohen, 2006; McKenzie et al., 2006).

The initial focus of McKenzie's work was physical education, using SOFIT to investigate the physical education behaviour of elementary and middle-school students in the standardized physical environment of gymnasia.

Using SOPLAY, McKenzie moved investigations outdoors to schoolyard environments, the large majority of which contain standardized, manufactured play equipment, surrounded by open areas of asphalt and mown grass, and used primarily during school recess. Most recently, using SOPARC, McKenzie and other investigators have begun to study community spaces such as parks and playgrounds where, unconstrained by schoolday schedules, populations are more varied and exhibit more diverse behaviours in both space and time. Each of McKenzie's instruments uses similar time sampling observational protocols and codes for physical activity level, activity type, and ratings for a limited number of environmental variables, such as 'accessible' and 'usable'. The SOPARC protocol subdivides the park into observational 'target areas', predefined by activity function (organized sports fields, playgrounds, social areas, and mobile activity such as walking and biking) (McKenzie and Cohen, 2006). SOPARC cannot be defined as a behaviour mapping tool as discussed here because it does not plot precise locations of observed individuals, and uses predefined, roughly sketched observation 'target zones' instead of more precisely delineated behaviour settings. However, as a reliable, validated tool most often cited in the literature, it was applied in the main I-PARK study. However, behaviour mapping was used to study more heavily used zones in three of the parks (Figure 2.5).

To capture a broad range of environmental variables, investigators have used Environmental Assessment of Public Recreation Spaces (EAPRS), developed by Saelens and colleagues (fifth edition), to code physical settings and attributes of public parks and playgrounds (Saelens et al., 2006).[7] This eighty-three-page 'environmental audit' instrument codes a vast range and number of park environment attributes (646 items in sixteen domains and six subscales). However, corresponding behavioural data must be gathered by some other means, and SOPARC is most commonly used by active living park researchers for this purpose. As behaviour and environment are coded separately using different instruments, complex statistical modelling must be used to search for possible relationships between a relatively small number of behavioural variables and a vast number of environmental attributes. Interpretation of results that may apply to design policy is potentially challenging.

These validated, reliable methods have been rapidly adopted in the active living research field; however, they lack coding protocols that link behaviour to environmental attributes at a level of physical precision necessary to produce outcomes that can be applied to built environment design policy and practice related to children. The SOPARC roughly sketched 'target areas', more than likely delineated in a mere outline sketch of the park area serve as systematic targets for observation. Accurate site base plans are often not available and must be generated by overlaying available GIS real property data with aerial photography. However, they cannot be considered as precisely defined behaviour setting boundaries corresponding to the items of direct relevance to users' behaviour and therefore useful to design professionals.

Behaviour mapping has the potential to overcome this limitation by defining empirically established behaviour setting boundaries, and by coding behaviour and environmental attributes simultaneously at the same spatial location so that environment and behaviour are directly linked to the same data point. By linking location and behaviour, detailed analyses can be conducted that include policy-sensitive outcome measures. Use/space ratio, for example, provides a direct measure of the efficiency of different behaviour settings in terms of amount of use relative to footprint size and construction cost – useful metrics for guiding park management decisions (Moore and Cosco, 2007).

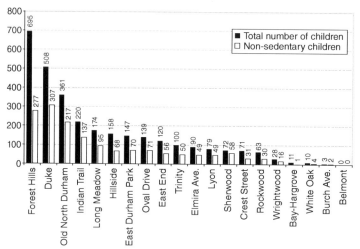

Figure 2.2

Children observed (N=3049) by park across 20 urban parks in Durham, North Carolina, USA. Physical activity data was gathered using the SOPARC three-point scale during eight weeks, summer 2007. Level of use was highly variable with the majority of parks underused. The proportion of children exhibiting non-sedentary physical activity varied between 81% and 40% (ignoring one outlier of 9%) with a mean of 54%. Just three parks accounted for 51% of total use by children across all 20 sites. In two of these parks, the playground had recently been replaced. The third site was adjacent to a school where summer programs used the park. Variability of total use and proportion of non-sedentary physical activity across the 20 parks may be due to neighbourhood physical factors (traffic levels, accessibility, etc.), neighbourhood perception of danger (crime, for example), or could be due to physical characteristics of the parks themselves (choice of facilities and activities, amount of shade, for example), or negative park perception (crime, rundown, unkempt landscape, for example). Interpretation presents a challenging task that may be assisted by results of in-park interviews (currently being analyzed) and/or by using statistical modelling.

SOPARC offers possible advantages in contexts where park sites are relatively large and density of activity is low. In the I-PARK study, SOPARC was used to gather data across twenty study sites, where the majority of 'target zones' were large compared with typical behaviour settings. Results (after eight weeks of observation) indicated low to very low levels of use of many parks (essentially nonuse in most: see Figure 2.2). In a small minority of sites where recent physical improvements had been made, use levels were far higher. Three of these 'high-use' park sites were studied further using behaviour mapping (one of which, Forest Hills, is presented here, Figures 2.3–2.9). Behaviour mapping, together with a measure of physical activity (SOPARC) and user interviews, were used to assist understanding why these parks were more heavily used, thereby helping to interpret the results of the larger study.

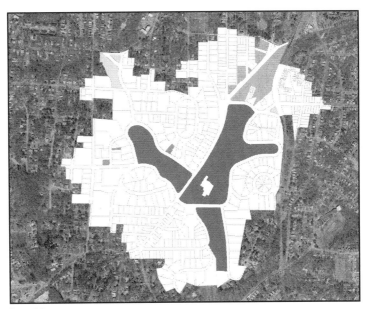

Figure 2.3
Forest Hills, Durham, North Carolina: One of the larger (45.86 acres) I-PARK sites shown in context of its surrounding older residential neighbourhood with ¼-mile network buffer (used in neighbourhood analysis of 'getting to the park'). The recently renovated playground case study site (white shape), accounted for almost 70% (68.8%) of observed children in Forest Hills Park (SOPARC data), which ranks the park as the most heavily used of the 20 in the I-PARK study. However, the playground occupied only 2% of the park area, resulting in a high use/space ratio of 34.4 (cf. Moore & Cosco, 2007).

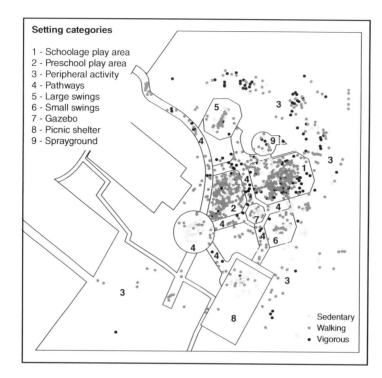

Figure 2.4
Forest Hills Park
playground
behaviour map:
Physical activity
level coded using
SOPARC codes
(pale grey –
sedentary activity,
mid grey – walking,
dark grey –
vigorous physical
activity). The
majority of activity
can be observed in
two main clusters
of children using
the school age
manufactured play
equipment area
(right) and the
preschool play area
containing three
small playhouses
and sand and water
play settings (see
Figures 2.6 and 2.7).

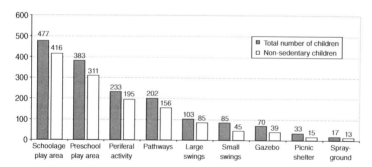

Figure 2.5
Forest Hills Park playground: Distribution of total and non-sedentary child activity across settings. In six of the total of nine behaviour settings, the proportion of non-sedentary behaviour was greater than three-quarters of all behaviour in the setting and in the school age and preschool play areas, the proportions were 87% and 81%, respectively. Across all settings (including those affording more sedentary social behaviour – gazebo and picnic shelter), non-sedentary behaviour was still high (72%). This easily accessible, well-used, recently renovated playground, offering a variety of play settings and comfortable, shady social settings, afforded a high proportion of non-sedentary activity, rising to a high of 87% in the school age play equipment setting. (Note: the low activity level in the spray ground was because data were gathered in the autumn season. In midsummer, this setting would have attracted more activity.

Figure 2.6
Forest Hills Park
playground:
Overall view of
playground.

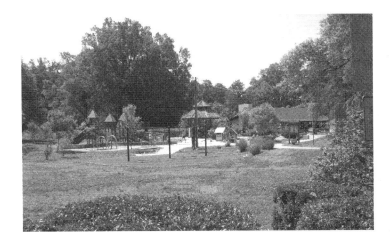

Figure 2.7
Forest Hills Park
playground: School
age manufactured
play equipment,
and social/sitting
affordances.

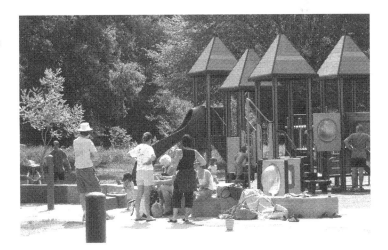

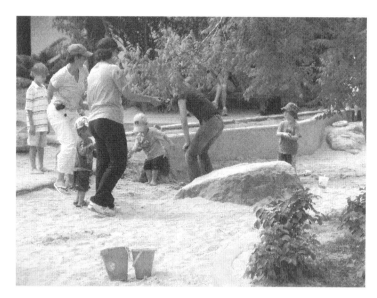

Figure 2.8
Forest Hills Park
playground:
Preschool sand
and water play
settings (the area
also included
three small
playhouses).

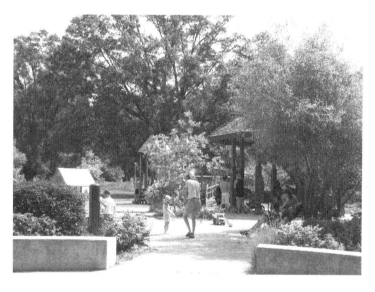

Figure 2.9
Forest Hills Park
playground:
Shady, central
favourite
gathering place for
families with
young children.

Main conclusion based on behaviour mapping

Children and their caregivers are more likely to be attracted to neighbourhood parks if they have up-to-date, well-maintained playground equipment. Particularly attractive playground settings include composite climbing structures, swings, water play and sand play. Comfortable, shady seating will attract caregivers and provide a viable social setting for adults, which may prolong the duration of park visits. These findings partly replicate those of the earlier study by Moore and Cosco (2007). Policies proposing neighbourhood parks as important active recreation destinations should recognize the need to provide a diverse choice of play and social settings, and also emphasize the critical management role of regular maintenance and periodic retrofitting to upgrade equipment.

Healthy outdoor settings for children's museums

Children's museums are 'places where children and adults can engage in interactive exploration, adventure, and learning together' (Frost, Wortham and Reifel, 2005: 83). They offer active community destinations that are particularly attractive to children and families, especially museums with outdoor environments. In the United States, more than 340 children's museums are members of the worldwide Association of Children's Museums (ACM). However, only eighty-three (24 per cent) extend their programmes into designed outdoor settings (Rajakaruna, 2006). To change this situation, the ACM has stressed the importance of designed outdoor settings in its member institutions (ACM, 2008).

At community level, museums and similar nonformal education institutions such as zoos and botanical gardens are potentially important family destinations for healthy outdoor activity. Design can make a difference in attractiveness and therefore increase the likelihood of repeat visits, which are good for the sustainability of the museum as well as the health of visitors of all ages.

As the US National Science Foundation (NSF) funded construction of the BADM outdoor areas (accommodating young children, three to eight years old), research focused on 'early science learning'. However, results show that children's play is the primary vehicle for science learning – indeed, BADM could be called a successful play museum in relation to its outdoor environment. As healthy child development through play is cloaked in the language of science learning, research findings offer a new message, 'come and learn science through healthy outdoor play'. The study of the museum's outdoor exhibits identifies environmental attributes more likely to support such a message. As this type of design-based research is sparse, the results will provide valuable guidance to children's museums and other nonformal education institutions interested in designing successful outdoor early childhood spaces.

The lack of research literature helps explain the undeveloped state of the art in design of early childhood outdoor spaces in community institutions (besides childcare centres, discussed later). Empirical findings are still lacking. For example, in the well-documented national report on early childhood pedagogy by Bowman, Donovan and Burns (2000), the outdoors is not mentioned even though science-related learning was a central topic.

Robin C. Moore and Nilda G. Cosco

However, we know from play environment research that diverse outdoor environments motivate spontaneous interaction by children and freely accommodate a broad range of individual differences (Moore and Wong, 1997). Such environments motivate exploration, assembly and reassembly of parts, and in the process provide a multitude of cues or affordances that encourage active play (Cosco, 2007). We know that diverse outdoor environments can be designed to motivate learning through play. In this regard, the BADM behaviour mapping study was an attempt to link physical attributes of settings to particular types of play behaviour.

Part of BADM, Lookout Cove occupies a dramatic location on the shoreline of San Francisco Bay in sight of the famed Golden Gate Bridge (Figure 2.10). The layout of Lookout Cove contains a variety of exhibits (settings), each one of which is intended to convey a science-related aspect of the Bay Area region to young visitors and accompanying adults (Figure 2.11). Children using the area had a median age of five years (according to an online survey of museum members conducted as part of the overall study).

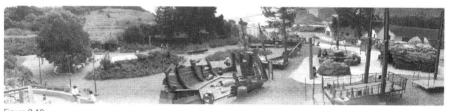

Figure 2.10
Bay Area Discovery Museum, Lookout Cove: Gravel Pit (far left), Shipwreck, 'Sunken Digs' (mid-foreground), the real Golden Gate Bridge (far distance, against sky), Fishing Boat (below Golden Gate Bridge), Tide Pools and Sea Cave (far right), Golden Gate Bridge manipulable play and learning setting (foreground right).

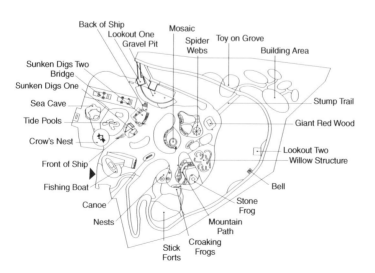

Figure 2.11
Lookout Cove:
Exhibit (setting)
layout.

Two linked behaviour mapping studies were conducted. First, data were gathered on a paper base map (to record spatial location) in multiple rounds of observation, timed at equal intervals of twenty minutes. Results were used to define behaviour settings and their boundaries, which defined target areas for coding the second study of play and learning behaviours using codes developed through a pilot project conducted by the authors at the North Carolina Botanical Garden, Chapel Hill, North Carolina.[8] Appendix A presents the full coding scheme demonstrating the possibility of creating an extensive database of independent and moderator variables to study hypothesized relationships with a dependent variable (in this case, early science learning).

For the second study, two observers moved in timed circuits in opposite directions (clockwise and anticlockwise) around Lookout Cove and coded the behaviour of each individual occupying the setting sequentially using PDAs with customized pull-down menus. By systematically scanning each setting and capturing snapshots of each child's behaviour, this method made it possible to gather multiple-coded data more easily and reliably than paper and pencil methods. Codes included early science learning activity (playing, observing, exploring, experimenting, and cause and effect), related environmental and social contextual codes, and interaction with accompanying adults.

The composite behaviour map shows a concentration of activity in behaviour settings close to the entrance area, on the left side of the drawing by Crow's Nest (Figure 2.12). Distribution of use across behaviour settings is highly varied (Figure 2.13). Almost three-quarters of use by children (74 per cent) is accounted for by just six of the twenty-one settings (fishing boat, gravel pit, shipwreck, bridge, willow structure and tide pools). Figure 2.14, which shows behaviour mapping data converted to density of use (average per round of observation), underscores the effectiveness of the two most densely used settings: the gravel pit and fishing boat. That is, they occupy a relatively small amount of space compared to the amount of use they afford or attract.

The success of the gravel pit may be explained by the affordance of its pile of gravel and large toy trucks which were especially attractive to preschoolers. The low wall containing the gravel afforded caregivers a convenient, comfortable place to sit near their children so they did not get bored and uncomfortable, ready to move on after a few minutes.

The attraction of the fishing boat may be explained by the large amount of dramatic play it stimulated. Larger proportions of observing, exploring, and cause and effect activity relative to other settings were afforded by its physical features. It was a 'real' boat and still retained accoutrements such as a wheel, various knobs and levers, a bell and a cooking galley, which afforded manipulation during fantasy play, helping children to pretend to go on voyages, battle storms at sea, navigate dangerous waters, and so on. The fishing boat was located with the Golden Gate Bridge in the background, which may have added to the dramatic play value of the setting.

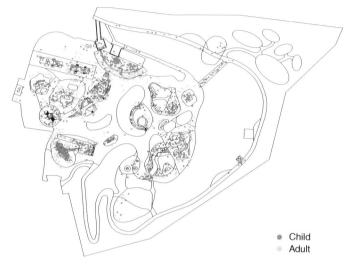

● Child
● Adult

Figure 2.12
Lookout Cove: Composite behaviour map (children, dark dots; adults, pale dots). In
several behaviour settings (Gravel Pit, Sunken Digs, Tide Pools, Fishing Boat) there is a
clear pattern of children clustered within the setting with caregivers distributed closely
around the setting – possibly because the settings were physically uncomfortable for
adults to be in. In other settings (Bridge, Willow Structure) children and caregivers were
more intermingled – possibly because the settings were comfortable for caregivers to
get inside to participate in the activity with their children (building a bridge with loose
parts, playing hide-and-go-seek in and around the structure).

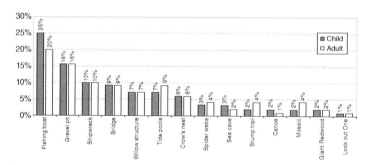

Figure 2.13
Lookout Cove: Distribution of child and adult users by setting. In the majority of settings,
child and adult use was roughly equal. As informally observed in verbal interactions
between adults and children, this may reflect the interest of educated middle class
caregivers in engaging with their children in enjoyable activities with perceived educational
benefits. Caregivers were also observed chatting with each other while their children
played. This observation underscores the importance of designing outdoor play and
learning settings to afford comfortable social gathering and interaction among adults.

Figure 2.14
Lookout Cove:
Average use
density of settings
(average per
round of
observation).
Density measures
such as this could
provide a useful
objective
parameter for
managing visitor
perception of
crowding.

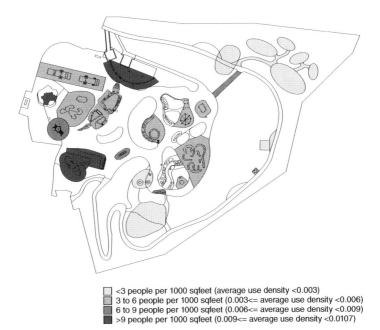

☐ <3 people per 1000 sqfeet (average use density <0.003)
▨ 3 to 6 people per 1000 sqfeet (0.003<= average use density <0.006)
▩ 6 to 9 people per 1000 sqfeet (0.006<= average use density <0.009)
■ >9 people per 1000 sqfeet (0.009<= average use density <0.0107)

With the exception of the willow structure, the other five high-use settings could be manipulated by children and/or contained loose parts. The willow structure, which in fact was a work of art constructed from 'living willow', attracted use because of the hide-and-seek and chase games afforded by its complex, exploratory, three-dimensional sculptural spaces. None of the remaining settings with relatively low proportions of use afforded manipulability or loose-parts play.

Main conclusion based on behaviour mapping

Nonformal education destinations with outdoor exhibit areas serving young children will be more attractive if they include settings with manipulable components and or loose parts. These attributes are more likely to increase both dramatic and active play and will provide a broader range of learning activity, particularly related to early science learning behaviour. Policies proposing non-formal education institutions as active recreation community destinations should recognise the need to provide a diversity of outdoor settings designed to stimulate dramatic and imaginative play and managed to offer manipulative, loose parts play.

Childcare outdoor environments: Investigating setting attributes and preschool physical activity

Current US policies for providing healthy children's environments are based on childcare quality assessment scales used for licensing (Harms, Cryer and Clifford,

1990). Increased knowledge of play environment characteristics is needed to inform childcare licensing policy and accreditation regulations, and encourage the development of best practices to support physical activity. Researchers are making efforts to rectify the knowledge gap by identifying environmental characteristics that might be associated with children's health factors such as physical activity (Dowda et al., 2004, 2009).

The behaviour mapping study presented here is part of a study of thirty preschool play areas, the aim of which is to link behaviour setting attributes with early childhood activity affordances and to identify environmental features that might encourage different ranges of preschool physical activity. Behaviour mapping results illustrate how play settings may produce different physical activity outcomes.

Using the behaviour mapping methodology described above, outdoor behaviour settings were systematically and consecutively scanned using a paper map to locate subjects in space, and a handheld computer (PDA Dell Axim Pocket PC, Austin, Texas) to record gender, setting type, physical attributes where the target subject was observed, and physical activity level using the Children's Activity Rating Scale (CARS) (Puhl et al., 1990; DuRant et al., 1993). The scale allows trained observers to record children's activity on a scale 1–5 representing different levels of energy expenditure (1 = motionless; 5 = vigorous).

Eight behaviour maps were collected per play area (four from each observer) and processed using GIS software (Longley et al., 2005). The total number of children in the play area and the weather conditions were noted at the time of observation. The data were used to create the attribute tables in GIS to conduct analyses. Additional environmental variables that might contribute or hinder preschool activity were added to the GIS attribute table (setting square feet, ground surface material and amount of shade).

Study overview

To illustrate the method, behaviour maps of two childcare centres (Centre A, Figure 2.15; and Centre B, Figure 2.17) located in the Research Triangle Area, N.C., are presented here. Both centres were high-quality early childhood institutions and held a North Carolina licence that requires the highest performance in teacher training, environmental quality, safety and educational standards.

The outdoor areas were comparable in several key dimensions. They had a similar number of behaviour settings, similar square footage, and a comparable number of behaviour mapping observations in relation to the number of children (thirty and twenty-one, respectively). Children were observed during outdoor play in each centre. The composite behaviour maps are shown in Figures 2.16 and 2.18. However, the layout of the sites and the mix of settings were different (Figure 2.19). Settings in Centre A included four dramatic play areas, one

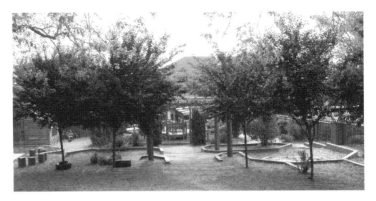

Figure 2.15
Centre A: The upper end of the site is a large open area shaded by several trees and surfaced with woodchips to protect against erosion. This area is gently sloping down away from the camera. A sand play setting is visible to the right. A concrete paved pathway is just visible looping around a central, custom-made timber play structure. The pathway was highly attractive to children using wheeled toys. The roof of the centre building can be seen rising in the background.

- ○ Sedentary
- ◌ Light
- ● MVPA

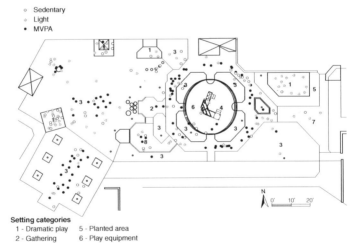

Setting categories
1 - Dramatic play   5 - Planted area
2 - Gathering   6 - Play equipment
3 - Open area   7 - Porch trans.
4 - Pathway   8 - Sandplay

Figure 2.16
Centre A: Behaviour map of physical activity. The moderate to vigorous physical activity (MVPA) 'affordance' of the circular pathway for wheeled toys is indicated by the higher density of observations, which may also be influenced by the synergetic effect of the number and diversity of settings adjacent to the circular pathway.

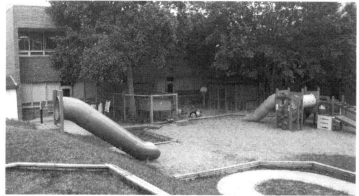

Figure 2.17

Centre B: One side of the site included a steep hill with, at the midpoint, a slide descending into a large area surfaced with woodchips. Two additional manufactured play equipment behaviour settings are visible as well as a narrow wheeled toy path in the lower right corner of the photograph.

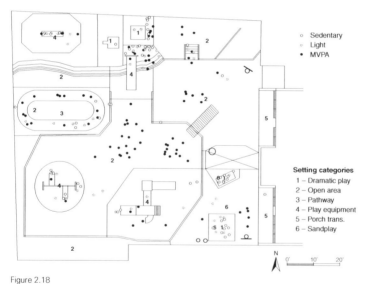

Figure 2.18

Centre B: Behaviour map of physical activity. Activity is spread evenly across the behaviour settings, all of which appear attractive. The central area contains several manufactured equipment settings, including swings. A large sand play area is located at the bottom right corner, which affords more sedentary activity than other settings.

	Play area sqft	Number of settings	Observations
Centre A	9,414.58	17	256
Centre B	8,265.72	18	207

Figure 2.19
Centre A: Physical activity related to ground surface material. The high level of moderate to vigorous physical activity (MVPA) on concrete reflects the wheeled toy affordance on the circular pathway. The higher MVPA on the woodchip surface reflects the 'runnable' affordance of the open areas, which were surfaced with a thin layer of woodchips for anti-erosion control in the shady zone under a large oak tree (as compared to a thick layer of woodchips used as a safety surface, which typically is less 'runnable').

gathering area, eight open areas, a multiple loop pathway, one planted area, one composite play structure, a porch/transition area, and a sand play area. Settings in Centre B included three dramatic play areas, six open areas, a looped pathway, four pieces of play equipment including a slide on a slope, and a large sand play area.

Results of behaviour mapping

The large majority of observations of activity occurred in three types of behaviour settings in Centre A: pathway, open areas and dramatic play. Most activity was also observed in the same type of settings in Centre B, with the addition of play equipment (Figure 2.20). However, the distribution of activity in the same type of setting was different in each centre (Figure 2.20). In Centre A, 87 percent of children's activity was observed in the three behaviour settings mentioned above: open areas (35 percent), pathway (33 percent) and dramatic play settings (19 percent). Two of these settings (open areas and multiple loop pathway) accounted for 92 percent of the moderate to vigorous activity (MVPA). In Centre B, most children were observed in the play equipment area (38 percent), open areas (26 percent), dramatic play areas (18 percent) and the looped pathway (13 percent). The open area and play equipment accounted in this case for 72 percent of MVPA.

Discussion

As in the previous examples, behaviour mapping can be used to identify *specific environmental features*, in this case associated with higher levels of physical activity, where behaviour setting is the unit of analysis. Results from these types of analyses may provide appropriate guidance to designers and policy makers to help them create healthier, active preschool playgrounds through environmental interventions. The illustrations presented here support the assumption that the different characteristics of play areas might influence children's behaviour and their level of physical activity related to *setting category*, *setting form*, and *ground surface*.

Centre	Dramatic play	Gathering	Open areas	Pathway
Centre A	4	1	8	1 (multiple loop)
Centre B	3	0	6	1 (loop)

Centre	Planted area	Play equipment	Porch / transition	Sand play
Centre A	1	1	1	1
Centre B	0	4	2	1

Figure 2.20
Centre B: Physical activity related to ground surface material. The wheeled toy path, which lacked the exploratory affordance of the larger pathway of Centre A, afforded less MVPA. On the other hand, the woodchip surface afforded a similar amount of MVPA as the woodchip surface of Centre A. Even though the woodchip setting was a thick safety surface and possibly less 'runnable', its central location adjacent to several other settings may have created a synergetic effect of children running between settings, which may explain the larger amount of MVPA.

Setting category

In these examples, children preferred specific behaviour settings (open areas, pathways, play equipment and sand play settings).

Setting form

Children are attracted by specific behaviour setting forms, pathways being a clear example (Cosco, 2006). The behaviour maps presented here show levels of play that appear to be influenced by the particular forms of pathway (Figure 2.21). In Centre A, the multiple looped pathway setting was used by children to run or ride around and to access the diverse settings connected to it. We could speculate that children 'read' the pathway affordance (circulation route and connector to other play nooks) and use it freely. Designers could apply this knowledge for creating active play settings.

In Centre B, we speculate that the narrow pathway had less influence on children's activity for several reasons: although looped, this pathway was unattractive because it was narrow, and was undifferentiated spatially, therefore lacking in exploratory appeal. It supported a limited number of play behaviours (a line of 'drivers' riding in one direction). The low number of adjacencies compared with Centre A may have reduced the potential synergetic effect of the pathway (as discussed below).

Ground surface

It was assumed that different ground surface materials would afford different levels of physical activity given the variability of responsive qualities to movement.

Centre A	Sedentary	Light	MVPA	Total
Dramatic play	22%	35%	1%	19%
Gathering area	2%	0%	1%	1%
Open area	36%	29%	41%	35%
Pathway	19%	25%	51%	33%
Play equip	16%	3%	3%	6%
Porch trans	2%	3%	0%	2%
Sandplay	5%	5%	3%	4%
Subtotal	25%	38%	37%	100%

Centre B	Sedentary	Light	MVPA	Total
Dramatic play	38%	17%	5%	18%
Gathering area	0%	0%	0%	0%
Open area	6%	13%	47%	26%
Pathway	11%	10%	15%	13%
Play equip	44%	56%	25%	38%
Porch trans	2%	0%	0%	.5%
Sandplay	%	4%	7%	4%
Subtotal	32%	24%	45%	100%

Figure 2.21

Centres A and B: Physical activity distribution by behaviour setting as recorded using 5-point CARS scale. Physical activity 'sedentary' represents levels 1 and 2; 'light' level 3; and 'MVPA' (moderate to vigorous physical activity) levels 4 and 5. The types of setting were similar in Centres A and B; however, the distribution of total activity and MVPA was variable across setting types. This may be interpreted in terms of affordance factors (layout, objects, and events). For example, the more engaging, exploratory layout of the pathway in Centre A could explain the larger amount of active use, particularly for wheeled toys, compared to Centre B. Conversely, the greater number and relative attraction of the Centre B play equipment could explain its higher level of active use compared to the Centre A play equipment.

In both centres, moderate to vigorous physical activity was found in settings with medium to hard ground surfaces such as concrete, decking, soil and woodchip (Figure 2.22 and Figure 2.23). Hard pathway surfaces such as the Centre A concrete pathway appear to support more moderate to vigorous activity, especially when wheeled toys are available, because they are easier to use on smooth surfaces. These findings have clear implications for design, since ground surface selection is considered a critical decision by designers, until now driven by safety criteria rather than by physical activity objectives. Harder ground surfaces have been identified as a predictor of higher levels of activity in preschool boys, suggesting ground surfaces could be a modifiable environmental factor to promote physical activity (Cardon et al., 2008).

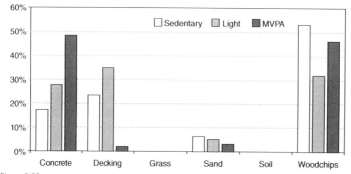

Figure 2.22

Centre A: Physical activity related to ground surface material. The high level of MVPA on concrete reflects the wheeled toy affordance on the circular pathway. The higher MVPA on the woodchip surface reflects the 'runnable' affordance of the open areas, which were surfaced with a thin layer of woodchips for anti-erosion control in the shady zone under a large oak tree (as compared to a thick layer of woodchips used as a safety surface, which typically is less 'runnable').

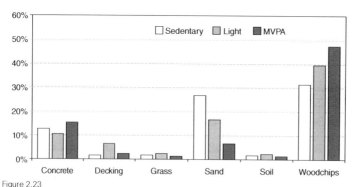

Figure 2.23

Centre B: Physical activity related to ground surface material. The concrete wheeled toy path, which lacked the exploratory affordance of the larger pathway of Centre A, afforded less MVPA. On the other hand, the woodchip surface afforded a similar amount of MVPA as the woodchip surface of Centre A. Even though the woodchip setting was a thick safety surface and possibly less 'runnable,' its central location adjacent to several other settings may have created a synergetic effect of children running between settings, which may explain the larger amount of MVPA.

In contrast, moderate to vigorous activity is negligibly supported by sand. It is very difficult to run through sand and yet it has been used frequently as a ground surface, sometimes covering the entire playground as a safety feature. This suggests that the prevailing practice of meeting safety standards using sand as a safety surface may inhibit higher levels of activity. Such knowledge may help designers and policy makers understand the need for tighter fall zones and diversified ground surfaces around play equipment. Ground surface treatments may support higher moderate to vigorous activity and encourage the use of wheeled toys, balls, and similar loose or moveable equipment.

Synergetic effect

Children's play behaviour can be highly dynamic in space and time, changing from one moment to the next, from vigorous to sedentary and vice versa. An important aim of health-promoting design is to create environments that support *sustained* moderate to vigorous activity. To achieve this policy objective, increased under-standing is required about how behaviour settings may be linked to one another to produce a synergetic effect that supports children's higher levels of activity (Cosco, 2006). This approach assumes that setting diversity, materials, and spatial arrangement or *layout* (a key attribute of affordance) may be combined (by design) to increase attraction for children, hold their day-to-day interest, and thereby encourage moderate to vigorous activity as they develop varied motor skills and capabilities.

For example, children were observed using a combination of play equipment, wheeled toy path, and vegetation that enticed them to collect leaves and twigs in carts, pull them around the path, move the cart's load onto the play equipment platform and make it fall down the slide only to collect it and start the cycle again. Behaviour mapping is able to capture such temporal sequences by coding both fixed features (platform and slide) and loose parts (leaves and twigs), which in combination can animate children's ranging behaviour across several settings.

Analysis of the childcare data currently underway indicates a signif-icant relationship between behaviour setting adjacency (the number of settings touching the target setting) and level of physical activity. This further reinforces the relevance of the potential synergetic effect in children's environments, and suggests that compact layouts affording more choice of activity at any given moment are likely to produce higher levels of physical activity than dispersed layouts. This is not to say that the layout of children's environments should always be compact. Domains of child development other than physical activity may be afforded by less compact settings that offer children more breathing space (for sociodramatic play, for example). Behaviour mapping is available to continue to explore such hypotheses.

Concluding discussion

Behaviour mapping is a relatively simple, versatile, objective research method processed with GIS that yields a relational database for performing statistical analyses and the ability to represent environment and behaviour data graphically. Designers may find spatial displays more meaningfully connected to their visual thinking styles than conventional data tables and charts, and therefore be moti-vated to apply environment–behaviour knowledge in evidence-based design.

67

Robin C. Moore and Nilda G. Cosco

The availability of small PDA devices and simple coding software with pull-down menus has opened up new possibilities for rapid data gathering using direct entry in the field. By using paperless digital 'coding sheets' for field data entry, data management can be more streamlined and less subject to error, therefore reducing the time devoted to data cleaning.

Behaviour mapping has been applied at many built environment scales ranging across early childhood spaces, school grounds, parks, neighbourhoods and urban downtown areas. The method is highly adaptable, allowing variables and codes to be tailored to different physical contexts, study objectives, research designs, and research investment including pilot studies, pre/post-interventions, post-occupancy evaluations of individual sites (Cooper Marcus and Francis, 1998), and larger-scale, multi-site studies to identify significant variables (such as the study of preschool outdoor environments reported here).

In any particular study, variables of interest may be added to the database to shed light on specific topics or issues such as the optimal size of behaviour settings, significant environmental characteristics for higher levels of activity, improved understanding of types of social interaction and environmental characteristics, empirical testing of safety standards, and the cost-effectiveness of different types of design or programmatic interventions.

The implications of refining and continuing to apply behaviour mapping in health-related community design holds promise for guiding best practice in the creation of high-quality environments for children, their families, and indeed all types of users of outdoor space. New data will continue to emerge that identify behaviour settings, objects, layouts and events that afford higher levels of health-promoting behaviour in children and adults. Over the course of time, such findings will help form the basis of healthy community design policy at levels of detail relevant to built environment regulations through which policy is implemented. Our hope is that design professionals will see this method as an aid for developing evidence-based policies that frame design problems as health interventions and allow designers to apply their creative skills to search for solutions that maximize the public health value of design outcomes.

Acknowledgements

Assistance with data gathering – Robert Massengale, Shirley Varela, and the I-PARK student team; data gathering and analysis – Evrim Demir, Orçun Kepez, Gary Kueber, Zaki Islam. GIS data analysis – Tom Danninger.

Notes

1 The authoritative source of his broad definition is the US National Institute of Environmental Health Sciences (NIEHS), published it in 2004 in a request for proposals for a research programme on obesity and the built environment. http://grants.nih.gov/grants/guide/rfa-files/rfa-es-04-003.html

2 This approach to conceptualizing the built environment is based on a model developed by Kevin Lynch, with whom the first author studied. Lynch conceived the urban environment as *adapted space* and *flow system*. He was the first urban designer to make the important, yet simple, theoretical distinction between space and human use. For further information, see Banerjee and Southworth (1990: 355).

3 Here we refer to formulations and distinctions of multidisciplinary, interdisciplinary and transdisciplinary articulated by Jantsch (1975) and Nicolescu (2008).

4 The goal of Investigating Parks for Active Recreation of Kids (I-PARK) was to explore relationships between neighbourhood environment, park physical environment and levels of physical activity in discrete age categories of children and youth. The N.C. State University research team in addition to the authors, included Perver Baran, Ph.D.; Jason Bocarro, Ph.D.; Myron Floyd, Ph.D.; Orçun Kepez, Ph.D. and William Smith, Ph.D. To better understand active neighbourhood environments for children and families, potential links were investigated between walkable characteristics of neighbourhoods such as connectivity, park location and park use; and park settings such as trails, bike paths, athletic facilities and playgrounds. The study was supported by the Robert Wood Johnson Foundation through Active Living Research, San Diego State University.

5 The goal of My Place by the Bay: Prepared Environments for Early Science Learning, was to investigate relationships between the design attributes of early childhood museum outdoor settings and early science learning behaviours of young children. The field research was conducted at the Bay Area Discovery Museum (BADM), Sausalito, California, outdoor exhibit areas, which opened between 2003 and 2004. The study was sponsored by the US National Science Foundation as part of a construction and research project developed by Catherine Eberbach.

6 The goal of Measuring Physical Activity Affordances in Preschool Outdoor Environments was to identify discriminatory environmental items in preschool play areas to be included in a pilot tool to rate their potential to produce physical activity when three to five-year-old children are exposed to them. In addition to the authors, the research team included Howard Frumkin, Ph.D.; Orçun Kepez, Ph.D.; Karen Mumford, Ph.D.; Stewart Trost, Ph.D. and co-PI Dianne Ward, EdD. The study characterized behaviour settings, their components and attributes in terms of the physical activity patterns in preschool outdoor areas in childcare centres. The study was supported by the US National Institute of Environmental Health Sciences.

7 In an effort to both reduce the number of variables and to define variables more closely tied to the needs of designers, co-author Moore and colleagues have developed a new park audit tool, Children and Families Park Audit Tool (CAFPAT). Although published results are not yet available, preliminary analyses are promising.

8 A pilot project was conducted at the North Carolina Botanical Garden in July 2004. Four family groups were observed visiting the Herb Garden. This particular garden had been enhanced to accommodate child and family interests. Play components included fairy figures placed among planters, a fairy playhouse, fairy mailbox, digging pit, signs with activity prompts, and a blueberry house. During the pilot session, children exhibited curiosity and engagement although some parents appeared to rush them through the settings. Dramatic play was commonly observed. Even when children were asked to leave the setting, they continued to observe and make comments about aspects of the environment and to ask questions. From the open-ended observations, a list of behaviours of children and caregivers was compiled and used as a source for drafting the BADM observation protocol.

Appendix A: Early science learning codes

With the purpose of assessing the impact of the designed environment on science learning, types of behaviours were defined to be observed and coded in My Place by the Bay, Tot Spot and Lookout Cove (reported in this chapter). Children learn about the environment and its properties by interacting with them. They explore and manipulate materials and create assumptions about phenomena

(National Research Council, 1996). Learning science implies also the ability to verbalize questions and to interact with others (children or adults) formalizing explanations or hypothesis. The possibility of being engaged allows children to learn from their own actions (Dyasi, 1999).

The following behaviours were selected to code for early science learning; engagement (Dyasi, 1999; Chermayeff, Blandford and Losos, 2001), child social interactions (Worth, 1999), interactions with the environment (Bowman et al., 2000; National Research Council, Science Education Standards, 1996), child expression of understanding/discovery (Bowman et al., 2000; National Research Council, 1996), and adult intervention (Bowman et al., 2000; Crowley et al., 2001).

The identified behaviours that support science learning follow a gradient of specificity from non-differentiated to intentional actions:

1   No science readiness behaviour.
2   Playing.
3   Observing.
4   Exploring.
5   Experimenting.
6   Cause and effect.

Although play is present in all of them (Wellington, 1990), for the purpose of behaviour coding by setting, play was coded when more specific behaviours could not be identified. Code descriptors are listed below.

No science readiness behaviour

'No science readiness behaviour' was coded when the child was not engaged in any activity or type of play, For example, the child was sitting on the lap of the caregiver, sleeping or eating.

Playing

'Playing' was coded when the child was performing pretend play or engaged in an activity that could not be considered as any other science learning behaviour. For example, at the moment of the scan the child was engaged and carrying a pail but the intentions of movement were not clear.

Observing

'Observing' was coded when the child was observing, examining closely but not engaged in in-depth inquiry. For example, the child was arriving at the setting but not yet performing a defined activity, or the child stopped acting to observe other children.

Figure 2.24
My Place by the
Bay (Bay Area
Discovery
Museum) code
structure and
descriptions.

Domain	No	Codes	Description of Codes
Science Learning Behaviour	1	Cause-effect	Making a deliberate action to produce a certain response to the action
	2	Experimenting	Making an intentional inquiry where there is a plan carried out
	3	Exploring	Making an explicit inquiry into something
	4	Observing	Watching closely
	5	Playing	Engaged in an activity that cannot be identified as any of the other science learning behaviours
	6	None	Not engaged in any activity or type of play
Engagement	1	Engaged	Sustained attention. Full concentration on the activity
	2	On looking	Moving between unrelated activities with scattered attention
	3	Disengaged	Not engaged with activity
	4	None	None of the three codes above describe the situation
Peer Interaction	1	Cooperative	Working together with other children during the activity
	2	Altercation	Signs of conflict, disagreement, or argument with peers
	3	None	None of the two codes above describe the situation
Environmental Interaction	1	Fixed manufactured	Manufactured (man-made) elements that are fixed and cannot change location (e.g. boat)
	2	Fixed natural	Natural elements that cannot be moved (e.g. tree)
	3	Loose manufactured	Manufactured (man-made) elements that are not fixed and can change location (e.g. toys)
	4	Loose natural	Natural elements that are not fixed and can change location (e.g. leaf, sand)
	5	None	Child is not in contact with any material or equipment
Child's Communication	1	No expression	When none of the conditions described below are present
	2	Converses	Any verbal communication by the child outside the activities that may initiate science learning behaviour
	3	Explains	Child explains his/her activity to others
	4	Listens	Child pays attention to explanations, answers, and conversations
	5	Questions	Child inquires verbally
	6	Demonstrates	Child demonstrates his/her discoveries
	7	Repeats	Child repeats words or phrases that are related to science learning experience
Adult Intervention	1	None	When none of the conditions described below are present
	2	Positive	Intervention that results in child's engagement in any of science learning behaviours
	3	Neutral	Intervention that is independent from initiating any science learning behaviour
	4	Observant	Keeping an eye on child's activities without interacting
	5	Negative	Intervention that stops any child behaviour

Exploring

'Exploring' was coded when the child was making an explicit inquiry about something. For example, the child was minutely examining a play object or natural material (gravel, an insect or a leaf).

Experimenting

'Experimenting' was coded when the child was making an intentional inquiry, when it was clear that there was a plan being carried out. For example, the child manipulated and combined objects in a functional manner to create piles or a series with loose materials.

Cause and effect

'Cause and effect' was coded when the child was making a deliberate action to produce a certain response: for example, hitting a bell or damming water.

References

Aboelata, M. J., Mikkelsen, L., Cohen, L., Fernández, S., Silver, M., Fujie Parks, L. et al. (2004) *The Built Environment and Health: 11 Profiles of Neighborhood Transformation*. Oakland, Calif.: Prevention Institute.

American Academy of Pediatrics (Committee on Environmental Health) (2009) 'The built environment: designing communities to promote physical activity in children', *Pediatrics* 123 (6): 1591–8.

American Society of Landscape Architects (ASLA) (nd) General information, ASLA, Washington, D.C., available at: <www.asla.org> (accessed 1 December 2009].

Andersen, L., Harro, M., Sardinha, L., Froberg, K., Elelund, U., Brage, S. and Anderssen, S. (2006) 'Physical activity and clustered cardiovascular risk in children: a cross-sectional study (The European Youth Heart Study)', *The Lancet*, 368: 299–304.

Association of Children's Museums (2008) *Kids Dig Dirt!* Green Paper, Washington, D.C.: Association of Children's Museums.

Banerjee, T. and Southworth, M. (eds) (1990) *City Sense and City Design: The Writings and Projects of Kevin Lynch*, Cambridge, Mass.: MIT Press.

Barker, R. (1976) 'On the nature of the environment', in H. Proshansky, W. Ittelson, and L. Rivlin (eds), *Environmental Psychology: People and their Physical Settings*, New York: Holt, Rinehart & Winston.

Berto, R. (2005) 'Exposure to restorative environments helps restore attentional capacity', *Journal of Environmental Psychology*, 25: 249–59.

Björklid, P. (1982) 'Children's outdoor environment. A study of children's outdoor activities in two housing estates from the perspective of environmental and developmental psychology', *Studies in Education and Psychology,* 11 (Stockholm Institute of Education, Department of Educational Research).

Bowman, B., Donovan, M. and Burns, S. (eds) (2000) *Eager to Learn: Educating our Preschoolers*, Washington, D.C.: National Academy Press.

Cardon, G., Van Cauwenberghe, E., Labarque, V., Haerens, L. and De Bourdeaudhuij, I. (2008) 'The contribution of preschool playground factors in explaining children's physical activity during recess', *International Journal of Behavioral Nutrition and Physical Activity*; 26 February: 5–11.

Centers for Disease Control and Prevention, National Center for Environmental Health (2008) 'Healthy community design, fact sheet', available at: <http://www.cdc.gov/healthyplaces/docs/Healthy%20Community%20Design.pdf> (accessed 31 July 2009).

Centers for Disease Control and Prevention, National Center for Environmental Health (nd) 'Children's health and the built environment', available at: <http://www.cdc.gov/healthyplaces/healthtopics/children.htm> (accessed 31 July 2009).

Chawla, L. (ed.) (2002) *Growing Up in an Urbanising World*, London: Earthscan.

Chermayeff, J., Blandford, R. and Losos, C. (2001) 'Working at play: informal science education on museum playgrounds', *Curator*, 44 (1): 47–60.

Cooper Marcus, C. and Francis, C. (1998) *People Places: Design Guidelines for Urban Open Space*, 2nd edn, New York: Wiley ('Post-Occupancy Evaluation,' Chapter 8: 346–56).

Cornell, E. H., Hadley, D. C., Sterling, T. M., Chan, M. A. and Boechler, P. (2001) 'Adventure as a stimulus for cognitive development', *Journal of Environmental Psychology*, 21: 219–31.

Cosco, N. (2006) *Motivation to Move: Physical Activity Affordances in Preschool Play Areas*, unpublished doctoral dissertation, Edinburgh College of Art, Heriot-Watt University, Edinburgh.

Cosco, N. (2007) 'Developing evidence-based design: environmental interventions for healthy development of young children in the outdoors', in C. Ward Thompson and P. Travlou (eds), *Open Space: People Space,* 125–35, London: Taylor & Francis.

Crowley, K., Callanan, M., Jipson, J., Galco, J., Topping, K. and Shrager, J. (2001) 'Shared scientific thinking in everyday parent–child activity', *Science Education,* 85(6): 712–32.

Dowda, M., Brown, W. H., McIver, K. L., Pfeiffer, K. A., O'Neill, J., Addy, C. L., et al. (2009) 'Policies and characteristics of the preschool environment and physical activity of young children', *Pediatrics,* 123: 261–6.

Dowda, M., Pate, R., Trost, S., Almeida, M. and Sirard, J. (2004) 'Influences of preschool policies and practices on children's physical activity', *Journal of Community Health,* 29 (3): 183–96.

Driskell, D. (2002) *Creating Better Cities with Children and Youth: A Manual for Participation,* London: Earthscan.

DuRant, R. H., Baranowski, T., Puhl, J., Rhodes, T., Davis, H., Greaves, K. A., and Thompson, W. O. (1993) 'Evaluation of the Children's Activity Rating Scale (CARS) in young children', *Medicine and Science in Sports and Exercise,* 25: 1415–21.

Dyasi, H. (1999) 'What children gain by learning through inquiry', *Foundations,* Arlington, Va.: National Science Foundation.

Faber Taylor, A. and Kuo, F. E. (2008) 'Children with attention deficits concentrate better after walk in the park', *Journal of Attention Disorders,* available at: <http://jad.sagepub.com/> (accessed 20 December 2008).

Frank, L., Engelke, P. and Schmid, T. (2003) *Health and Community Design: The Impact of the Built Environment on Physical Activity,* Washington, D.C.: Island Press.

Francis, M. (1984) 'Mapping downtown activity,' *Journal of Architecture and Planning Research,* 1 (1): 21–35.

Frost, J., Wortham S. and Reifel, S. (2005) *Play and Child Development.* Upper Saddle River, N.J.: Prentice Hall.

Frumkin, H., Frank, L. and Jackson, R. (2004) *Urban Sprawl and Public Health: Designing, Planning, and Building for Healthy Communities,* Washington, D.C.: Island Press.

Gibson, E. and Pick, A. (2000) *An Ecological Approach to Perceptual Learning and Development,* New York: Oxford University Press.

Gibson, J. (1979) *The Ecological Approach to Visual Perception,* Boston, Mass.: Houghton-Mifflin.

Harms, T., Cryer, D. and Clifford, R. (1990) *Infant/Toddler Environment Rating Scale,* New York: Teachers College Press.

Heft, H. (2001) *Ecological Psychology in Context: James Gibson, Roger Barker, and the legacy of William James's Radical Empiricism,* Mahwah, N.J.: Erlbaum.

Ittleson, W., Rivlin, L. and Proshansky, H. (1976) 'Use of behavior maps in environmental psychology', in H. Proshansky, W. Ittleson and L. Rivlin (eds), *Environmental Psychology: People and their Physical Settings,* 2nd edn, New York: Holt Rinehart & Winston.

Jackson, R. and Kochtitzky, C. (2001) 'Creating a healthy environment: the impact of the built environment on public health', Sprawl Watch Clearinghouse Monograph Series, available at: <http://www.sprawlwatch.org/health.pdf> (accessed 3 July 2009).

Jantsch, E. (1975) *Design for Evolution: Self-Organization and Planning in the Life of Human Systems,* New York: George Braziller.

Longley, P., Goodchild, M., Maguire, D. and Rhind, D. (2005) *Geographic Information Systems and Science,* London: Wiley.

Louv, R. (2005) *Last Child in the Woods: Saving our Children from Nature-Deficit Disorder,* Chapel Hill, N.C.: Algonquin.

Lynch, K. (1977) *Growing Up in Cities,* Cambridge, Mass.: MIT Press.

Lynch, K. (1981) *Good City Form,* Cambridge, Mass.: MIT Press.

Maller, C., Townsend, M., Pryor, A., Brown, P. and St. Leger, L. (2006) 'Healthy nature healthy people: 'Contact with nature' as an upstream promotion intervention for populations', *Health Promotion International,* 21 (1): 45–54.

McKenzie, T. and Cohen, D. (2006) 'SOPARC (System for Observing Play and Recreation in Communities)' *Description and Procedures Manual,* Department of Exercise and Nutritional Sciences, San Diego State University, San Diego.

Robin C. Moore and Nilda G. Cosco

McKenzie, T. L., Cohen, D., Sehgal, A., Williamson, S. and Golinelli, D. (2006) 'System for Observing Play And Recreation in Communities – SOPARC. Reliability and feasibility measures', *Journal of Physical Activity and Health*, 1: 203–17.

Mitchell, R. and Popham, F. (2008) 'Effect of exposure to natural environment on health inequalities: an observational population study', *The Lancet*, 372(9650): 1655–60.

Moore, R. (1974) 'Patterns of activity in time and space: the ecology of a neighborhood playground', in D. Canter and L. Lee (eds), *Psychology and the Built Environment*, 118–31, London: Architectural Press.

Moore, R. (1986) *Childhood's Domain: Play and Place in Child Development*, London: Croom Helm.

Moore, R. and Cooper Marcus, C. (2008) 'Healthy Planet, Healthy Children: Designing Nature into the Daily Spaces of Childhood', in S. Kellert, J. Heerwagen and M. Mador, *Biophilic Design: The Theory, Science, and Practice of Bringing Buildings to Life*, Hoboken, N.J.: Wiley.

Moore, R. and Cosco, N. (2007) 'What makes a park inclusive and universally designed? A multimethod approach', in C. Ward Thompson and P. Travlou (eds), *Open Space: People Space*, 85–110, London: Taylor & Francis.

Moore, R., Cosco, N., Kepez, O. and Demir, E. (2008) *My Place by the Bay: Prepared Environments for Early Science Learning*, Bay Area Discovery Museum (BADM), Sausalito, California. Final report to the National Science Foundation, project #0125740.

Moore, R. and Wong, H. (1997) *Natural Learning: Creating Environments for Rediscovering Nature's Way of Teaching*. Berkeley, Calif.: MIG Communications.

Moore, R. and Young, D. (1978) 'Childhood outdoors: towards a social ecology of the landscape', in I. Altman and J. Wohlwill (eds), *Human Behavior and Environment, vol. 3: Children and the Environment*, 83–130, New York: Plenum Press.

National Institute of Environmental Health Sciences (NIEHS), http://grants.nih.gov/grants/guide/rfa-files/rfa-es-04-003.html (accessed 2 December 2009).

National Research Council (1996) 'National Science Education Standards', *National Research Council*, available at: <http://books.nap.edu/openbook.php?record_id=4962&page=R2> (accessed 4 May 2009).

Nicolescu, B. (ed.) (2008) *Transdisciplinarity – Theory and Practice*, Cresskill, N.J.: Hampton Press.

Olmsted, F. L., Jr. (1911) 'The city beautiful', *The Builder*, 101, July 7, 1911: 15–17, formatted as a web document by John W. Reps, available at: <http://www.library.cornell.edu/Reps/DOCS/olmst_11.htm> (accessed 31 May 2009).

Ogden, C., Carroll, M. and Flegal, K. (2008) 'High body mass index for age among US children and adolescents, 2003–2006' *Journal of the American Medical Association*, 299 (20): 2401–05.

Puhl, J., Greaves, K., Hoyt, M. and Baranowski, T. (1990) 'Children's Activity Rating Scale (CARS): description and calibration', *Research Quarterly for Exercise and Sport*, 61 (1): 26–36.

Rajakaruna, C. (ed.). (2006) *2006 Membership Directory*, Washington, D.C.: Association of Children's Museums.

Reps, J. (nd) 'Writing about Frederick Law Olmsted, Jr', available at: <http://www.library.cornell.edu/Reps/DOCS/olmst_11.htm> (accessed 31 May 2009).

Roemmich, J. N., Epstein, L. H., Raja, S., Yin, L., Robinson, J. and Winiewicz, D. (2006) 'Association of access to parks and recreational facilities with the physical activity of young children', *Preventive Medicine*, 43: 437-41.

Rose, K. A., Morgan, I. G., Ip, J., Kifley, A., Huynh, S. and Smith, W. (2008) 'Outdoor activity reduces the prevalence of myopia in children', *Ophthalmology*, 115 (8): 1279–85.

Saelens, B. E., Frank, L. D., Auffrey, C., Whitaker, R. C., Burdette, H. L. and Colabianchi, N. (2006) 'Measuring physical environments of parks and playgrounds: EAPRS instrument development and inter-rater reliability', *Journal of Physical Activity and Health*, 3 (1): 190–207.

Sallis, J., Nader, P. R., Broyles, S. L., Berry, C. C., Elder, J. P., McKenzie, T. L. and Nelson, J. A. (1993) 'Correlates of physical activity at home in Mexican–American and Anglo-American preschool children', *Health Psychology*, 12 (5): 390-98.

Staempfli, M. B. (2009) 'Reintroducing adventure into children's outdoor play environments', *Environment and Behavior*, 41 (2): 268–80.

Van Andel, J. (1984-1985) 'Effects on children's behavior of physical changes in a Leiden neighborhood', *Children's Environments Quarterly*, 1 (4): 46–54.

Watanabe, M., Nakamura, K., Fukuda, Y. and Takano, T. (2006) 'Association of parental and children behaviors with the health status of preschool children', *Preventive Medicine*, 42: 297–300.

Webster's Third International Dictionary (1981), Springfield, MA.: Merriam-Webster, Inc.

Wellington, J. (1990) 'Formal and informal learning science: the role of interactive science centres', *Physical Education*, 25: 247–52.

Wells, N. M. and Evans, G. W. (2003) 'Nearby nature: a buffer of life stress among rural children', *Environment and Behavior*, 35: 311-30.

Williams, C. H. (2007) 'The built environment and physical activity: what is the relationship?' New Jersey: Robert Wood Johnson Foundation., available at: <http://www.rwjf.org/pr/product.jsp?id=20112> (accessed 21 December 2008).

Worth, K. (2000) 'The power of children's thinking', *Foundations*, 2: 25–32, available at: <http://www.nsf.gov/pubs/2000/nsf99148/> (accessed 31 July 2009).

Part II

Evidence on the relationship between landscape and health

Chapter 3

Nearby nature and human health:

looking at mechanisms and their implications

Sjerp de Vries

Introduction

In the past centuries human health tended to be primarily threatened by infectious diseases. At present our health seems to be increasingly threatened by so-called lifestyle-related diseases (Nilsson, Baines and Konijnendijk, 2007). Partly this may be due to a broader view on health, as exemplified by the definition adopted by the World Health Organization (WHO) in 1946 (to which I too will adhere): 'Health is a state of complete physical, mental and social well-being and not merely the absence of disease or infirmity.'

One could argue that, especially in the developed world, health standards have gone up, as well as that in general, lifestyles have become less healthy. Either way, there has been a growing interest in the factors that influence people's lifestyle, especially in its health-related aspects. In ecological models of lifestyle and health (for example, Swinburn, Egger and Raza, 1999) the physical environment is an important component. In this chapter I shall focus on the residential environment, and more specifically on the availability of green space within this environment.

As more and more people live (and work) in cities, having green space nearby and/or coming into contact with nature on a regular basis cannot be taken for granted. Although few people doubt that green spaces and natural elements benefit human health, such insights are not commonly applied in policy making in relevant sectors such as nature conservation, spatial planning and public health.

Sjerp de Vries

There appear to be other, more pressing reasons leading policy makers to opt for concentrated urbanisation and compact cities: preventing urban sprawl from fragmenting habitats or spoiling the countryside, limiting car use and creating a solid user base for public facilities and transport (Van den Berg, Hartig and Staats, 2007). The possible negative health consequences of living in a compact city with a low amount of green space may partly be overlooked because, according to the Health Council of the Netherlands, the scientific evidence for the beneficial effects of nearby nature is as yet very limited (GR/RMNO, 2004).

Nevertheless, earlier Dutch research (De Vries et al., 2003; Maas et al., 2006) has shown a relationship between the amount of nearby green space and self-reported health. Studies in other countries have shown similar relationships. Table 3.1 gives an overview of a number of such studies, classified by whether the environmental characteristic and/or the health status were measured as perceived by inhabitants or more objectively assessed. Studies using more objective measurements are assumed to provide more substantial evidence regarding the importance of the actual physical aspects of the environment. This is relevant because the physical aspects themselves, rather than the way they are perceived, are more directly influenced by spatial planning and design.

Most of these studies took place in northwest European countries: Denmark, England, the Netherlands and Sweden. So the positive relationship between easy access to green space and health seems well established, at least for this part of Europe. However, this does not necessarily imply that greening the urban environment will improve public health: correlation does not equal causation. Selective migration might be at work, with healthier people moving into greener neighbourhoods, and/or less healthy people moving out (Verheij, Maas and Groenewegen, 2008). Most studies have tried to rule out this type of explanation by correcting statistically for differences in the composition of the population. But, although such corrections can make causality more plausible, they cannot prove it.

Table 3.1 Classification of studies showing a positive relationship between nearby green space and human health.

| | | Natural environment | |
		Residents' perceptions	More objective measures
Human health	Self-report	Grahn & Stigdotter (2003) Nielsen & Hansen (2007; stress)	De Vries et al (2003) Maas et al (2006) Mitchell & Popham (2007)
	More objective measures	Takano et al (2002) Nielsen & Hansen (2007; overweight)	Mitchell & Popham (2008) Maas et al (2009b)

Linked to the issue of causality is the question about the mechanism behind the relationship between nearby green space and health. Up until now it has been largely unclear which type of green space will most benefit the health of local residents. How many green areas and natural elements of what size and type are needed, and where, to achieve certain health benefits? And for whom? This also has implications for the best way to assess the local situation. For example, the exclusion of small green areas, such as gardens and street trees, in most geographical information system (GIS)-based measures may be undeserved. On the other hand, distance criteria that are relevant for adults may be too inclusive for children, because of the smaller action radius of the latter. If the green-space indicators that have been used in previous studies are not optimal, the relationship between (the right types of) nearby nature and health might not be measured accurately; the relationship might be even stronger than observed thus far.

In this chapter I address the following questions:

If the relationship between nearby green space and human health is causal in nature, then: a) what is the most likely causal mechanism behind this relationship, and b) what are the implications of this mechanism regarding the most effective green infrastructure?

The relevance of a mechanism may differ between segments of the population. Moreover, more than one mechanism might be involved. I will also briefly look into the matter of the compatibility of different mechanisms in terms of their requirements for an optimal green infrastructure. Furthermore green space may also (need to) serve functions that are not health-related, for example, water retention. Issues of multifunctionality in a broader perspective fall outside the scope of the present chapter. However, specifying the health-related requirements may help to assess which combinations of functions are likely to be successful and which are not.

Mechanisms linking nearby nature to health

Based on a review of the scientific and policy literature, possible mechanisms that are frequently mentioned in connection to the favourable effects of green spaces on local public health have been identified. Four mechanisms were selected for further study:

- improving air quality, especially by filtering fine particulate matter from the air
- reducing stress and restoring people's power of concentration

- stimulating physical activity, whether in a recreational context or otherwise
- facilitating social contacts and social cohesion among residents.

This selection is partly based on the importance of the associated health problems in present Western societies: health problems caused by air pollution, in particular high concentrations of fine dust; stress-related health problems, such as cardio-vascular diseases; diseases related to overweight and obesity, such as diabetes mellitus type II; and depression. In part, the selection is also based on the availability of studies and evidence on the mechanisms involved. Mechanisms that have not been selected are other improvements in air quality or the micro-climate; increasing satisfaction with one's residential environment and place attachment; and reducing aggression and crime, and thereby fear of crime. This does not necessarily mean that these mechanisms are less relevant, merely that they are less well documented in the literature to date.

I shall examine, or in most cases try to argue, what requirements local green spaces have to meet to optimise the operation of each of the four selected mechanisms. In addition, I shall try to identify which sections of the population are most likely to benefit from a particular mechanism. Furthermore, I offer an indication of how important the mechanism is likely to be in explaining the observed relationships between nearby nature and human health. Below, the main conclusions for each of the four mechanisms are presented.

Improving air quality

The deleterious effects of fine particulate air pollution have been sufficiently proven, even though the precise effects of long-term exposure are still unclear (Singels, Klooster and Hoek, 2005; MNP/RIVM, 2005). It is also generally accepted that green elements can filter fine particulate pollution from the air. Trees, in particular coniferous ones, have proved effective in filtering very small soot particles (PM2.5), which are thought to be very harmful (Wesseling et al., 2004). In terms of structure, fairly open linear structures appear to be more effective than closed planar structures. The polluted air should be able to flow through the vegetation, rather than passing overhead. The sections of the population that benefit most seem to be those spending much time near the filtering green structures. Furthermore, certain groups can be identified that are particularly in need of clean air, such as people with respiratory problems. In addition, people may be extra vulnerable to fine dust during strenuous physical activity: because of the deeper inhalation, the dust will penetrate further into the lungs (Van Wijnen et al., 1995).

Quite another matter is to what extent the air filtering capacity of trees can explain the health benefits of local green spaces. To begin with, the severity of fine particulate air pollution varies considerably across areas, and the filtering capacity of vegetation is especially important in areas with a severe air quality problem. Even with filtering by trees, however, the remaining levels of fine particulate matter may be higher than in areas where the problem was less severe to begin with. An additional issue is that it may be difficult to achieve air filtration by trees in the urban environment itself, as the trees may actually impede airflows. Fine dust could thus be 'trapped' in places where many people live.

Nowak, Crane and Stevens (2006) estimated improvements of air quality by trees for a number of cities in the United States. The highest improvement in terms of a reduction of fine dust was 1 per cent, and this was in a city with a tree cover of 42 per cent. In a similar vein McDonald and colleagues (2007) concluded that the effect of the maximum obtainable increase in tree cover within the Glasgow conurbation, from 4 to 21 per cent (almost 3,800 hectares), would lower the level of fine dust in the centre of the city by no more than 2 per cent. A recent report by the Dutch National Institute for Public Health and the Environment (Wesseling, Beijk and Van Kuijeren, 2008) concludes that the effect of vegetation (trees and shrubs) on air quality in and around cities appears to be not only limited, but also variable (positive or negative).

All in all, the filtering of fine dust by vegetation does not seem a very likely causal explanation of the relationship between nearby green space and human health. It seems more plausible that there is a negative relationship between the presence of emission sources of fine particulate matter (such as busy roads and industry) and the presence of green elements. Although this is not a causal relationship related to the filtering qualities of the vegetation, it would be worthwhile to investigate this correlation, in order to be able to determine whether or not it offers an alternative explanation for the relationship between the amount of green space and health.

Reducing stress and mental fatigue

Experimental research has clearly established that contact with nature reduces levels of stress in humans. Much of this research on restoration is inspired by either Ulrich's psycho-evolutionary theory of stress reduction (1983) or the attention restoration theory (ART) of the Kaplans (Kaplan and Kaplan, 1989). However, in most studies stress is induced as a part of the experiment and the focus is on short-term effects. Less is known about the long-term effects of a 'daily dose' of exposure to green elements on stress-related health complaints (see also Hartig, 2007). But the few studies on everyday environments that are available tend to show positive relationships (see, for example, Kaplan, 2001; Grahn and Stigsdotter, 2003).

Few studies have focused on which type of green space works best. Usually only a rough distinction is made between urban areas and nature areas

(Velarde, Fry and Tveit, 2007). Parsons and colleagues (1998) found more positive effects for a golf course than for woodland. The influence of the spatial structure on the effects achieved is not clear either. One potentially beneficial option would be to maximise people's visual contact with green elements. This would argue for planting trees and shrubs along frequently used routes, such as those that people take to work, school or shops. Based on findings of (mostly experimental) research, showing stress-reducing effects of many types of green elements, and even of images of parks and green landscapes, one could conclude that 'vertical green elements', such as building facades overgrown with creepers and climbers, would present a very efficient way to implement this first option, that of maximising visual contact.

Another option would seem to be ensuring easy access to green 'oases', to which people can go when they feel stressed. Within this option the quality of the experience is assigned more importance than within the first option. De Kort and colleagues (2006) have coined the term 'immersion' with regard to this quality. It seems conceptually related to the concepts 'extent' and 'being away', which are used in the Kaplans' ART. In a similar vein, Korpela and Hartig (1996) talk about deep restoration. However, they see this most strongly linked to another ART concept, 'compatibility'.

An important question relating to the 'green oases' option is whether people will actually go and visit such oases at times they would benefit most from them: that is, whether visits to quiet green areas would actually be used more intensively as a conscious strategy for coping with stress if more of them were made locally available. A study by Korpela and Ylen (2007) suggests that this might not be the case. People with health complaints had a stronger preference for natural environments and benefited more from visiting such an environment, but they did not visit natural environments more frequently. It should be noted that Korpela and Ylen did not take differences in the availability of or access to natural environments into account.

A relevant question is to what extent the restorativeness of natural environments is universal, and whether there are alternatives for natural environments in this respect. There have been some studies on cultural differences in landscape preferences, showing that differences tend to be small (Stamps III, 1999; Herzog et al., 2000). However, it is unclear to what extent attractiveness ('scenic beauty') and restorativeness of landscapes are causally linked, and if so, by what process. A study by Chang (2004) showed no cultural differences in landscape preference, but did find differences in perceived restorativeness. Chang proposes that an environment is more restorative to the degree that it is more familiar. Interestingly, if this is true then 'being away' could also be taken too far: new and unfamiliar surroundings may demand too much attention to be restorative. In a similar vein more natural may not always be more restorative (see the 1998 study by Parsons and colleagues mentioned earlier).

As for the uniqueness of nature as a restorative environment, Karmanov and Hamel (2008) concluded that a well-designed and attractive urban environment had stress-reducing and mood-enhancing effects similar to that of an attractive natural environment. Pretty and colleagues (2005) concluded that, in the context of exercise, unpleasant rural scenes had an even worse effect on self-esteem and mood than unpleasant urban scenes. Both pleasant urban and pleasant rural scenes had a positive effect. According to Kaplan and Kaplan (1989), the qualities needed for an environment to be restorative are not unique to nature, but natural environments tend to possess them to a high degree. This would imply that well-designed and attractive urban environments are rarer than attractive natural environments.

The people for whom stress reduction is a relevant mechanism are likely to be those who have high stress levels prior to coming into contact with nature. An experimental study by Morita and colleagues (2007) supports precisely this assumption, and so do field studies by Wells and Evans (2003) and Ottosson and Grahn (2008). Population segments that are likely to benefit most from nearby nature in their residential environment would be people exposed to chronic stressors, or those otherwise in danger of falling victim to chronic high stress levels. Single parents with a full-time job might be one such category. Quite another category is people experiencing stressful life events, such as the death of a close relative or the loss of their job. Such events may have long-term effects if coping is unsuccessful.

To what extent stress reduction and restoration mediate the earlier observed relationship between nearby nature and health is still uncertain. I identified one study on the possible buffering effect of nearby green space with regard to stress. Maas and colleagues (in Maas, 2008) concluded that the impact of a stressful life event on the number of health-related complaints was smaller in residential areas with more green space within a 3 km radius. However, a similar conclusion could not be drawn for two other health indicators, perceived mental and general health. The earlier mentioned studies by Wells and Evans and by Ottosson and Grahn could also be interpreted as supporting stress reduction as a mechanism, depending on whether the dependent measure they used in their study is considered an indicator of the level of stress, or a more general (mental) health indicator. Either way, in neither of the studies have both stress levels and general health been measured. A straightforward analysis of the extent to which the effect of nearby green space on health is mediated by stress levels has not been performed thus far.

At this point it should be noted that I interpret 'buffering' here quite generally as preventing the effect of a stressor leading to chronically high stress levels. This may operate in different ways. The first way is that the impact of semi-permanent (mild) stressors or incidental (major) life events is smaller to begin with. The second way is that more and quicker restoration occurs after stress is experienced. The first way opens up the possibility that green space can also be effective at times when someone is not stressed, preventing them from being thrown out of balance. It seems to argue for the importance of frequent (casual) encounters with green space. The second way is more about resilience, the ability to bounce back when out of balance. It is the difference between what Hartig (2007: 164) calls 'instorative' versus restorative benefits. The experimental research thus far has focused almost exclusively on this latter path, reducing stress once it has occurred.

So although restoration is one of the most researched and plausible links between nature and health, there are still some important questions unanswered. They deal largely with to what extent stress levels actually do mediate the relationship between nearby nature and health, the quality of restorative experience associated with different green structures, and the importance of this quality with regard to health benefits.

Stimulating physical activity

The benefits of exercise have been well established, for both physical (GR/RMNO, 2004) and mental health (Fox, 1999). I focus here on physical activity as a means to help prevent people being overweight. So the main question is whether more green space and natural elements in the neighbourhood are likely to lead to more physical activity, preferably of at least moderate intensity, and in this way increase energy expenditure. Unlike stress reduction, this is a topic of study that does not have an experimental research tradition. Based on reviews of studies on environmental correlates of physical activity, several authors propose that studies should be specific with regard to the activity under investigation, and focus on environmental aspects that may be expected to be relevant with regard to the selected activity (Ball, Timperio and Crawford, 2006; Giles-Corti et al., 2005; Wendel-Vos et al., 2005). As for types of physical activity that might be influenced by the greenness of the neighbourhood environment, a rough distinction can be made between exercise achieved through active transport (on foot or by bicycle) and that through recreational activities.

Nowadays, many adults in West European countries get most of their physical activity in the form of active transport, more so than in the form of leisure activities (WHO Europe, 2002). The main factors influencing the choice of mode of transport (modal split) appear to be the distance to be travelled and the infrastructure and facilities that are present for this mode of transport. Many European cities score rather well in these respects, compared with cities in the United States (Pucher and Buehler, 2008). According to the framework provided by Pikora and colleagues (2006), the contributions made by green areas and natural elements seem to be predominantly in the aesthetic domain. Therefore theoretically, it seems likely that their influence on the modal split is minor. In line with this, based on a systematic review, Wendel-Vos and colleagues (2005) conclude that there is little empirical support for the importance of the aesthetic quality of the environment with regard to overall physical activity.

When it comes to recreational activities, people do usually appreciate the presence of green spaces in the local area, and will use them for recreation, provided they are regarded as accessible and safe. The same holds for attractive streetscapes (Giles-Corti and Donovan, 2002). This does not mean, however, that people will not engage in recreational activities if green elements are not locally available. There are two reasons why more visits to parks and other green areas, or spending more time there, does not necessarily equal more physical activity. Not only can people be physically active during leisure time outside green areas, but also being in a green area does not necessarily imply physical exercise of at least moderate intensity. The design of green spaces seems to be a major factor in this respect, as some green spaces invite exercise while others invite more passive forms of recreation.

Kaczynski and Henderson (2007) reviewed studies focusing on parks and recreational settings and physical activity. They concluded that the nearness of parks and recreation settings in general was positively related to the amount of physical activity. With regard to the type of park or setting, the results were rather mixed. However, it should be noted that the physical activity measures in the studies that were reviewed were sometimes quite limited. In some cases the measure was simply restricted to the frequency of use of a newly developed trail. In line with what was said above, with regard to energy expenditure the total amount of physical activity is what is relevant (taking the intensity into account as well). So there may be a drawback to studying activities in isolation. With regard to positive health effects by way of increased energy expenditure, such studies tend to ignore the possibility of negative interrelationships between different types of activity. Wilkin and colleagues (2006), for example, suggest that children who receive more hours of physical education at school are less physically active outside school. Activity or location substitution may be more likely than an overall increase in physical activity.

When it comes to segments of the population for which nearby nature might be especially relevant with regard to physical activity, I would like to draw attention to children. There is growing evidence that the greenness of the environment is related to the amount of time spent on outdoor play and/or the amount of energy expended by this type of activity. This is an important category of activity for this age group (De Vries et al., 2008). Roemmich and colleagues (2006) studied the relationship between the percentage of park plus recreation area within half a mile of home, and physical activity as measured by an accelerometer for four to seven-year-old children (n = 59). After statistically controlling for sociodemographic characteristics there was a positive correlation. A similar study for eight to twelve-year-old children (n = 88) showed a similar relationship between the percentage of park area and physical activity, but for boys only (Roemmich et al., 2007). Neither study has data on where the (extra) physical activity took place, but it seems reasonable to assume that the parks were involved.

The latter finding is more or less replicated in a recent Dutch study (De Vries et al., 2008). This study is based on data gathered on over 4,500 children between six and twelve years of age by a municipal health service in a quite rural part of the Netherlands. Time spent on outdoor play, BMI and the health of the child were all reported by parents. The dataset was enriched with a green space indicator, namely whether or not there was at least on average 75 m^2 of public green space per dwelling available within 500 metres of the postcode area. This 75 m^2 is a guideline on green space that is provided by the national government. Secondary analyses showed that meeting the guideline was associated with more outdoor play. But only for boys was the time spent on outdoor play negatively related to being overweight. This makes it likely that it is the type of activity that is performed while playing outdoors that differs between boys and girls in the age category. As one would expect, being overweight was negatively related to the health of the child, although not very strongly so. It is interesting to note that, even after correcting for the overweight status of the child, the time spent on outdoor play still showed a considerable relationship with health. This suggests that outdoor play may have beneficial effects that do not rely on increased energy expenditure.

Another segment of the population for which nearby nature might be especially important with regard to physical activity is elderly people. Li and colleagues (2005) reported that the total amount of green and open spaces for recreation in the neighbourhood showed a significant predictive contribution to self-reported walking activity. The intensity of the activity is unclear and may not be very high on average. But even at low intensities, neighbourhood walking may still be important. This is because of the social contacts and cohesion it may bring about, something I turn to in the next section.

As for the extent to which physical activity levels mediate the relationship between the amount of nearby green space and health, two studies have explicitly investigated this question. Sugiyama and colleagues (2008) found that walking for recreation could fully explain the relationship between perceived neighbourhood greenness and physical health, while it contributed to explaining the somewhat stronger relationship between perceived neighbourhood greenness and mental health. Walking for transport had no such role: it was related to neither greenness nor to the health scores. On the other hand, Maas and colleagues (2008) concluded that overall physical activity was not an important mediator of the 'effect' of the quantity of nearby green space on perceived general health. Moreover, people with more green space in their living environment walked and cycled less during leisure time in this study.

The difference in outcome with regard to recreational walking may have something to do with the way the environmental characteristic was assessed in different studies: the perception of the resident himself versus a GIS-based measure for at least a 1 km zone. Using the first type of measurement in combination with analyses conducted at the individual level may lead to a same source reporting bias (Raudenbush and Sampson, 1999), in this case, enhancing the relationship between the greenness of the neighbourhood and the level of activity. The aforementioned study on children by De Vries and colleagues (2008) could also be included with regard to physical activity as mediator. However, in this study there was no direct relationship between the greenness of the neighbourhood and the health of the child as perceived by the parent to begin with. Additional analyses suggest that this might be because of the crudeness of the environmental indicator that was used.

All in all, the evidence for the importance of nearby green space for overall physical activity levels, and thereby energy expenditure, does not seem very promising thus far, with the possible exception of outdoor play by children. This makes it less plausible that energy expenditure is an important link in a causal chain between the nearby nature and the health of the adult population. With regard to children, questions might be raised regarding whether more natural playgrounds, or playgrounds in a green setting, have an advantage over other types of playgrounds (Potwarka, Kaczynski and Flack, 2008).

Facilitating social contacts and cohesion within the neighbourhood

Although the evidence is not as overwhelming as in the case of physical activity, social contacts, social cohesion and/or social capital do appear to enhance health and well-being (Kawachi, Kennedy and Glass, 1999; Berkman, Glass and Brisette, 2000; Leyden, 2003). Here I focus on contacts with neighbourhood members and (perceived) cohesion within the neighbourhood. These might especially be expected to be influenced by the physical characteristics of the neighbourhood, such as the availability of green space and the presence of natural elements.

There is even less research on the relationship between nearby nature, and social contact and cohesion within the neighbourhood. Studies by Coley, Kuo and Sullivan (1997), Kuo, Sullivan and Wiley (1998) and Kweon, Sullivan and Wiley (1998) indicate that green space very close at hand may contribute to social contacts and cohesion between neighbourhood members. However, these studies have predominantly focused on the same and quite specific setting: a very poor segment of the population of a large city (Chicago), living in high-rise apartment buildings. The comparisons that are made involve a neighbourhood environment without any vegetation and one with a small patch of grass and a few trees. Notwithstanding the high quality of at least some of the studies (almost perfect natural experiments), this raises questions regarding the generalisability of the conclusions. In a more recent study by the same research group (Sullivan, Kuo and DePooter, 2004), arriving at the same conclusion regarding nearby greenery and social contacts, the authors themselves discuss to what extent their conclusions are also valid in the greener and/or wealthier part of the spectrum.

Which type of green space would be most effective in terms of this particular mechanism is likely to depend on the type of social contact to be facilitated. If the aim is to stimulate casual encounters, a good option would seem to be to improve the 'walkability' of the neighbourhood (Leyden, 2003). Green elements can be used to make certain routes more attractive, which would seem to be favourable especially for recreational strolls. More intensive social contacts could probably be stimulated better by creating small neighbourhood parks catering for local areas. In general social contacts, especially the more intensive ones, are more likely to be stimulated by stationary activities than by activities such as skating and cycling, especially when the latter involve relatively high speeds.

On the other hand, there is growing evidence that relatively superficial contacts, such as greeting people one passes in the street, are enough to help create a sense of community (Blokland-Potters, 2006; Cattell et al., 2008). This is an important issue since the physical characteristics of residential areas may have a greater impact on such superficial contacts (very weak ties) than on the development of more intensive relations with neighbours (strong ties). Some studies have observed a positive relationship of the quality and amenities of the public space within the neighbourhood, including green and/or recreational elements, with the sense of community and/or social cohesion. At the same time these environmental characteristics were not related to the amount of contact between neighbourhood members (Skjaeveland, 2001; Flap and Völker, 2004).

A segment of the population for whom the social side of the neighbourhood, and thereby this mechanism, may be particularly relevant is the elderly, especially those living alone and less mobile people (Bertera, 2003; Glass et al., 2006). This segment requires high-quality options in terms of infrastructure (such as comfortable and well-kept paths and benches) and physical and social safety, for both the site itself and the access routes (Loukaitou-Sideris, 2006; Sugiyama and Ward Thompson, 2007, 2008).

As for explicit tests of the mediation of the nearby nature–health relationship by social contacts and/or cohesion, two studies have been identified. In the study mentioned earlier, Sugiyama and colleagues (2008) found that the relationship between perceived neighbourhood greenness and mental health was partially accounted for by walking for recreation and social coherence. Interestingly, they did not observe a similar finding for the amount of social contact with neighbours. This seems in line with previously mentioned results, questioning the importance of (serious) social contacts as an intermediate step. However, Sugiyama and colleagues did also include superficial contacts, such as waving to a neighbour. Maas and colleagues (2009b) concluded that loneliness and perceived shortage of social support partially explained the relationship between the objectively assessed amount of green space and self-reported health indicators. In the case of mental health, mediation by shortage of social support was shown to be complete: after including the social support variable in the analysis there was no longer a significant direct relationship between the amount of green space and mental health. However, they also concluded that the frequency of (more than superficial) social contacts had no such mediating role.

Summarising the above, social cohesion seems to be an important mediator of the relationship between nearby nature and human health. This is somewhat surprising, since it is the least studied of the four mechanisms discussed in this chapter. The relationship between actual social contacts and the sense of social cohesion within the neighbourhood merits further research attention. Superficial contacts might already be enough to create a sense of social cohesion. The number of chance meetings is more likely to be influenced by the physical characteristics of the neighbourhood than the number of strong social ties usually associated with social capital.

Synthesis, conclusions and questions remaining

The first question I started out with was to what extent each of the selected four possible mechanisms was likely to be an important cause of the relationship between the availability of green space in a residential area and the health of its inhabitants. Based on the available evidence thus far, stress reduction and the facilitation of social cohesion are likely to be more important than improving air quality and stimulating physical activity (increasing energy expenditure). The consequences of this conclusion depend largely on the answer to the second question: do the four mechanisms differ in terms of what the accompanying optimal green infrastructure might be?

Space is scarce (or expensive) in the urban context, and open space is likely to become even more scarce, since at present policies tend to favour densi-fication of the urban fabric (for example, VROM, 2008). In other words, there is a strong pressure to use urban space efficiently. To the extent that the green space requirements for the mechanisms are not compatible, it makes sense to give priority to the mechanism that produces the most health benefits (at the lowest costs). With the exception of improving the air quality by means of filtering fine dust out of the air, relatively little is known with certainty about the optimal green infrastructure per mechanism. The evidence base is small in this regard. I have

Sjerp de Vries

tried to argue what type of infrastructure would fit best with each of the other mechanisms. Rather than summarising the conclusions per mechanism, I briefly discuss the issue of the compatibility of the different mechanisms. This also includes the question whether the four mechanisms can operate simultaneously at the same green sites, and might even reinforce each other, or whether they will actually interfere with one another. Table 3.2 gives an overview of the assumed compatibility (or lack of it), based on the arguments developed above. In this overview, two pathways are distinguished for stress reduction: maximising visual contact with green elements (green routes), and offering high-quality, immersive restorative experiences in green space (green oases).

Linear structures of coniferous trees seem optimal with regard to the filtering of fine dust. They should be located between emission sources and places where people live, without obstructing airflows and without keeping the dust trapped at places where it is most likely to be damaging to human health. Green structures accompanying busy roads could also be very effective in maximising visual contact with natural elements, especially since the quality of the experience is not deemed very important in the green route option for stress reduction. For the other option, green oases, the quality of the experience is considered important. In this case coniferous trees are less likely to be the optimal choice. Also, a location close to busy roads does not seem optimal: traffic noise will not contribute to the restorativeness of the experience. Vice versa, green oases are unlikely to be highly effective locations with regard to filtering the air.

With regard to physical activity near any linear elements such as roads with air filtering street trees, despite this filtering there is still likely to be a rather high concentration of fine dust, which is undesirable for healthy activity. As indicated earlier, a higher level of activity implies taking deeper breaths; fine dust will get deeper into the lungs, with more detrimental health consequences (Van Wijnen et al., 1995).

Table 3.2 Compatibility of green structures required by different mechanisms.

	Stress: green routes	Stress: green oases	Physical activity	Social cohesion
Fine dust filtering	+	−	−	−
Stress: green routes		−	+	+
Stress: green oases				+
Physical activity				−/+

Furthermore, especially for recreational activity, the pleasantness of the environment is likely to be important for the choice of location. The same holds for social contacts. If the source of air pollution is busy traffic, it will demand attention, while at the same time the noise of motorised traffic may hinder communication. So, although in the latter cases they may help to make the environment more pleasant, planting trees along busy streets may not be enough to make those streets attractive locations for recreational walking or 'hot spots' for casual meetings with neighbourhood members.

As for the two options with regard to stress reduction, they were distinguished precisely because of their different spatial implications. The green routes could to some extent be combined with settings for physical activity. However, the optimal routes are likely to differ from those where planting trees can effectively contribute to the filtering of fine dust. Quiet roads are more suitable for physical activity than busy roads, although this implies that fewer people will be using them. Perhaps such routes are even better suited for (superficial) social contacts with neighbourhood members. A residential area with little traffic, in which streets are lined with trees and/or front gardens, may be an attractive area for walking, in which people frequently encounter neighbours.

Green oases, at least in the form of pocket parks or courtyards, seem less suited for physical activity. There is little room for activity and it is unlikely that there will be special facilities for sports and play activities. Conversely, physical activity may lead to a dynamic and noisy environment, which may not be very conducive to a restorative experience. Green oases might go well together with social contacts. This depends on whether a possible need for privacy will be respected. Conversation that is forced upon a person is more likely to induce stress than to reduce it. It could also be a matter of timing: a green space might be quiet and suited for stress reduction in the morning, and busier, so good for social contacts, during lunchtime.

Stimulating physical activity and facilitating social contacts may not always go hand in hand. This has already been suggested with regard to green oases. For green routes this is a little more complicated. In principle, the same green infrastructure may work for both mechanisms. That is not to say that this can happen simultaneously. When something like Nordic walking, running, skating, or cycling is the dominant activity, people may be less inclined to seek contact: they are busy. A quick nod or hello in passing may be all that can be expected under such circumstances. On the other hand, when such superficial contacts are enough, practically all forms of simultaneous presence may help, as long as the different uses do not conflict; the casual contacts should be positive in nature.

Mechanisms may not only interfere with one another, they might also strengthen each other. A higher level of social cohesion might help to enhance restoration in public green spaces, because it reduces the fear of crime. And with regard to physical activity and social contacts, there may also be positive exceptions. For example, the playing together of very young children under the supervision of their parents may give these parents an opportunity for social contact and restoration; as long as the children have fun with each other, they might demand almost no attention. Furthermore, the children themselves are also engaged in social contact.

In conclusion, this chapter is more intended to raise awareness of the fact that the health benefits that one might want a local green space to produce bring different requirements for that same green space, rather than offering a single, definitive design solution. To unthinkingly assume that one small green space can fulfil several functions in an optimal way at the same time may be too optimistic.

Finally, as indicated earlier, many of the conclusions in this chapter are based on theoretical considerations rather than empirical evidence. This means that they primarily offer a framework for further research, rather than providing definite answers to the question of the relative importance of each of the four mechanisms. This is even truer for the question regarding the optimal green infrastructure per mechanism. Although attempts to specify the effective or optimised availability of green elements for each of the mechanisms are an important intermediate step, they are no more than that.

Studies on the quality of nearby green space and health or well-being, such as that by Agyemang and colleagues (2007) and Björk and colleagues (2008) may be one way forward. However, I would argue that the desirable qualities of green space might differ by mechanism. In my opinion, future research on nearby nature and health should involve the development and use of indicators of the availability of suitable nearby green spaces and natural elements for each of the mechanisms. Although Hartig and colleagues (1997) developed a scale for perceived restorativeness, to rate (green) areas, this is also not exactly what is meant here. What I propose is to develop, for example, an instrument to assess the restorative potential of a (green) environment based solely on its physical characteristics.

It should also be taken into account that suitability for a given function may differ by population segment. For example, children may require different settings than adults to stimulate physical activity. In addition, any such research should preferably include mediating factors that can tell us more about the process at work. This type of research could establish the health benefits of each mechanism under optimal conditions, and hence the type of green elements that would be most effective or efficient. It would allow policy makers and spatial planners to take nature for health in an urban residential context as seriously as it deserves to be taken, however serious that is.

References

Agyemang, C., van Hooijdonk, C., Wendel-Vos, W., Lindeman, E., Stronks, K. and Droomers, M. (2007) 'The association of neighborhood psychosocial stressors and self-rated health in Amsterdam, the Netherlands', *Journal of Epidemiology and Community Health*, 61: 1042–9.

Ball, K., Timperio, A. F. and Crawford, D. A. (2006) 'Understanding environmental influences on nutrition and physical activity behaviors: where should we look and what should we count?', *International Journal of Behavioral Nutrition and Physical Activity*, 3: 33–41.

Berkman, L. F., Glass, T. and Brissette, I. (2000) 'From social integration to health: Durkheim in the new millennium', *Social Science and Medicine*, 51: 843–57.

Bertera, E. M. (2003) 'Physical activity and social network contacts in community dwelling older adults', *Activities, Adaptation and Aging*, 27 (3–4): 113–27.

Björk, J., Albin, M., Grahn, P., Jacobsson, H., Ardö, J., Waldbro, J., Östergren, P.-O. and Skärbäck, E. (2008) 'Recreational values of the natural environment in relation to neighbourhood satisfaction, physical activity, obesity and wellbeing', *Journal of Epidemiology and Community Health*, 62: e2.

Blokland-Potters, T. V. (2006) 'Het sociaal weefsel van de stad: cohesie, netwerken en korte contacten' [The social fabric of the city: cohesion, networks and brief contacts], *Oratie Erasmus Universiteit*, The Hague: Dr Gradus Hendriks Stichting.

Cattell, V., Dines, N., Gesler, W. and Curtis, S. (2008) 'Mingling, observation, and lingering: everyday public spaces and their implications for well-being and social relations', *Health and Place*, 14: 544–61.

Chang, C. (2004) 'Psychophysiological responses to different landscape settings and a comparison of cultural differences', *Acta Horticulturae (ISHS)*, 639: 57–65.

Coley, R., Kuo, F. and Sullivan, W. (1997) 'Where does community grow? The social context created by nature in urban public housing', *Environment and Behavior*, 29 (4): 468–92.

De Kort, Y. A. W., Meijnders, A. L., Sponselee, A.-M. and IJsselsteijn, W. A. (2006) 'What's wrong with virtual trees?', *Journal of Environmental Psychology*, 26: 309–20.

De Vries, S., Verheij, R., Groenewegen, P. and Spreeuwenberg, P. (2003) 'Natural environments – healthy environments? An exploratory analysis of the relation between nature and health', *Environment and Planning A*, 35: 1717–31.

De Vries, S., Van Winsum-Westra, M., Vreke, J. and Langers, F. (2008) 'Jeugd, overgewicht en groen; nadere beschouwing en analyse van de mogelijke bijdrage van groen in de woonomgeving aan de preventie van overgewicht bij kinderen' [Youth, overweight and green space: elaborating on and analysis of the possible contribution of green space in the residential environment to the prevention of overweight among children], *Alterra-rapport* 1744. Wageningen: Alterra.

Flap, H. and Völker, B. (2004) 'Gemeenschap, informele controle en collectieve kwaden' [Community, informal control and collective ills], in B. Völker (ed.), *Burgers in de buurt; samenleven in school, wijk en vereniging* [Citizens in the neighbourhood; living together in school, neighbourhood and club], Amsterdam: Amsterdam University Press. pp. 41–67.

Fox, K. R. (1999) 'The influence of physical activity on mental well-being', *Public Health Nutrition*, 2(3a): 411–18.

Glass, T. A., De Leon, C. F. M., Bassuk, S. S. and Berkman, L. F. (2006) 'Social engagement and depressive symptoms in late life – longitudinal findings', *Journal of Aging and Health*, 18 (4): 604–28.

Giles-Corti, B., Broomhall, M. H., Knuiman, M. et al. (2005) 'Increasing walking: how important is distance to, attractiveness, and size of public open space?', *American Journal of Preventive Medicine*, 28 (2S2): 169–76.

Giles-Corti, B. and Donovan, R. J. (2002) 'The relative influence of individual, social and physical environment determinants of physical activity', *Social Science and Medicine*, 54: 1793–812.

GR/RMNO (2004) *Nature and Health; The Influence of Nature on Social, Psychological and Physical Well-being*, The Hague: Health Council of the Netherlands (GR) and Advisory Council for Research on Spatial Planning, Nature and the Environment (RMNO).

Grahn, P. and Stigsdotter, U. (2003) 'Landscape planning and stress', *Urban Forestry and Urban Greening*, 2: 1–18.

Hartig, T. (2007) 'Three steps to understanding restorative environments as health resources', in C. Ward Thompson and P. Travlou (eds), *Open Space: People Space*, London/New York: Taylor & Francis.

Hartig, T., Korpela, K., Evans, G. W. and Garling, T. (1997) 'A measure of restorative quality in environments', *Scandinavian Housing and Planning Research*, 14 (4): 175–94.

Herzog, T. R., Herbert, E. J., Kaplan, R. and Crooks, C. L. (2000) 'Cultural and development comparison of landscape perception and preferences', *Environment and Behavior*, 32 (3): 323–46.

Kaczynski, A. T. and Henderson, K. A. (2007) 'Environmental correlates of physical activity: a review of evidence about parks and recreation', *Leisure Sciences*, 29 (4): 315–54.

Kaplan, R. (2001) 'The nature of the view from home', *Environment and Behavior*, 33 (4): 507–42.

Kaplan, R. and Kaplan, S. (1989) *The Experience of Nature; A psychological perspective*, Cambridge: Cambridge University Press.

Karmanov, D. and Hamel, R. (2008) 'Assessing the restorative potential of contemporary urban environment(s): beyond the nature versus urban dichotomy', *Landscape and Urban Planning*, 86 (2): 115–25.

Kawachi, I., Kennedy, B. P. and Glass, R. (1999) 'Social capital and self-rated health: a contextual analysis', *American Journal of Public Health*, 89: 1187–93.

Korpela, K. and Hartig, T. (1996) 'Restorative qualities of favorite places', *Journal of Environmental Psychology*, 16 (3): 221–33.

Korpela, K. and Ylen, M. (2007) 'Perceived health is associated with visiting natural favorite places in the vicinity', *Health and Place*, 13 (1): 138–51.

Kuo, F. E., Sullivan, W. C. and Wiley, A. (1998) 'Fertile ground for community: innercity neighborhood common spaces', *American Journal of Community Psychology*, 26: 823–51.

Kweon, B., Sullivan, W. and Wiley, A. (1998) 'Green common spaces and the social integration of inner-city older adults', *Environment and Behavior*, 30 (6): 832–58.

Leyden, K. (2003) 'Social capital and the built environment; the importance of walkable neighborhoods', *American Journal of Public Health*, 93 (9): 1546–51.

Li, F., Fisher, K. J., Brownson, R. C. and Bosworth, M. (2005) 'Multilevel modeling of built environment characteristics related to neighbourhood walking activity in older adults', *Journal of Epidemiology and Community Health*, 59: 558.

Loukaitou-Sideris, A. (2006) 'Is it safe to walk? Neighborhood safety and security considerations and their effects on walking', *Journal of Planning Literature*, 20 (3): 219–32.

Maas J., Verheij R. A., Groenewegen P. P., De Vries S. and Spreeuwenberg, P. (2006) 'Green space, urbanity, and health: how strong is the relation?', *Journal of Epidemiology and Community Health*, 60: 587–92.

Maas, J. (2008) 'Vitamin G, green environments – healthy environments', doctoral dissertation, Utrecht University. Utrecht: NIVEL.

Maas, J., Verheij, R. A., Spreeuwenberg, P. and Groenewegen, P. P. (2008) 'Physical activity as a possible mechanism behind the relationship between green space and health: A multilevel analysis', *BMC Public Health*, 8: 206.

Maas, J., Van Dillen, S., Verheij, R. and Groenewegen, P. P. (2009b) 'Social contacts as a possible mechanism behind the relation between green space and health', *Health and Place*,15: 586–92.

Maas, J., Verheij, R. A., De Vries, S., Spreeuwenberg, P., Schellevis, P. G. and Groenewegen, P. P. (2009a) 'Morbidity is related to a green living environment', *Journal of Epidemiology and Community Health*, 63: 967–73.

McDonald, A. G., Bealey, W. J., Fowler, D. et al. (2007) 'Quantifying the effect of urban tree planting on concentrations and depositions of PM10 in two UK conurbations', *Atmospheric Environment*, 41 (38): 8455–67.

Mitchell, R. and Popham, F. (2007) 'Greenspace, urbanity and health: relationships in England', *Journal of Epidemiological and Community Health*, 61: 681–3.

Mitchell, R. and Popham, F. (2008) 'Effect of exposure to natural environment on health inequalities: an observational population study', *The Lancet*, 372 (9650): 1655–60.

MNP/RIVM (2005) 'Fijn stof nader bekeken; de stand van zaken in het dossier fijn stof' [Fine dust examined more closely; the state of affairs of the file on fine dust], *MNPrapport 500037008*,

Bilthoven: Netherlands Environmental Assessment Agency (MNP)/National Institute for Public Health and the Environment (RIVM).

Morita, E., Fukuda, S., Nagano, J. et al. (2007) 'Psychological effects of forest environments on healthy adults: Shinrin-yoku (forest-air bathing, walking) as a possible method of stress reduction', *Public Health*, 121: 54–63.

Nielsen, T. S. and Hansen, K. B. (2007) 'Do green areas affect health? Results from a Danish survey on the use of green areas and health indicators', *Health and Place*, 13: 839–50.

Nilsson, K., Baines, C. and Konijnendijk, C. C. (eds) (2007) 'Final report of the COST Strategic Workshop on Health and the Natural Outdoors', Larnaca Cyprus, 19–21 April, 2007, available at: <http://www.umb.no/statisk/greencare/general/strategic_workshop_final_report.pdf> (accessed 19 August 2009).

Nowak, D. J., Crane, D. E. and Stevens, J. C. (2006) 'Air pollution removal by urban trees and shrubs in the United States', *Urban Forestry and Urban Greening*, 4: 115–23.

Ottosson, J. and Grahn, P. (2008) 'The role of natural settings in crisis rehabilitation: how does the level of crisis influence the response to experiences of nature with regard to measures of rehabilitation?' *Landscape Research*, 33: 51–70.

Parsons, R., Tassinary, L., Ulrich, R., Hebl, M. and Grossman-Alexander, M. (1998) 'The view from the road; implications for stress recovery and immunization', *Journal of Environmental Psychology*, 18: 113–40.

Pikora, T., Giles-Corti, B., Knuiman, M. W., Bull, F. C., Jamrozik, K. and Donovan, R. J. (2006) 'Neighborhood environmental factors correlated with walking near home: using SPACES', *Medicine and Science in Sports and Exercise*, 38 (4): 708–14.

Potwarka, L. R., Kaczynski, A. T. and Flack, A. L. (2008) 'Places to play: association of park space and facilities with healthy weight status among children', *Journal of Community Health*, 33: 344–50.

Pretty, J., Peacock, J., Sellens, M. and Griffins, M. (2005) 'The mental and physical health outcomes of green exercise', *International Journal of Environmental Health Research*, 15 (5): 319–37.

Pucher, J. and Buehler, R. (2008) 'Making cycling irresistible – lessons from the Netherlands, Denmark and Germany', *Transport Reviews*, 28 (4): 495–28.

Raudenbush, S. and Sampson, R. (1999) 'Ecometrics: toward a science of assessing ecological settings, with application to the systematic social observation of neighbourhoods', *Sociological Methodology*, 29, 1–41.

Roemmich, J. N., Epstein, L. H., Raja, S. and Yin, L. (2007) 'The neighborhood and home environments: disparate relationships with physical activity and sedentary behaviors in youth', *Annals of Behavioral Medicine*, 33 (1), 29–38.

Roemmich, J. N., Epstein, L. H., Raja, S., Yin, L., Robinson, J. and Winiewicz, D. (2006) 'Association of access to parks and recreational facilities with the physical activity of young children', *Preventive Medicine*, 43, 437–41.

Singels, M., Klooster, J. P. G. N. and Hoek, G. (2005) 'Luchtkwaliteit in Nederland; gezondheidseffecten en hun maatschappelijke kosten' [Air quality in the Netherlands; health effects and their social costs], Delft: CE.

Skjaeveland, O. (2001) 'Effects of street parks on social interactions among neighbors: a place perspective', *Journal of Architectural and Planning Research*, 18 (2): 131–47.

Stamps III, A. E. (1999) 'Demographic effects in environmental aesthetics, a meta-analysis', *Journal of Planning Literature*, 14 (2): 155–75.

Sugiyama, T., Leslie, E., Giles-Corti, B. and Owen, N. (2008) 'Associations of neighborhood greenness with physical and mental health: do walking, social coherence and local social integration explain the relationships?', *Journal of Epidemiological and Community Health*, 62 (e9).

Sugiyama, T. and Ward Thompson, C. (2007) 'Outdoor environments, activity and the well-being of older people: conceptualising environmental support', *Environment and Planning A*, 39: 1943–60.

Sugiyama, T. and Ward Thompson, C. (2008) 'Associations between characteristics of neighbourhood open space and older people's walking', *Urban Forestry and Urban Greening*, 7: 41–51.

Sullivan, W., Kuo, F. and DePooter, S. (2004) 'The fruit of urban nature; vital neighborhood spaces', *Environment and Behavior*, 36 (5): 678–700.

Swinburn, B., Egger, G. and Raza, F. (1999) 'Dissecting obesogenic environments: the development and application of a framework for identifying and prioritizing environmental interventions for obesity', *Preventive Medicine*, 29: 563–70.

Takano, T., Nakamura, K. and Watanabe, M. (2002) 'Urban residential environments and senior citizens' longevity in megacity areas: the importance of walkable green spaces', *Journal of Epidemiology and Community Health*, 56 (12): 913–18.

Ulrich, R. S. (1983) 'Aesthetic and affective response to natural environment', in I. Altman and J. F. Wohlwill (eds), *Behavior and the Natural Environment*, 85–125, New York: Plenum Press.

Van den Berg, A., Hartig, T. and Staats, H. (2007) 'Preference for nature in urbanized societies', *Journal of Social Issues*, 63 (1): 79–96.

Van Wijnen, J. H., Verhoeff, A. P., Jans, H. W. A. and Van Bruggen, M. (1995) 'The exposure of cyclists, car drivers and pedestrians to traffic-related air pollutants', *International Archives of Occupational and Environmental Health*, 67: 187–274.

Velarde, M. D., Fry, G. and Tveit, M. (2007). 'Health effects of viewing landscapes – landscape types in environmental psychology', *Urban Forestry and Urban Greening*, 6 (4): 199–212.

Verheij, R. A., Maas, J. and Groenewegen, P.P. (2008) 'Urban–rural health differences and the availability of green space', *European Urban and Regional Studies*, 15: 307–16.

VROM (2008). *Structuurvisie Randstad 2040; naar een duurzame en concurrerende Europese topregio* [Strategic policy document Randstad 2040; towards a sustainable and competitive top region], The Hague: Ministry of Housing, Spatial Planning and the Environment.

Wells, N. and Evans, G. (2003) 'Nearby nature, a buffer of life stress among rural children', *Environment and Behavior*, 35 (3): 311–30.

Wendel-Vos, W., Droomers, M., Kremers, S., Brug, J. and Van Lenthe, F. (2005) 'Potential environmental determinants of physical activity in adults', in J. Brug and F. Van Lenthe (eds), *Environmental Determinants and Interventions for Physical Activity, Nutrition and Smoking*, Rotterdam: Erasmus MC.

Wesseling, J. P., Duyzer, J., Tonneijck, A. E. G. and Van Dijk, C. J. (2004) *Effecten van groenelementen op NO2 en PM10 concentraties in de buitenlucht* [Effects of green elements on NO2 and PM10 concentrations in the outdoor air], Apeldoorn: TNO.

Wesseling, J., Beijk, R. and Van Kuijeren, N. (2008) *Effecten van groen op de luchtkwaliteit; status 2008* [Effects of greenery on air quality; status 2008] (with summary in English), RIVM-rapport 680705012/2008. Bilthoven: RIVM.

World Health Organization (WHO) Europe (2002) *A Physically Active Life Through Everyday Transport with a Special Focus on Children and Older People and Examples and Approaches From Europe*, Copenhagen: WHO, Regional Office for Europe.

Wilkin, T. J., Mallam, K. M., Metcalf, B. S., Jeffery, A. N. and Voss, L. D. (2006) 'Variation in physical activity lies with the child, not his environment: evidence for an 'activitystat' in young children (EarlyBird 16)', *International Journal of Obesity*, 30: 1050–5.

Chapter 4

Active landscapes:
the methodological challenges in developing the evidence on urban environments and physical activity

Fiona Bull, Billie Giles-Corti and Lisa Wood

Introduction

Increasing participation in physical activity can make an important contribution to the health and well-being of individuals, communities and society. There is a strong and well-accepted evidence base demonstrating the key role an active lifestyle can play in the prevention of most major diseases responsible for premature death and disability (US DHHS, 2008; DoH, 2004). Inactivity is a central risk factor for many of the most common chronic diseases, notably heart disease, stroke, cancers, and type 2 diabetes. Moreover, an active lifestyle can improve mental health, and reduce the risk of depression, prevent falls in older people, and may enhance cognitive function and improve academic performance in children (Kelty, Giles-Corti and Zubrick, 2008). Accumulating at least 30 minutes of at least moderate intensity physical activity, on most days of the week, is sufficient for adults to achieve benefits (DoH, 2004). Thus, this recommended amount of activity forms the basis of many of the current national, regional and international guidelines for the promotion of physical activity in the general population (US DHHS, 1996; Haskell et al., 2007; WHO, 2004, 2006; DoH, 2004, 2009). For children, a higher volume (60 minutes), and including some vigorous intensity activity, is recommended (US DHHS, 2008; CDCP, 2008; DHA, 2004).

In recent years there has been increased recognition of a broader focus of physical activity. In Europe this is often known as 'health-enhancing physical activity' (HEPA). This is the antithesis of a 'one size fits all' prescription for physical activity, and is based on evidence that various different types of activity can be beneficial, and that many adults and children may prefer to accumulate activity through a variety of structured and nonstructured modalities. This shift has opened up scope for promotional activities beyond those aimed at traditional 'exercise' and 'sports' usually undertaken in leisure time, or for children at school, to include the promotion of 'active transport' (such as walking or cycling for all or part of travel trips) and programmes aimed at maintaining active participation in cultural activities and dance. This broader focus necessitates working beyond the traditional health and sport sectors, and has increased the range of settings that are now of interest for the promotion of physical activity.

A population health-based approach to the promotion of physical activity seeks to increase community levels of participation by influencing the personal, educational, social and environmental factors that support or hinder physical activity behaviour (Bull et al., 2006). To most effectively maximize disease prevention, there is increasing recognition that it is through population-based approaches rather than medical interventions aimed at individuals with, or at high risk of, chronic disease that success is likely to be achieved. For example, there is now a major focus in research and practice looking at the everyday environments in which we live, work and play, as it is these that shape people's everyday experiences and their opportunities to be active or not. Such a focus offers potential for important new partnerships with transport, landscape design and urban planning sectors and disciplines.

This chapter presents a brief summary of the research developments aimed at understanding and influencing the factors determining participation in physical activity, particularly in adults, and the role of the urban landscape and the physical environment in shaping opportunities and choices to be active. This field of research is relatively new, and we explore some of the challenges and methodological issues as well as presenting a case study example of a large, longitudinal research study that is under way to test the effectiveness of a government urban design policy to support increased physical activity levels in Australia.

The importance of creating a supportive landscape for physical activity

Despite the wide range of positive benefits accruing from regular participation in even relatively modest levels of activity, participation rates are low. In England only one-third of men and one quarter of women are sufficiently active to benefit their health (DoH, 2004; Craig and Mindell, 2008) and the estimated costs of physical inactivity in England are £8.2 billion annually (Butland et al., 2007). This has considerable consequences for the healthcare budget. In 2007, the direct cost of physical inactivity, considering only the impact through coronary heart disease, stroke, diabetes mellitus and breast and colon cancers, was estimated at £1.06 billion (Allender, 2007). However, this is an underestimate, as it excludes benefits from the prevention of falls (through maintaining strength and flexibility, especially for older adults) and improvements in social and mental health.

The levels of activity in the United Kingdom are lower than neighbouring European countries; for example, in the Netherlands (44 per cent), Germany (40 per cent) and Luxembourg (36 per cent) of adults meet recommendations, yet in the study by Sjöström et al. (2006) this level was achieved by only 28 per cent of British adults. Similarly, activity levels in the United States, Canada and New Zealand are also higher than in the United Kingdom (Craig et al., 2004) although, even in these countries, physical activity levels are still far from ideal. Data from other UK sources reveal alarming downward trends in specific modes of activity, for example, walking and cycling for transport (DoT, 2007). Yet again levels of walking and cycling are much higher in many other European countries. For example, 28 per cent and 18 per cent of trips are undertaken by cycling and walking respectively in the Netherlands, while in England and Wales the figures are 4 per cent and 12 per cent respectively (Pucher and Dijkstra, 2003).

Very few countries can show sustained success in increasing activity levels. Although this may, in part, be because of limitations in data collection, much of the culpability seems to lie in changes relating to where and how we lead our day-to-day lives. Indeed, the modern urban landscape is making it more difficult to maintain an active lifestyle (Giles-Corti et al., in press a). Globally, the World Health Organization (WHO) has recognized inactivity as one of the key contributors to the global burden of ill health, and in 2004 launched a Global Strategy on Diet, Physical Activity and Health to encourage national-level action in all countries (WHO, 2004). This has commenced in many countries including in the United Kingdom (DoH, 2009; SEPATF, 2003; Welsh Assembly, 2006). In most of these policies and elsewhere (Kopelman, Jebb and Butland, 2007; NICE, 2008) there is a strong call for cooperation and partnership with other sectors to help create and sustain the environments that support active lifestyles for all ages.

What factors influence physical activity?

Although there is a long history of research on physical activity, much of the early work focused on participation in formal sports and traditional modes of exercise, usually undertaken for the purpose of increasing cardio-respiratory fitness. The findings consistently showed that adults who were more confident in their abilities, were more motivated and perceived more positive benefits with fewer barriers, and those who felt supported by friends or family, were more likely to be more active (Trost et al., 2002). Women, older adults, and adults with dependent children are less likely to be active (Department of Health, 2004).   Much earlier research was underpinned by theories of health behaviour from behavioural psychology, which focused on intra- and inter-individual determinants (Sallis, 2009). Although social cognitive theory highlighted the reciprocal relationship between individuals and their environment, it was only in the last decade that the importance of the study of the environmental factors really emerged along with the development of socio-ecological models (Sallis, 2009; Story et al., 2009; Sallis and Owen, 1997; Giles-Corti et al., 2005b). Findings from early studies during the 1990s identified aspects of the urban landscape that were associated with higher levels of activity (Transportation Research Board, 2005; Owen et al., 2004).

Although the initial measures were crude, these studies provided the starting point for targeted research efforts involving more diverse measures of the environment, as well as better assessment of physical activity behaviours, and in a variety of populations. What followed next might best be described as an explosion of individual, cross-sectional research studies and a rapid succession of review papers aimed at capturing emerging results across multiple disciplines (Bauman and Bull, 2007). Fuelled by an injection of funding in the United States by the Robert Wood Johnson Foundation (for more detail, see http://www.active-livingresearch.org/), in just over a decade there have been well over 200 studies examining the impact of the urban environment on physical activity, particularly walking, with contributions from a variety of disciplines (Saelens and Handy, 2008; Owen et al., 2004; Humpel, Owen and Leslie, 2002).

Overall, these studies show a growing and consistent evidence base indicating that the design of the built environment (land use and transportation systems as well as landscape and urban design) influences patterns of physical activity and the transport-mode choices of adults (Transportation Research Board, 2005) and young people (McMillan, 2005). Urban landscapes characterized by poorly connected street networks, low levels of mixed-use planning, poor access to shops and services, and low density are associated with lower levels of physical activity, and specifically walking. In addition, urban sprawl (Ewing et al., 2003; Sugiyama et al., 2007) or areas of low 'walkability' (Saelens et al., 2003) are associated with obesity. This may be partly because of long commuter trips, which decrease opportunities for local walking, but may also be the result of additional time spent being sedentary while driving. The presence of necessary infrastructure such as footpaths and the level of perceived personal safety and attractiveness of the landscapes have been shown to be associated with levels of walking (Pikora et al., 2006).

Thus, the quality of the landscape is one factor that appears to influence physical activity (Ellaway, Macintyre and Bonnefoy, 2005). Access to large, attractive public open space was found to be associated with higher levels of walking (Giles-Corti et al., 2005a). In addition to encouraging physical activity, the attractiveness of open space may result in other health benefits since exposure to nature is said to be restorative, reducing mental fatigue and improving well-being (Kaplan and Kaplan, 1989). Walking locally also increases opportunities for casual interactions with neighbours, and has the potential to increase the sense of community (Lund, 2002) and social capital (Wood et al., 2007; Wood and Giles-Corti, 2008). While the mechanisms remain under investigation, creating landscapes and neighbourhoods that encourage interactions between neighbours and create a sense of community and social capital may influence the mental health of residents and contribute to the enhancement of social and cultural vibrancy and civic life (Jackson, 2003). Many forms of physical activity can be undertaken in natural landscapes such as parks and open space, providing an opportunity for contact with nature which is itself protective for mental health (Louv, 2008; Maller et al., 2002).

As research into the urban environment evolves, there are some interesting differences in the emerging findings, with apparent associations not always consistent across different health-related behaviours. For instance, neighbourhood aesthetics and safety have been found to be associated with walking for recreation but not walking for transport (Ball et al., 2007). Conversely, neighbourhood connectivity has been found to be associated with transport but not leisure-time walking (Ball et al., 2007). Inconsistent relationships between features of the urban landscape and different types of physical activities have also been reported elsewhere (Ball, Timperio and Crawford, 2006). Such variances in findings highlight the complexities of research in this area, and the need for careful selection of the environmental factors under investigation, the specificity of both the independent and dependent variables, and the articulation of a coherent conceptual framework matching the behaviour with the setting (Giles-Corti et al., 2005b).

One of the major limitations in the evidence base to date is that it relies extensively on cross-sectional study design; this limits conclusions about causality, in part because of issues of self-selection. Central to this concern is that people who desire to be active might simply choose neighbourhoods that match this predisposition (for example, they elect to live in neighbourhoods that are more walkable), rather than the environment influencing their behaviour per se. In recognition of this, there have been calls for more experimental designs, longitudinal studies (Ewing et al., 2003) and natural experiments (Cummins et al., 2005; Ogilvie et al., 2007) using opportunistic interventions such as policy reforms, new site developments or redevelopments and urban areas earmarked for regeneration, and assessing change over time (Handy, Cao and Mokhtarian, 2005; Ewing et al., 2003; Ogilvie et al., 2007; Ogilvie et al., 2006). This is particularly relevant given that randomized controlled trials are impractical for studies of this kind (Ogilvie et al., 2007; Ogilvie et al., 2006).

In response to the concerns identified above, an example of one opportunistic evaluation of urban policy and development is the longitudinal RESIDential Environment study (RESIDE), which commenced in 2003. RESIDE is a natural experiment evaluating the West Australian state government's new subdivision design code called the 'Liveable Neighbourhood Community Design Code' (WAPC, 2000). This code aimed to create pedestrian-friendly neighbourhoods through design to increase local walking, cycling and public transport use. The trial provided a unique opportunity for a natural experiment to examine the extent to which a government planning policy could influence the behavioural outcomes of residents. The Liveable Neighbourhood code is based on 'New Urbanism' principles (Calthorpe, 1993; Katz, 1994; McCormack et al., 2003; Jones, 2001) and, accordingly, combines connected street networks, higher densities, mixed-use zoning (that is, a combination of commercial and residential development) and access to public transport (Dutton, 2001; Hall and Giles-Corti, 2000). By creating more 'liveable' neighbourhoods, with greater access to services and more efficient use of land, it was hoped that walking, cycling and public transport use would be increased and car use would be reduced (McCormack et al., 2003). (See Box 4.1 below for an outline of Project RESIDE study design.)

> *Box 4.1* Project RESIDE: A case study example of a longitudinal, quasi-experimental study of state urban design policy.
>
> The RESIDential Environments Project (RESIDE) commenced in 2003 as a longitudinal natural experiment evaluating the West Australian state-government's subdivision design code 'Liveable Neighbourhood (LN) Guidelines.' The principal aim of RESIDE is to study the impact of the state government's Liveable Neighbourhood guidelines on the walking, cycling and public transport use behaviour of local residents (Giles-Corti et al. 2008).
>
> RESIDE involves a study of people building homes in 73 new housing developments in metropolitan Perth, surveyed three times: at baseline before moving into their new homes (in 2003-5) and then again at 12 months (2004-6) and 36 months (2006-8). On each occasion, participants complete a self-complete questionnaire and wear a Yamix Digi-walker pedometer for seven days. The pedometer is a small motion sensor worn on the belt that measures the number of steps taken. It provides an objective measure of overall physical activity behaviour irrespective of the type and where it takes place. The questionnaire measures a range of individual-level (for example, demographic and health-related characteristics, attitudes, perceptions); social environmental (for example, social support for physical activity); and physical environmental (for example, perceptions of the local neighbourhood) factors that might influence participation in physical activity, walking and cycling (Giles-Corti et al. 2007). Overall, 33 per cent of those eligible to participate agreed to take part, while 83 per cent and 73 per cent of those still eligible remained in the study at first and second follow-up.

All housing developments in the metropolitan area released during the study time period were considered for inclusion in RESIDE. All developments assessed by the Department for Planning and Infrastructure as 'liveable' were included along with all those assessed as 'hybrid' developments (i.e., meeting all but not all of the liveable criteria). A sub sample of 'conventional' developments were also included in the study, the latter matched to the liveable and hybrid developments, where possible, in terms of stage of development, lot value and proximity to the ocean.

RESIDE has several unique features: it is evaluating a current government policy designed to create pedestrian-friendly environments; it provides the opportunity to explore the role of self-selection because participants are surveyed before moving into their new home; and it provides a rare opportunity to study the impact of a changing environment on residents over time, given that randomized controlled trials in this area are not feasible (prior research has relied on retrospective reporting on behaviour prior to moving, which is open to bias recall (Handy, Cao & Mokhtarian 2006)).

The RESIDE project developed a comprehensive Geographic Information Systems (GIS) platform, used to develop objective measures of the neighbourhood built environment. This included: road network and Euclidean (as the crow flies) distance to destinations relevant for walking for transport and walking for recreation (including shops, public transport stops, newsagents, post offices, schools, cafes, public open space, beaches, the river); as well as the density of destinations within 1.6km of study participants' homes; the presence, size and quality of public open space (the latter supplemented by a survey of public open spaces using the POST tool (Broomhall, Giles-Corti & Lange 2004; Giles-Corti et al. 2005a); and a measure of neighbourhood walkability (an index that combines the connectivity of street networks, the intensity and diversity of mixed use planning and population density). These data complement subjective measures of the neighbourhood obtained from survey respondents. The GIS data has been sourced from a wide range of government sources. Final data collection was completed in 2009 and analyses are under way.

To read more about the research, go to: **http://www.sph.uwa.edu.au/ research/cbeh/projects/reside**

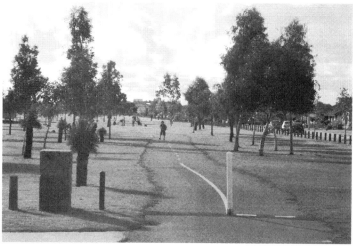

Figure 4.1
RESIDE study estate: Parkland with shared use path. Element 1 of WA's Liveable Neighbourhoods addresses 'community design' and guidance on 'public parkland', states that layout should provide well-distributed parkland that contributes to the legibility and character of the development, provides for a range of uses and activities; major linear, district or regional open spaces and drainage should be located to define the boundaries of neighbourhoods rather than dissect them.

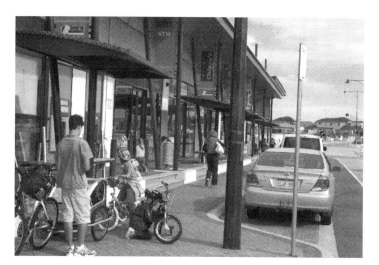

Figure 4.2
RESIDE study estate: Local shopping strip. Element 7 of WA's Liveable Neighbourhoods specifies 'neighbourhood and local centres' where neighbourhood centres should be located and distributed to provide a centre for most residents in a 400–500m walk and the minimum requirements of a neighbourhood centre are to be a small convenience shop, a public transport stop and a post box.

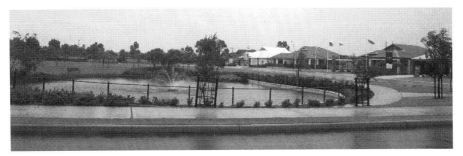

Figure 4.3
RESIDE study estate: Parkland with water feature. Element 3 of WA's Liveable
Neighbourhoods addresses 'lot layout', stating that lots must be orientated to front
parkland and natural areas to enhance amenity while contributing to personal and property
security and deterrence of crime and vandalism.

Methodological challenges and future directions

Obtaining baseline data in 'natural' or 'opportunistic' studies

For natural experiments, it is important to survey study participants prior to exposure
to the environmental interventions. In the RESIDE project, the targeted participants
were building new homes in new neighbourhoods, thus it was necessary to
identify, recruit and survey them prior to their move to their new home (Giles-Corti
et al., 2008). This was achieved by working with the statewide water supply
authority (the Water Corporation) to obtain contact details of customers purchasing
land and building new homes in the study area. To overcome privacy issues, the
Water Corporation agreed to write to all these customers to invite their participation in the study, and those who did not wish to participate were asked to return
a reply-paid card. After two weeks, the Water Corporation provided the contact
details of customers who had (by default) agreed, and they were contacted by the
University of Western Australia's Survey Research Centre, either by telephone or
by letter (if after six attempts they could not be contacted by telephone). This
method was deemed successful as it achieved an overall recruitment of 34 per
cent of those eligible, not insignificant given the survey demands made on the
participants. It is, however, important in a longitudinal study to maintain engagement
of participants and maximize response rates over time, and this also requires strategic attention in the framing and implementation of the study.

Maintaining response rates

In longitudinal studies it is necessary to develop a recruitment and retention
protocol to minimize loss to follow-up. In RESIDE, numerous strategies were
implemented including:

- small incentives were offered as a 'token of appreciation' for participation
- contact details of two people who knew the study participants' whereabouts were collected
- an annual newsletter was used to maintain contact with participants.

Tokens of appreciation are often used effectively in studies to maximize response rates (Chapman and Wong, 1991). We undertook an unpublished study (Lange et al., 2005) which found that offering small material incentives upfront (for example, a free video voucher) was more effective than chances to win prizes.

The follow-up protocol is also critical in terms of maximizing response rates. RESIDE used a modified protocol proposed by Dillman (2000) which included sending postcards to inform prospective study participants that they would be contacted, as well as providing second copies of questionnaires to nonresponders. We believe these strategies have assisted in maximizing participation over the three data-collection phases of the study.

Measurement of the dependent variable: physical activity

A good measure of physical activity is central to research in this field, but this behaviour is complex and it can be measured in a number of different ways (Bauman and Phongsaven, 2006). Pedometers provide an objective measure of overall behaviour, but these data are not context-specific, providing no information on the type and location of activity undertaken. Self-report measures of activity are frequently used to address this issue but there are well-reported concerns about validity because of recall bias and measurement error. Further, until recently there has been no self-report measure that adequately addressed the issue of specificity of purpose for this particular field of study, where context is important.

The Neighbourhood Physical Activity Questionnaire (NPAQ) was developed as part of RESIDE, and specifically aimed to overcome a range of methodological problems observed in other instruments (Giles-Corti et al., 2006). For example, NPAQ was designed for use in longitudinal studies of the impact of urban design on physical activity. Thus, rather than measuring behaviour in the last seven days, it measures 'usual' behaviour. While this may slightly overestimate behaviour, it was felt that usual behaviour would be a more stable measure over time (Giles-Corti et al., 2006). Importantly, NPAQ is a behaviour-specific and context-specific tool, measuring walking and cycling behaviours that take place 'within' and 'outside' the neighbourhood, thus matching the intended scale of interest (the neighbourhood) and impact of the government's Liveable Neighbourhood Community Design Code. Finally, the NPAQ measures the frequency and duration of walking and cycling as well as other moderate and vigorous-intensity physical activity. Thus, in addition to providing behaviour-specific and context specific measures, it also provides an overall measure of active behaviour. An assessment of NPAQ's reliability shows it to have acceptable reliability which is as good as, or better than, other tools commonly used in physical activity studies, and it is now being used in other countries (Van Dyck et al., 2009).

Measures of the urban environment

The development and modification of methods to measure the urban environment has been a significant feature of research in this field. Sallis recently reviewed the history of relevant measures and noted the rapid shift from self-report instruments to objective measures made possible by the use of geographic information systems (GIS) (Sallis, 2009). Many studies now integrate both a self-report measure of perceptions of the environment along with objective measures derived from GIS, as they measure different attributes. Yet to date there has been no standardized approach to either, making comparisons of findings between studies quite complex. One of the earliest examples of collecting street-level data on the urban landscape was the environmental audit SPACES (Systematic Pedestrian and Cycling Environmental Scan), an instrument designed to capture data on features related to function, safety, aesthetics and destinations based on an explicit model of environmental influences (Pikora et al., 2006). Other instruments have subsequently been developed. NEWS is a measure for use to assess perceptions of the local community environment (Cerin et al., 2006), while more specific audit tools have been developed for certain settings. CHEW was designed for the workplace environment (Oldenburg et al., 2002) and POST is an assessment tool for capturing details of public open space (Broomhall, Giles-Corti and Lange, 2004). Each measure differs in the items, scope and response scales and setting for which it is used, thus results from any study must be appraised carefully to fully understand the measures and comparability of data. This point is illustrated well in a recently published review by Foster and Giles-Corti (2008) of studies investigating the relationship between neighbourhood safety and physical activity, where much of the prima facie inconsistency of findings is explained by issues of measurement specificity.

Many of the tools to date have been developed in North America and Australia, and there is an urgent need for the development and testing of appropriate tools for use in other regions. Work is under way in Europe (Project ALPHA), which includes adapting, and testing a modified NEWS (Cerin et al., 2006) in a subset of countries. Other examples include the development of a Scottish Walkability Index (Millington et al., 2009). However, much work remains to be done in other regions. A large number of different audit tools addressing a variety of purposes are now in use, and can be accessed via the Active Living Research website (http://www.activelivingresearch.org/resourcesearch/toolsandmeasures).

Fiona Bull, Billie Giles-Corti and Lisa Wood

Challenges in using GIS

Objective measures of the environment capture different aspects from self-reported assessments, and address some of the weaknesses of self-report (Ball et al., 2008; Kirtland et al., 2003; Giles-Corti et al., in press b), such as respondent burden and measurement bias caused by recall. But they do present other demands, such as the need for extensive training to establish high inter-rater reliability and the high cost of onsite street audit data collection. Advances in GIS hardware and software used to store, analyse and display spatial information have provided enormous benefits, some of which can reduce the burden of on-site data collection. In the last decade there has been a rapid uptake in its use in physical activity research, but it too presents some challenges (Giles-Corti and Donovan, 2002; Frank et al., 2005; Owen et al., 2007). GIS is highly technical, and familiarity with the software and specific data sets is essential, as is access to high-quality data, including base maps. A major factor in using GIS data is that the data were generally developed for purposes other than research, so before using them, extensive data manipulation is often required. It is therefore often time-consuming to build and integrate new data layers for any specific geographical area of interest, and often requires a large investment of human resources which can exceed typical research funding budgets. Collaboration with local and national government agencies to establish access to data is essential, and yet these partnerships can take time to develop. Often relevant data is not available. For instance, RESIDE (see Box 4.1) uncovered the absence of adequate data on the presence of footpaths in the metropolitan area. In this study, additional resources were allocated to fill the data gap and develop the GIS layer using a combination of digital and paper-based sources from local government authorities as well as satellite imagery. This is clearly not always possible, thus research efforts can be limited by the data availability and suitability.

Another challenge in using GIS is the validity of the dataset, in terms of both accuracy and correspondence with the time period of interest. One recent study reported substantial inconsistencies in GIS layers of information provided by a commercial database of physical activity facilities (Boone et al., 2008). The authors conducted on-the-ground validation after concerns were raised, and their results on physical activity showed errors in both the presence of a facility being correctly recorded and the type of facility recorded. As access to, and possibly type of, destinations feature as important correlates of physical activity levels, valid measures are essential. There is a clear need, therefore, to consider incorporating some testing for validity of GIS data into research study protocols, budgets and timelines.

Finally, critical in using GIS is obtaining data that is temporally the same as the population survey data that is being used. In longitudinal studies, it is necessary to source GIS data that is dynamic rather than static, in order to ensure the GIS data matches each population survey data time point. At this stage, there is no reported evidence that GIS databases are sensitive to change, so that these data can be used to predict changes in behaviour as a result of a changing environment.

The question of observation scale: what is a 'neighbourhood'?

Using GIS data raises both methodological and theoretical issues which impact on measurement error and the predictive capacity of models (Giles-Corti et al., 2005b). Particularly difficult is the question of what scale to use. Many studies define the 'neighbourhood' using administrative definitions such as postcodes, local government boundaries or other census-based units, yet it is well recognized that these may have no bearing on the behaviours of interest. Other approaches include using buffer zones based on Euclidean distances either derived from estimating walking distance in a set time (for example, 10–15 minutes' walk is approximately 1.6 km) (Van Dyck et al., 2009), and taking a measure from previous studies to allow for comparison. A further complication is that, as Ball and colleagues (2007) note, not only do most people live lives that cross multiple contexts and settings, these are often nested within each other (Ball et al., 2007). Our research has shown that the scale of analysis affects the strength of relationships between the built environment and walking for transport (Learnihan, 2007). Learnihan compared three scales: suburb, collector's census districts (a spatial unit developed by the Australian Bureau of Statistics that contains around 200 households), and a 15-minute network distance walk from each participant's neighbourhood, and found that the predictive capacity of models was best at the 15-minute network distance scale level (Learnihan, 2007). Although a 15-minute network scale avoids methodological weaknesses associated with using fixed scales, as yet researchers in this field have not yet reached any consensus, nor is there likely to be a single 'right way' to define the appropriate neighbourhood for different behaviours and population groups of interest. It is therefore reasonable to expect and recommend that multiple definitions should continue to be explored, a position taken within other areas of investigation (Flowerdew, Manley and Sabel, 2008).

Another important aspect of 'scale' is that it is likely to vary depending on the target group. For example, the walkable neighbourhood for a child or an older adult may be somewhat different to a walkable distance for a healthy, young to middle-aged adult. More studies are required to better understand the impact of scale on different target groups.

Street network versus pedestrian network

Most studies that use GIS use the street network rather than the pedestrian network to assess proximity to destinations and to create 'walkability' indices.

The street network follows the road network, while the pedestrian network includes informal routes such as cut-throughs as well as allowing pedestrians to cross parks and thoroughfares. This is important because it is likely to present a very different assessment of the urban landscape. This difference was shown in a study by Chin and colleagues, which found that using the pedestrian network rather than street network enhanced the connectivity of neighbourhoods with cul-de-sacs (Chin et al., 2008). Whilst this difference is obviously important for studies that focus on pedestrian activity, the data on footpaths, cut-throughs and informal paths across open public space and green space within the urban land-scape are often not available in existing electronic data sets. Digitizing aerial photographs of landscapes of interest is one solution, but is expensive and time-consuming (Chin et al., 2008).

Explaining variance needs sufficient variability

One of the more challenging practical aspects to undertaking studies in this field is the need for sufficient variance in the urban landscape to be able to detect and explain any associations or causal pathways. To date, much of the research has come from North America and Australia, and mostly from urban areas with often limited heterogeneity. Although more research is now under way in the United Kingdom, Europe and elsewhere, exploring research questions in landscapes based on different, older design principles and values, they too may suffer from insufficient variation in form. This highlights the need for international and multi-centre research initiatives with shared research protocols and tools. One early example of this work is the International Prevalence Study (Bauman et al., 2009; Sallis et al., 2009), which included a shortened form of NEWS (Cerin et al., 2006) in an eleven-country comparative study. In addition to looking at absolute levels of physical activity in these countries, associations between activity and features of the environment were explored. Results are now in press, and this study demonstrates that these kinds of research projects on an international scale are possible (Sallis et al., in press).

Following along these lines, a large collaborative network for similar studies is under way, and represents an important platform for research devel-opment and applications in other regions of the world (International Physical Activity and the Environment Network, 2004). It is notable that much of the published research has focused on urban (often metropolitan) settings, and this is important given the large proportion of the world's population that currently live in cities (approximately 49 per cent in 2005) and the rapid increase in the rate of urbanization. Global estimates project that 60 per cent of the world's population will live in cities by 2030 (United Nations, 2004). In developed coun-tries this movement, combined with an increase in car ownership, has led to 'urban sprawl' (Frumkin, Frank and Jackson, 2004). However, it is worth noting that there are likely to be important differences in the influence of the landscape on health and physical activity in peri-urban and rural areas, and these should receive research attention.

The role of the social environment

Along with the growth of research and policy interest in the urban environment there has been mounting evidence around the nexus between the social and physical environments and the combined context these form for various health behaviours. Street layout, perceptions of safety and the presence or absence of places for human interaction are among factors that may impact on physical activity directly, but are also implicated in the shaping of sense of community and social capital (Bothwell, Gindroz and Lang, 1998; Joongsub and Kaplan, 2004; Wood et al., 2007), which in turn can influence the propensity of residents to be active in their community (Leyden, 2003; Lund, 2002). For example, a higher presence and level of vehicle traffic and car parking not only deters physical activity (Mullen, 2003), but also has been shown to negatively affect perceptions of area friendliness, safety and helpfulness (Mullen, 2003). Safety and perceived friendliness can impact on the extent to which people get out and about actively within their community (Foster and Giles-Corti, 2008), perpetuating a downward spiral of effects on both social and physical health outcomes. Thus, studies that focus only on urban form or only on the social realm do not capture the full story, and research would benefit from studies that incorporate measures of both the urban and social environments, along with physical activity and psychological health outcomes. One of the methodological challenges this presents, however, is that existing instruments and scales developed to study a particular behaviour (for example, physical activity), social outcome (for example, social support) or environment design (for example, neighbourhood attributes) are often quite detailed, and become onerous or impractical to administer if a number of them are combined. This problem was faced in the RESIDE study, which had to balance the need for comprehensive measures across various behaviours, settings and outcomes with the need to avoid overburdening participants with data collection.

Understanding the relative influence of different aspects of the total environment

The use of ecological models has been proposed with a view to developing a research agenda aimed at identifying potentially high-leverage interventions in relevant settings (Sallis and Owen, 2007). Such multi-level models seek to capture and enable the study of the complex interactions between the multitude of individual, cultural and social, physical and policy environmental factors in settings in which people live, work and play, in an attempt to better predict physical activity behaviour. Nevertheless, few studies have reported the relative influence of these factors on behaviour concurrently (Ball et al., 2007). One of the earliest studies (Giles-Corti and Donovan, 2002) found that the relative influences of psychosocial and environmental factors on walking were nearly of equal importance. More recently, De Bourdeaudhuij and colleagues (2005) found that urban landscape features (including a measure of walkability) explained much less variance in physical activity than psycho-social factors (10 per cent and approximately 42 per cent, respectively). This is consistent with an Australian study, which found that cognitive factors (self-efficacy, enjoyment and behavioural intentions) remained the strongest predictors of leisure time and transport-related walking, with features of the environment (including aesthetics and safety) modifying the relationship (Ball et al., 2007).

Another feature, demonstrated in these studies and others, is that the relative contribution may differ for different behaviours and for different population groups. This reaffirms previous calls for greater use of clear, well-conceptualized models of the behaviour and context, matched with the appropriate scale and measurement of variables to test the interactions and pathways among personal, social and environmental factors (Giles-Corti et al., 2005b; Ball, Timperio and Crawford, 2006). Recently there has been a notable shift in focus to understanding transport behaviours (walking and cycling), yet it is important and necessary to continue to explore and better understand recreational activities as well.

Research informing policy

Despite the challenges noted above in this emerging field of research, over the last five years leading US, UK, Canadian and Australian health and transport organizations have published position papers on the importance of the urban landscape and its impact on various health behaviours or outcomes, particularly physical activity and obesity (Transportation Research Board, 2005; NICE, 2008; Heart and Stroke Foundation of Canada, 2007; Kopelman, Jebb and Butland, 2007; National Preventative Health Taskforce, 2008). Each of these recognize that land use patterns, transportation systems, building design and social infra-structure can create conditions that optimize conditions for positive health and positive health behaviours, and vice versa. In England, the new national strategy for physical activity, Be Active, Be Healthy: A plan for getting the nation moving, reports that the design and layout of towns and cities can encourage or discourage access on foot or by bike, while building design can encourage (or discourage) the use of stairs (DoH, 2009). Furthermore, access to parks, the countryside and other green space, as well as specific features of green space, are recognized as helping people to be more active (DoH, 2009).

Similarly, in the United States the 'Community Guide for Preventative Services' includes recommendations on the design of urban landscapes, including zoning regulations, street connectivity, residential density and street-scale, factors such as lighting, ease and safety of street crossing, footpath continuity, traffic-calming measures and aesthetic enhancements (Heath, Brownson and Kruger, 2006). It is therefore evident that the research findings to date have already found their way into informing policy and recommendations for future practice.

As the evidence base continues to develop, both policy makers and practitioners are likely to continue to look for clear guidance from researchers. This represents an opportunity for public health, landscape architecture, civil engineering and planning academics, practitioners, and policy makers to work collaboratively with the aim of improving health (Corburn, 2004). However, to avoid unintended consequences, it is important for researchers to take a broad view beyond their own area of research. All too often, researchers consider only one population group (for example, adults or children) or setting (school or neighbourhood), and fail to take into account the implications of their research recommendations on groups other than their own study population (Giles-Corti and King, 2009). Recently, Giles-Corti and King (2009) noted that to optimize environments that encourage an active lifestyle across the life course, there is a need for researchers to think 'outside the square' and consider in tandem multiple forms of physical activity, settings and population groups. This is more likely to produce a comprehensive set of policy and programme strategies, as well as research directions, that will advance our knowledge, and in so doing, improve population health while avoiding unintended negative consequences.

Summary

In summary, the multidisciplinary nature of this research field has paved the way for unparalleled opportunities for health and physical activity researchers to work with sectors outside of health, including transportation, planning, urban design, and environmental protection. New methods and technologies are being combined to address challenging and complex questions about the relationships between where people live, and how healthy, and particularly active, lifestyles can be sustained and supported. There is a large base of cross-sectional studies providing some clear directions to the most promising attributes of the urban landscape that promote more active communities, but there is also wide scope for more avenues of enquiry.

The methodological challenges discussed in this chapter range from the conceptual through to the practical and even financial. Potential solutions and the scope for innovation were explored with examples from recent studies. Alongside strengthening the methods used in the descriptive research agenda, the next phase of this research field should combine a greater focus on interventions, evaluating at different scales both physical improvements and policy implementation. There is also great potential for research focused on physical activity to combine with other areas of interest, and to use large, linked datasets, to study the types, quantity and design of the urban landscapes most conducive to positive mental health, including sense of belonging (Baumeister and Leary, 1995), social capital (Baum and Palmer, 2002), social ties (Kawachi and Berkman, 2001) and community involvement (Donovan et al., 2006).

Acknowledgements

All funding bodies are gratefully acknowledged. RESIDE was funded by grants from the Western Australian Health Promotion Foundation (Healthway) (#11828) and the Australian Research Council (ARC) (#LP0455453). Giles-Corti is supported by an NHMRC Senior Research Fellowship (#503712) and Wood by an NHMRC Capacity Building Grant (#458668). The authors would like to thank Paula Hooper at UWA for her assistance in the preparation of this chapter and Catharine Ward Thompson for her review.

References

Allender, S. (2007) 'The burden of physical activity related ill health in the UK', *Journal of Epidemiology and Community Health*, 61: 344–8.

Ball, K., Jeffrey, R., Crawford, D., Roberts, R., Salmon, J. and Timperio, A. (2008) 'Mismatch between perceived and objective measures of physical activity environments', *Preventive Medicine*, 47 (3): 294–8.

Ball, K., Timperio, A. and Crawford, D. (2006) 'Understanding environmental influences on nutrition and physical activity behaviours: where should we look and what should we count?', *International Journal of Behavioural Nutrition and Physical Activity*, 26 (3): 33.

Ball, K., Timperio, A., Salmon, J., Giles-Corti, B., Roberts, R. and Crawford, D. (2007) 'Personal, social and environmental determinants of educational inequalities in walking: a multilevel study', *Journal of Epidemiology and Community Health*, 61 (2): 108–14.

Baum, F. and Palmer, C. (2002) '"Opportunity Structures": urban landscape, social capital and health promotion in Australia', *Health Promotion International*, 17 (4): 351–61.

Bauman, A. and Bull, F. C. (2007) *Environmental Correlates of Physical Activity and Walking in Adults and Children: A Review of Reviews*, London: National Institute for Health and Clinical Excellence (NICE).

Bauman, A., Bull, F. C., Chey, T., Craig, C., Ainsworth, B., Sallis, J., Boweles, H., Sjostrom, M., Pratt, M. and Hagstromer, M. (2009) 'The international prevalence study on physical activity: results from 20 countries', *International Journal of Behavioural Nutrition and Physical Activity*, 6:21 dci: 10.1186/1479-5868-6-21.

Bauman, A. and Phongsaven (2006) 'Physical activity measurement – a primer for health promotion', *Promotion and Education*, 13: 92–103.

Baumeister, R. F. and Leary, M. R. (1995) 'The need to belong: desire for interpersonal attachments as a fundamental human motivation', *Psychological Bulletin*, 117 (3): 497–529.

Boone, J. E., Gordon-Larsen, P., Stewart, J. D. and Popkin, B. M. (2008) 'Validation of a GIS facilities database: quantification and implications of error', *Annals of Epidemiology*, 18 (5): 371–7.

Bothwell, S., Gindroz, R. and Lang, R. (1998) 'Restoring community through traditional neighbourhood design – a case study of Diggs Town public housing', *Housing Policy Debate,* 9 (1): 89–114.

Broomhall, M., Giles-Corti, B. and Lange, A. (2004) *Quality of Public Open Space Tool (POST),* Perth, Western Australia patent.

Bull, F. C., Shepherd, R., Pratt, M. and Lankenau, B. (2006) 'Implementing national population-based action on physical activity – challenges for action and opportunities for international collaboration', *IUHPE: Promotion and Education*, 13 (2): 43–9.

Butland, B., Jebb, S., Kopelman, P., McPherson, K., Thomas, S., Mardell, J. and Parry, V. (2007) *Foresight Tackling Obesities: Future Choices – Project Report,* London: Government Office for Science.

Calthorpe, P. (1993) *The Next American Metropolis: Ecology and Urban Form*, New Jersey: Princeton Architectural Press.

Centers for Disease Control and Prevention (CDCP) (2008) *How Much Physical Activity Do Children Need?* 5 November, available at: <http://www.cdc.gov/physicalactivity/everyone/guidelines/children.html> (accessed 5 May 2009).

Cerin, E., Saelens, B., Sallis, J. and Frank, L. (2006) 'Neighborhood Environment Walkability Scale: validity and development of a short form', *Medicine and Science in Sports and Exercise*, 38 (9): 1682–91.

Chapman, S. and Wong, W. (1991) 'Incentives for questionnaire respondents', *Australian Journal of Public Health*, 15 (1): 66–7.

Chin, G., Van Niel, K., Giles-Corti, B. and Knuiman, M. (2008) 'Accessibility and connectivity in physical activity studies: the impact of missing pedestrian data', *Preventive Medicine*, 46: 41–5.

Corburn, J. (2004) 'Confronting the challenges in reconnecting urban planning and public health', *American Journal of Public Health*, 94 (4): 541–6.

Craig, C., Russel, S., Cameron, C. and Bauman, A. (2004) 'Twenty-year trends in physical activity among Canadian adults', *Canadian Journal of Public Health*, 95 (1): 59–63.

Craig, R. and Mindell, J. (2008) *Health Survey for England 2006: CVD and Risk Factors in Adults*, London: Joint Health Surveys Unit: National Centre for Social Research, Department of Epidemiology and Public Health at the Royal Free and University College Medical School.

Cummins, S., Petticrew, M., Higgins, C., Findlay, A. and Sparks, L. (2005) 'Large scale food retailing as an intervention for diet and health: quasi-experimental evaluation of a natural experiment', *Journal of Epidemiology and Community Health*, 59 (12): 1035–40.

De Bourdeaudhuij, I., Teixeira, P., Cardon, G. and Deforche, B. (2005) 'Environmental and psychosocial correlates of physical activity in Portuguese and Belgian adults', *Public Health Nutrition*, 8 (7): 886–95.

Department for Transport (DoT) (2007) *Transport Trends: 2006 Edition*, London: DoT.

Department of Health (DoH) (2004) *A Report of the Chief Medical Officer: At Least Five a Week – Evidence on the Impact of Physical Activity and its Relationship to Health*, London, DoH.

Department of Health (DoH) (2009) *Be Active, Be Healthy: A Plan for Getting the Nation Moving*, London, DoH.

Department of Health and Ageing (2004) *Active Kids are Healthy Kids: Australia's Physical Activity Guidelines For 5–12 Year Olds*, Canberra: Australian Government.

Dillman, D. A. (2000) *Mail and Internet Surveys: The Tailored Design Method*, New York: Wiley.

Donovan, R., James, R., Jalleh, G. and Sidebottom, C. (2006) 'Implementing mental health promotion: the Act–Belong–Commit Mentally Healthy WA campaign in Western Australia', *International Journal of Mental Health Promotion*, 8 (1): 33–42.

Dutton, J. (2001) *American New Urbanism: Re-Forming the Suburban Metropolis*, UK: Skira.

Ellaway, A., Macintyre, S. and Bonnefoy, X. (2005) 'Graffiti, greenery, and obesity in adults: secondary analysis of European cross sectional survey', *British Medical Journal*, 331 (7517): 611–12.

Ewing, R., Schmid, T., Killingsworth, R., Zlot, A. and Raudenbush, S. (2003) 'Relationship between urban sprawl and physical activity, obesity and morbidity', *American Journal of Health Promotion*, 18 (2): 47–57.

Fiona Bull, Billie Giles-Corti and Lisa Wood

Flowerdew, R., Manley, D. and Sabel, C. (2008) 'Neighbourhood effects on health: does it matter where you draw the boundaries?', *Social Science and Medicine*, 66: 1241–55.

Foster, S. and Giles-Corti, B. (2008) 'The built environment, neighborhood crime and constrained physical activity: an exploration of inconsistent findings', *Preventive Medicine*, 47 (3): 241–51.

Frank, L., Schmid, T., Sallis, J., Chapman, J. and Saelens, B. (2005) 'Linking objectively measured physical activity with objectively measured urban form: findings from SMARTRAQ', *American Journal of Preventive Medicine*, 28 (2, Supp 2): 117–25.

Frumkin, H., Frank, L. and Jackson, R. (2004) *Urban Sprawl and Public Health: Designing, Planning and Building for Healthy Communities*, Washington: Island Press.

Giles-Corti, B., Broomhall, M., Knuiman, M., Collins, C., Douglas, K., Ng, K., Lange, A. and Donovan, R. (2005a) 'Increasing walking: how important is distance to the attractiveness and size of public open space?' *American Journal of Preventive Medicine*, 28 (2S2): 169–76.

Giles-Corti, B. and Donovan, R. (2002) 'The relative influence of individual, social and physical environmental determinants of physical activity', *Social Science and Medicine*, 54: 1793–1812.

Giles-Corti, B., Kelty, S., Zubrick, S. and Villaneuva, K. (in press a) 'Encouraging walking for transport and physical activity in children and adolescents: how important is the built environment?', *Journal of Sports Medicine*.

Giles-Corti, B. and King, A. C. (2009) 'Creating active environments across the life course: "thinking outside the square"', *British Journal of Sports Medicine*, 43 (2): 109–113.

Giles-Corti, B., Knuiman, M., Pikora, T. J., Van Neil, K., Timperio, A., Bull, F.C., Shilton, T. and Bulsara, M. (2007) 'Can the impact on health of a government policy designed to create more liveable neighbourhoods be evaluated? An overview of the RESIDential Environment Project', *New South Wales Public Health Bulletin*, 18 (11–12): 238–42.

Giles-Corti, B., Knuiman, M., Timperio, A., Van Neil, K., Pikora, T., Bull, F.C., Shilton, T. and Bulsara, M. (2008) 'Evaluation of the implementation of a state government community design policy aimed at increasing local walking: design issues and baseline results from RESIDE, Perth Western Australia', *Preventive Medicine*, 46 (46): 54.

Giles-Corti, B., Robertson-Wilson, J., Wood, L. and Falconer, R. (in press b) 'The role of the changing built environment in shaping our shape', in J. W. Pearce (ed.), *Geographies of Obesity: Environmental Understandings of the Obesity Epidemic*, London: Ashgate.

Giles-Corti, B., Timperio, A., Bull, F.C. and Pikora, T. (2005b) 'Understanding physical activity environmental correlates: increased specificity for ecological models', *Exercise and Sports Science Reviews*, 33 (4): 175–81.

Giles-Corti, B., Timperio, A., Cutt, H., Pikora, T. J., Bull, F. C., Knuiman, M., Bulsara, M., Van Neil, K. and Shilton, T. (2006) 'Development of a reliable measure of walking within and outside the local neighborhood: RESIDE's Neighborhood Physical Activity Questionnaire', *Preventive Medicine*, 42: 455–99.

Hall, K. and Giles-Corti, B. (2000) 'Complementary therapies and the general practitioner: a survey of Perth GPs', *Australian Family Physician*, 29 (6): 602–6.

Handy, S., Cao, X. and Mokhtarian, P. (2006) 'Self-selection in the relationship between the built environment and walking', *Journal of the American Planning Association*, 72 (1): 55–74.

Handy, S., Cao, X. Y. and Mokhtarian, P. (2005) 'Correlation or causality between the built environment and travel behavior? Evidence from Northern California', *Transportation Research Part D-Transport and Environment*, 10 (6): 427–44.

Haskell, W., Lee, I., Pate, R., Powell, K., Blair, S., Franklin, B., Macera, C., Heath, G., Thompson, P. and Bauman, A. (2007) 'Physical activity and public health: updated recommendation for adults from the American College of Sports Medicine and the American Heart Association', *Circulation*, 116: 1081–93.

Heart and Stroke Foundation of Canada (2007) *Position Statement: The Built Environment, Physical Activity, Heart Disease and Stroke*, available at: < http://www.heartandstroke.com/atf/cf/%7B99452D8B-E7F1-4BD6-A57D-B136CE6C95BF%7D/Built_Environment_PS-ENGLISH-07.pdf> (accessed 15 August 2009).

Heath, G., Brownson, R. and Kruger, J. (2006) 'The effectiveness of urban design and land use and transport policies and practices to increase physical activity: a systematic review', *Journal of Physical Activity and Health*, 3: 55-S71.

Humpel, N., Owen, N. and Leslie, E. (2002) 'Environmental factors associated with adults' participation in physical activity: a review', *American Journal of Preventive Medicine*, 22 (3): 188–99.

International Physical Activity and the Environment Network (2004) *International Physical Activity and
the Environment Network*, available at: <http://www.ipenproject.org/> (accessed 5 May 2009).

Jackson, L. E. (2003) 'The relationship of urban design to human health and condition', *Landscape
and Urban Planning*, 64 (4): 191–200.

Jones, E. (2001) 'Liveable neighbourhoods', *World Transport Policy and Practice*, 7 (2): 38–42.

Joongsub, K. and Kaplan, R. (2004) 'Physical and psychological factors in sense of community:
new urbanist Kentlands and nearby Orchard Village.', *Environment and Behaviour*, 36 (3):
313–40.

Kaplan, R. and Kaplan, S. (1989) *The Experience of Nature: A Psychological Perspective*, New York:
Cambridge University Press.

Katz, P. (1994) *The New Urbanism: Toward an Architecture of Community*, New York: McGraw
Hill.

Kawachi, I. and Berkman, L. (2001) 'Social ties and mental health', *Journal of Urban Health*, 78 (3):
458–67.

Kelty, S., Giles-Corti, B. and Zubrick, S. R. (2008) 'Healthy body, healthy mind: Why physically
active children are healthier physically, psychologically and socially', in N. Beaulieu (ed.), *Physical
Activity and Children: New Research*, Hauppauge, N.Y.: Nova Science.

Kirtland, K., Porter, D., Addy, C., Neet, M., Williams, J., Sharpe, P., Neff, L., Kimsey, C. J. and
Ainsworth, B. (2003) 'Environmental measures of physical activity supports: perception versus
reality', *American Journal of Preventive Medicine*, 24 (4): 323–31.

Kopelman, P., Jebb, S. and Butland, B. (2007) 'Executive summary: Foresight 'Tackling Obesities:
Future Choices' project', *Obesity Reviews*, 8 (Supp 1): vi–ix.

Lange, A., Francis, J., Knuiman, M. and Giles-Corti, B. (2005) 'Recruiting by mail: do incentives
make a difference?' poster presented at Fifth National Physical Activity Conference, Melbourne,
October 2005.

Learnihan, V. (2007) *The Physical Environment as an Influence on Walking in the Neighbourhood:
Objective Measurement and Validation*, Perth: University of Western Australia.

Leyden, K. (2003) 'Social capital and the built environment: the importance of walkable neighbourhoods', *American Journal of Public Health*, 93 (9): 1546–51.

Louv, R. (2008) *Saving Our Children from Nature-Deficit Disorder: Revised and Updated Edition*,
Chapel Hill, N.C.: Algonquin Books.

Lund, H. (2002) 'Pedestrian environments and sense of community', *Journal of Planning Education
and Research*, 21: 301–12.

Maller, C., Townsend, M., Brown, P. and St Leger, L. (2002) *Healthy Parks, Healthy People: The
Health Benefits of Contact with Nature in a Park Context*, Melbourne: Deakin University.

McCormack, G., Milligan, R., Giles-Corti, B. and Clarkson, J. (2003) *Physical Activity Levels of
Western Australian Adults 2002: Results from the Adult Physical Activity Survey*, Perth:
Government of Western Australia.

McMillan, T. (2005) 'Urban form and a child's trip to school: the current literature and a model for
future research', *Journal of Planning Literature*, 19 (4): 440–56.

Millington, C., Ward Thompson, C., Rowe, D., Aspinall, P., Fitzsimons, C., Nelson, N. and Mutrie,
N. (2009) 'Development of the Scottish Walkability Assessment Tool (SWAT)', *Health and
Place*, 15: 474–81.

Mullen, E. (2003) 'Do you think that your local area is a good place for young people to grow up?
The effects of traffic and car parking on young people's views', *Health and Place*, 9: 351–60.

National Institute for Health and Clinical Excellence (NICE) (2008) *Promoting or Creating Built or
Natural Environments that Encourage and Support Physical Activity*, London: NICE.

National Preventative Health Taskforce (2008) *Australia: The Healthiest Country by 2020 – A
Discussion Paper*, Canberra: Commonwealth of Australia Government.

Ogilvie, D., Foster, C., Rothnie, H., Cavill, N., Hamilton, V., Fitzsimons, C. and Mutrie, N. (2007)
'Interventions to promote walking: systematic review', *British Medical Journal*, 334 (7605): 1204.

Ogilvie, D., Mitchell, R., Mutrie, N., Petticrew, M. and Platt, S. (2006) 'Evaluating health effects of
transport interventions methodologic case study', *American Journal of Preventive Medicine*, 31
(2): 118–26.

Oldenburg, B., Sallis, J., Harris, D. and Owen, N. (2002) 'Checklist of Health Promotion Environments at Worksites (CHEW): development and measurement characteristics', *American Journal of Health Promotion*, 16 (5): 288–99.

Owen, N., Cerin, E., Leslie, E., duToit, L., Coffee, N., Frank, L. D., Bauman, A. E., Hugo, G., Saelens, B. E. and Sallis, J. F. (2007) 'Neighborhood walkability and the walking behavior of Australian adults', *American Journal of Preventive Medicine*, 33 (5): 387–95.

Owen, N., Humpel, N., Leslie, E., Bauman, A. and Sallis, J. (2004) 'Understanding environmental influences on walking: review and research agenda', *American Journal of Preventive Medicine*, 27 (1): 67–76.

Pikora, T., Giles-Corti, B., Knuiman, M., Bull, F., Jamrozik, K. and Donovan, R. (2006) 'Neighborhood environmental factors correlated with walking near home: using SPACES', *Medicine and Science in Sports and Exercise*, 38 (4): 708–14.

Pucher, J. and Dijkstra, L. (2003) 'Promoting safe walking and cycling to improve public health: lessons from the Netherlands and Germany', *American Journal of Public Health*, 93: 1509–16.

Saelens, B. and Handy, S. (2008) 'Built environment correlates of walking: a review', *Medicine and Science in Sports and Exercise*, 40 (7): 550–66.

Saelens, B. E., Sallis, J. F., Black, J. B. and Chen, D. (2003) 'Neighborhood-based differences in physical activity: an environment scale evaluation', *American Journal of Public Health*, 93 (9): 1552–8.

Sallis, J. (2009) 'Measuring physical activity environments: a brief history', *American Journal of Preventive Medicine*, 36 (4): 86–92.

Sallis, J. F., Bowles, H. R., Bauman, A., Ainsworth, B. E., Bull, F. C., Craig, C. L. et al. (2009), 'Neighborhood environments are related to physical activity among adults in 11 countries', *American Journal of Preventive Medicine*, 36(6): 484–90.

Sallis, J. and Owen, N. (1997) 'Ecological models', in K. Glanz, F. Lewis and B. Rimer (eds), *Health Behavior and Health Education. Theory, Research, and Practice*, 2nd edn, San Francisco, Calif.: Jossey-Bass.

Sallis, J. and Owen, N. (2007) 'Ecological models of health behaviour', in K. Glanz, F. Lewis and B. Rimer (eds), *Health Behaviour and Health Education: Theory, Research and Practice*, 3rd edn, San Francisco, Calif.: Jossey-Bass: 403-24.

Scottish Executive Physical Activity Task Force (SEPATF) (2003) *Let's Make Scotland More Active: A Strategy for Physical Activity*, Edinburgh: Scottish Executive.

Sjöström, M., Oja, P., Hagströmer, M., Smith, B. and Bauman, A. (2006) ' Health-enhancing physical activity across European Union countries: the Eurobarometer study', *Journal of Public Health*, 14: 291–300.

Story, M., Giles-Corti, B., Yaroch, A., Cummins, S., Frank, L., Huang, T.-K. and Lewis, L. (2009) 'Work Group IV: future directions for measures of the food and physical activity environments', *American Journal of Preventive Medicine*, 36 (4, supp 1): 182–8.

Sugiyama, T., Salmon, J., Dunstan, D. W., Bauman, A. E. and Owen, N. (2007) 'Neighborhood walkability and TV viewing time among Australian adults', *American Journal of Preventive Medicine*, 33 (6): 444–9.

Transportation Research Board (TRB) (2005) *Does the Built Environment Influence Physical Activity? Examining the Evidence*, Washington, D.C.: TRB.

Trost, S., Owen, N., Bauman, A., Sallis, J. and Brown, W. (2002) 'Correlates of adults' participation in physical activity: review and update', *Medicine and Science in Sports and Exercise*, 34 (12): 1996–2001.

United Nations (2004) *World Urbanization Prospects: The 2003 Revision*, New York: Department of Economic and Social Affairs, Population Division.

US Department of Health and Human Services (DHHS) (2008) *2008 Physical Activity Guidelines for Americans: Be active, Healthy and Happy!* Washington D.C, USA. www.health.gov/paguidelines

US DHHS, CDCP (1996) *Physical Activity and Health: A Report of The Surgeon General*, Atlanta, Ga.

Van Dyck, D., Deforche, B., Cardon, G. and De Bourdeaudhuij, I. (2009) 'Neighbourhood walkability and its particular importance for adults with a preference for passive transport', *Health and Place*, 15: 496–504.

Welsh Assembly Government (2006) Climbing Higher: next steps, Cardiff: Welsh Assembly Government.

Western Australian Planning Commission (2000) *Liveable Neighbourhoods: a Western Australian Government sustainable cities initiative*, edition 2.Western Australian Planning Commission, Western Australia.

Wood, L. and Giles-Corti, B. (2008) 'Is there a place for social capital in the psychology of health and place?', *Journal of Environmental Psychology*, 28 (2): 154–63.

Wood, L., Shannon, T., Bulsara, M., Pikora, T., McCormack, G. and Giles-Corti, B. (2007) 'The anatomy of the safe and social suburb: an exploratory study of the built environment, social capital and residents' perceptions of safety', *Health and Place*, 14: 15–31.

World Health Organization (WHO) (2004) *Global Strategy on Diet, Physical Activity and Health*, Geneva: WHO.

WHO (2006) 'Promoting physical activity for health: a framework for action in the WHO European Region', in *WHO European Conference on Counteracting Obesity: Diet and Physical activity for Health, Istanbul, Turkey*, available at: <http://www.euro.who.int/Document/NUT/Instanbul_conf_edoc10.pdf> (accessed 5 May 2009).

Chapter 5

Using affordances as a health-promoting tool in a therapeutic garden

Patrik Grahn, Carina Tenngart Ivarsson, Ulrika K. Stigsdotter and Inga-Lena Bengtsson

Stress-induced illnesses have become a huge global problem. According to the World Health Organization (WHO), mental health disorders and cardiovascular diseases – both of which are clearly affected by stress – are expected to be the two major contributors to illnesses in all parts of the world, with mental health disorders calculated for all age groups and both sexes, by the year 2020 (WHO, 2008). Stress is not an illness per se; rather, stress reactions are natural and necessary – they serve to sharpen our senses and make us more efficient. In the event of a perceived threat, stress reactions trigger our 'fight or flight' reflexes that helped our early ancestors survive (Atkinson et al., 1996). During stress, our body organs react in many different ways, and if stress is sustained for an inappropriately long time without the possibility of recovery, these reactions become dysfunctional and harmful, with the risk of causing serious and harmful effects on all vital organs (Aldwin, 2007). For early humankind, who lived on nature's terms, the body's own adaptation mechanisms were suited to their purpose. Today, many psychiatric diseases in particular are strongly associated with prolonged and incorrect stress reactions, the foremost being depression and fatigue syndromes (Aldwin, 2007). The widespread exhaustion and fatigue reactions caused by prolonged stress that we now face in Europe are a serious problem. In its latest report, the European Working Conditions Survey states that 'Work-related stress is one of the most common work-related health problems, affecting 22 per cent of European workers, and the sectors most at risk are health and social service and education' (Parent-Thirion et al., 2007). The WHO has rated stress as one of the major causes of death in the developed world, and consequently has made stress-related diseases a priority health prevention area (WHO, 2008).

All people, at some point during their lifetime, find themselves in extreme stressful situations. Without a refuge, personal adversity can develop into a life crisis, resulting in severe depression and/or pain and burnout syndrome (Aldwin, 2007). Depression is already the leading cause of disability as measured by years lived with disability (WHO, 2008). The connection between stress, a life crisis, ill health and premature death may be seen in light of the WHO's definition of health: 'Health is a state of complete physical, mental and social well-being and not merely the absence of disease or infirmity' (WHO, 1948). Thus, health encompasses the individual's entire life situation: housing, friends, work, recreation and so on. Today, there seem to be very few places in our everyday environment where people can recover from stress and crises (Grahn and Stigsdotter, 2003).

In the mid-1980s, some interesting research findings were published in the United States. It appeared that gardens, parks and areas of natural greenery have beneficial effects on people's mental health and capacity (Kaplan and Kaplan, 1989; Ulrich, 1984). The researchers called these effects 'restorative'. The above-mentioned health effects were connected to restoration from either 'mental fatigue' (Kaplan, 2001) or acute symptoms of stress (Ulrich, 1999). Accordingly, some results suggest that a stay in a natural environment can reduce harmful stress for people who are affected by mental fatigue (Nordh, et al., 2009). In addition, in the United States, several decades of research have shown good outcomes from treating post-traumatic stress symptoms with horticultural therapy (Hewson, 1994).

Stress and mental fatigue

In Sweden, stress-related illnesses – such as mental fatigue, burnout, stress-related pain and depression – had reached the level of a national disease by the mid-1990s. At the same time, at SLU Alnarp, we had started to study the connections between human health and the use of urban green areas (Grahn, 1994, 1996). We set out to develop a new kind of therapy that combines the use of restorative natural areas with horticultural therapy and traditional occupational therapy, physiotherapy and psychotherapy.

Patients seeking rehabilitation at Alnarp all suffer from stress-related mental fatigue and tiredness: the disease *exhaustion syndrome* (Nordh et al., 2009; Socialstyrelsen, 2003). Exhaustion syndrome often starts with a dramatic collapse, with the exhausted person chiefly sleeping during the first sick-leave period and feeling fatigued and lacking energy between sleep episodes (Hallsten,

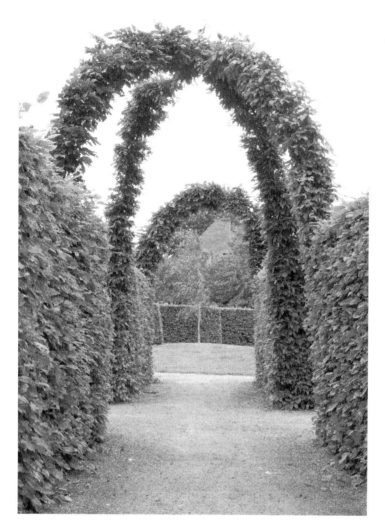

Figure 5.1
Entrance to the
Welcoming
Garden in Alnarp.
Photograph:
Elisabeth von
Essen

2001; Maslach, 2001). Interest in getting back to work gradually increases, but returning to work too early may lead to a relapse and bring about a very long period of sick leave. During this time, the individual is often hypersensitive to stress (Hallsten, 2001; Maslach, 2001). Family members and work colleagues may feel that these individuals have undergone a personality change, have become more self-centred, and feel less empathy for the people around them.

Rehabilitation needs

First of all, we should consider some important characteristics of the group of people being rehabilitated in the therapeutic garden, that need to be considered in the design of the garden rooms, the activities we offer and the behaviour of the staff:

- *Demands of the design of the therapeutic setting*: Some people afflicted with exhaustion syndrome state that they find it difficult to listen to music, others that they can hardly stand the smell of perfume. When at their worst, they feel almost electrified, so that the slightest odour, bright colour, sound or even sense of 'unbalance' or unattractiveness in the room they stay in seems unbearable (Hallsten, 2001; Ulrich, 1999).
- *Demands concerning activities in the therapeutic setting*: Individuals stricken with exhaustion syndrome are typically accustomed in their regular lives to being efficient, are often verbal, find it easy to express themselves, and may sometimes be regarded as critical of the people around them. Their harshest criticism, however, is usually of their own abilities (Maslach, 2001). They are often intelligent and creative. If they feel that they are ensnared in trivialities and find no outlet for their skills, or if they feel that their work is not appreciated, they may react by increasing their efforts to levels far beyond their actual strength. Very often, exhausted individuals are afraid of not being able to meet wholly the demands confronting them. However, even the slightest demand may trigger reactions of irritation and immense tiredness (Maslach, 2001).
- *Demands of the staff and other participants in the group*: Exhausted individuals find it increasingly difficult to understand, sympathize with and tolerate other people (Hallsten, 2001). However, the people around exhausted individuals must make demands on them. Otherwise, they will not be able to return to society. Vagueness and obscurity on the part of their superiors and workmates as to whether they have done enough or been efficient may play an important part concerning their disease. A healthy approach involves making demands that these individuals feel they can meet within a short period of time, and that they are able to cope with. Exhausted individuals and others susceptible to stress have a much better chance of recovering their self-confidence when they are able to cope with a task (Hallsten, 2001).

The idea of the design

First, our aim was to merge theories focusing on horticultural therapy and restorative nature. However, we have continued to integrate knowledge and other

Patrik Grahn, Carina Tenngart Ivarsson, Ulrika Stigsdotter and Inga-Lena Bengtsson

theories from environmental psychology, landscape architecture, medicine, occupational therapy, physiotherapy and psychotherapy:

- *Horticultural therapy* has a strong focus on the healing effects of activities in the garden, such as weeding, raking and sowing (Relf, 1999). The theory starts from the idea that human beings like to be active, they like to perform meaningful activities that interest them and give them the energy needed to exert themselves. If people have the opportunity to use their body and mind in the pursuit of pleasurable and meaningful occupations, they will feel rewarded. And working in a garden can be particularly rewarding (Relf, 1992; Kielhofner, 1997).
- *Restoring health* by experiencing nature, on the other hand, focuses on certain health-promoting characteristics in the environment, referring to the two theories below:
  - *Attention-Restoration Theory (ART)*: The theory is that people process information through two types of attention, directed attention and fascination (Kaplan, 2001). The directed attention system sorts information we have to use: for example, to focus on complex problems we have to solve in our everyday life, and to inhibit undesirable information, like noise, litter and certain problems we do not want to dwell on. Directed attention is a highly limited resource, which we can easily exhaust if we do not have opportunities for recovery. The demands of modern society mostly involve complex visual and auditory impressions, which may be difficult to interpret and overcome. This is particularly true when people are under great stress. People recover best in environments where this system can rest, and where they can use our other information system – involuntary attention or fascination. We use this kind of attention to explore the environment, to detect a glimpse of water, a rustle in a bush or a flower in a forest. Nature environments do not demand complicated decisions from visitors; they do not have to sort information, prioritize, plan and so on, and hence directed attention can be restored (Kaplan, 2001).
  - *The Aesthetic-Affective Theory (AAT)* considers that the healing effects of nature are a matter of unconscious processes and affects located in the oldest, emotion-driven parts of the brain (Ulrich, 1999). These processes or reflexes tell us when we can rest or when we should be active, including being prepared to flee or fight. The theory concerns special information in nature that can tell us when it is possible to rest, which results in decreased stress. This, Roger Ulrich (1999) argues, is an unconscious feeling of security which occurs in environments like those humans lived in originally. According to this evolutionary theory, our original environments were open pastoral landscapes with wooded meadows and a few larger trees. Nature, Ulrich (1993) claims, has an

ability to rapidly reduce, or induce, stress on an affective-symbolic level which Ulrich defines and labels as 'aesthetic'. Thus, in fractions of a second we get basic information about the whole context in the surrounding environment via our senses and our primitive emotions: our affects (Tomkins, 1995; Ulrich, 1993). Ulrich (1999) argues that the visual impact of the environment itself may signal danger or safety, and that this is most important when 'persons experience high levels of stress' (Ulrich, 1999).

Developing the therapeutic garden

During autumn 2001, the garden was designed and laid out at the SLU Alnarp campus outside Malmö in southern Sweden (Stigsdotter and Grahn, 2003). Today the garden covers about two hectares, and offers both nature-like areas with restorative qualities and more traditional cultivation areas with plant beds and qualities focusing on more demanding activities. We constructed the garden based on earlier research at SLU Alnarp and theories related to horticultural therapy, ART and AAT. The design is based on variation and contrasts, providing different garden rooms for different purposes, and the senses constituted an important aspect. The visitors can come close to the vegetation, stones and water, and thus are able to touch things, taste berries and smell flowers (Stigsdotter and Grahn, 2003), which are intended to maintain and strengthen experiential value. Activities are tailored to the entire garden, including social meeting places and areas planned for cultivation, as well as for tending nature, such as clearing and thinning the forest stands. For the therapist, it is important to get the individual to participate and become engaged in their thoughts, feelings, body and will. One way to achieve this is to inspire fascination and arouse curiosity in relation to different tasks. Most important is the fact that the garden contains areas for rest and contemplation, as well as for activities and work.

Research shows that experiences of nature affect people differently, largely depending on their life situation (Ottosson and Grahn, 2008). Therefore, the garden had to be designed to make different demands to suit participants at all levels. Demands can involve a participant simply coming to Alnarp. On a more strenuous level, it can involve cultivating a plant bed that requires considerable care. On an even more demanding level, it may involve working together with other people. There are garden rooms to which participants can retire privately and also rooms they can share with several individuals at the same time. All garden rooms should arouse participants' curiosities and tempt them to feel and smell the water, grass, flowers and soil, and encourage them to partake in all activities. We have also taken pains to create transitional stages between very demanding rooms and undemanding rooms.

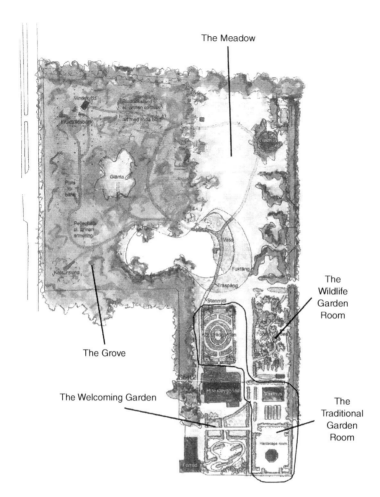

The Meadow

The Wildlife Garden Room

The Grove

The Welcoming Garden

The Traditional Garden Room

Figure 5.2
Illustrated plan of the therapeutic garden at Alnarp. Photograph: Elisabeth von Essen

Eight experienced dimensions

A therapeutic garden must be able to communicate with the visitor on many levels, through sights, smells, sounds and so on. Research shows that there exist eight main dimensions of experience that constitute the fundamental building blocks of parks and gardens (Grahn, Stigsdotter and Berggrern Bärring, 2005). These dimensions manifest themselves through many different sensations – sight, hearing, locomotion, etc. (Grahn and Stigsdotter, 2010). We believe that these eight dimensions constitute a basic foundation, and that some of them are more necessary than others. In the therapeutic garden at Alnarp, all eight dimensions have been included in the design.

Table 5.1 Dimensions of the nature/garden rooms.

The eight experienced nature dimensions	Description of the dimension
1. Serene	Peace, silence and signs of care. Sounds of wind, water, birds and insects. No rubbish, no weeds, no disturbing people, safe and secure. In its most distinct form, this can be described as having the character of a restful church interior.
2. Nature	Fascination with wild nature. Plants seem self-sown. Lichen- and moss-grown rocks, old paths. Something created not by humans, but by the power of something mightier.
3. Rich in species	A room offering a variety of species of animals and plants.
4. Space	A room offering a restful feeling of 'entering another world'. A coherent whole, like a beech forest.
5. Prospect	A green, open place with room for vistas and a place that invites you to stay.
6. Refuge	A sanctuary, an enclosed, safe, secret and secluded place, where you can relax and be yourself and also experiment and play.
7. Social	A meeting place for festivity and pleasure. A social arena or meeting place.
8. Culture	A place offering fascination through evidence of people's values, beliefs, efforts and toils, and perhaps with the passage of time.

The rehabilitation garden in Alnarp can be divided into two large areas, *the Nature Area*, which has a nature-oriented character and offers restorative experiences relating to the AAT and ART-hypotheses, and the *Cultivation and Gardening Area*, related to horticultural therapy. In the Nature Area we find two rooms: the *Grove* and the *Meadow*, both of which are examples of cherished parts of the Swedish landscape. The dominant dimensions experienced are Space, Serene, Nature, Rich in Species and (in the Meadow) Prospect.

In the Cultivation and Gardening Area we find the more demanding *Traditional Garden Room* and the much less demanding *Wildlife Garden Room*. Most of the Traditional Garden Room is designed like a traditional garden, focusing on cultivation. The room is elongated from north to south where the verdure dominates, but is confined to strict rows. The room closely and clearly resembles the common Swedish allotment garden. The dimensions Social, Culture, and

Rich in Species can be found in this room. In the south end, however, we find the more modern, progressive and less green *Hardscape Room*, where the cultivation is carried out in plant beds of different heights.

The Wildlife Garden Room offers great cultivation possibilities in a small area, and its organic and nature-like design is markedly different from the straight and strict lines of traditional gardening. In the Wildlife Garden Room, the landscape architects envision opportunities for cultivation in organic forms. Here, there is room for several dimensions, such as Rich in Species, Space and, most of all, Refuge. One purpose is that people can eat almost every plant in this area, or their fruits. This should trigger their senses. Considering that participants may sometimes wish to experiment with cultivation on their own, it seems a good idea to allow them to work in an environment that offers small private rooms as well as opportunities to consider what individual plants need in terms of light, heat, water and so on. These factors may lead to a more creative and playful contribution. People suffering from exhaustion syndrome are very often creative, but they are also plagued by a desire to be clever, capable and efficient. They may be more sensitive than others to the demands of the environment. The Wildlife Garden Room is more bohemian in its appearance, and hence there is more potential for these people to be creative in cultivation. It is also here that our two English lop-eared rabbits and chickens live, although during the day they may also run free in the other garden rooms.

The *Welcoming Garden* is the first garden room visitors enter. It is therefore important that the room does not make too many demands on the visitor, so that even those with little strength of mind can cope with it. At the same time, it should be experienced as interesting and attractive. Visitors should

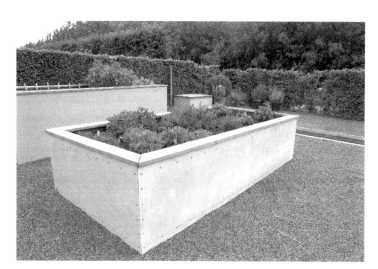

Figure 5.3
Photograph of the Hardscape Room: raised beds. This area is less preferred by our participants. Photograph: Elisabeth von Essen

Figure 5.4
Photograph of the
Hardscape Room:
water. This area is
less preferred by
our participants.
Photograph:
Elisabeth von
Essen

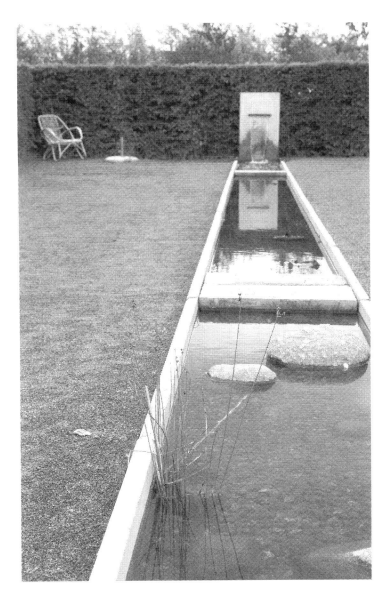

feel welcome, safe and secure here, and that they can be themselves. The dimension that dominates the whole garden room is Serene. Close to the entrance of the main building, the dimension Social is more prominent, while Refuge, Rich in Species and Culture are the dominant dimensions in the rest of the Welcoming Garden.

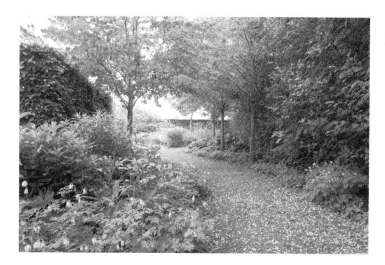

Figure 5.5
A path leading in
to the Welcoming
Garden.
Photograph:
Elisabeth von
Essen

The treatment programme

The treatment programme starts from a cluster of theories, maintaining that health effects are derived on the basis of experiences of the garden room as such, the activities in the garden room, staff members' knowledge, and the treatment measures and coaching they carry out. And, of course, the patient's background and character has a great influence. The qualities of the garden are used for different health-promoting activities. The first patients arrived in July 2002, since when we have treated 130 patients.

People visiting the garden for the purpose of rehabilitation are called therapy participants, not patients. The intention is to strengthen their image of themselves as nonpatients. These participants have been referred to the therapeutic garden at Alnarp from hospitals, social insurance offices, insurance companies and the industrial health service. They participate in a programme which lasts for twelve weeks, for three and a half hours per day. The schedule varies from one half day to four half days a week:

- First week: one half day.
- Second week: two half days.
- Third to tenth week: four half days.
- Eleventh week: two half days.
- Twelfth week: one half day.

We have a maximum of eight participants in each group. We treat one group in the morning and one in the afternoon. Three occupational therapists and a curative educational teacher work full time in the garden; a physiotherapist works half time and a psychotherapist works 40 per cent of the time. The therapists working part time in the garden work in ordinary hospitals on other days of the week. The landscape architect responsible for the garden works full time.

Environmental factors can supply more or less favourable opportunities for garden activities and also determine the outcome of these activities. Our participants are part of a behaviour setting (Barker, 1968): the Rehabilitation Garden. Activities in the garden can be passive (like resting) or active (like weeding). They can be obviously focused, purposeful and goal-directed ('molar'), or they may seem to be unfocused ('molecular') (Baum, 2002). Thus, one can identify specific units (that is, areas for walking, resting and cultivating) and their association with different levels of physical and mental activity. This is essential for understanding the impact of therapeutic design and horticultural therapy on people's behaviour, experiences and the resulting health effects. From the theories mentioned above (ART: Kaplan, 2001; AAT: Ulrich, 1999; horticultural therapy: Relf, 1992) we hypothesized that experiences of different qualities in therapeutic gardens, relating to different activities, have the potential to restore people suffering from stress and in this way promote health.

Four phases of rehabilitation

The participants in the garden have been ill for a long time, on average four and a half years, and during that time they have not been able to work or study. Women make up 85 per cent of the participants, most often in their thirties and early forties. At the beginning of rehabilitation, the participants are in a very prominent phase of exhaustion syndrome; they are hypersusceptible to stress and show a marked lack of mental energy. They feel guilt and even disgrace because of their highly reduced capacity. We find a strong emotional seclusion in the participants, and they have difficulties with social communication. In addition, our participants have difficulties with focusing attention, short-term memory, tiredness and physical pain. However, many also have problems with physical awareness: they are not aware of the boundaries of their own body and often feel dizzy when moving around. Sometimes the person is so closed off that the entire body is 'quiet', almost paralysed. For such individuals, pain may be experienced after several treatments. These participants sometimes report more physical pain after being in the garden for 12 weeks than they did when they arrived, but they still report feeling better in general.

Phase 1. Contact

The participants experience that they can no longer interact, like they used to do, with their social and physical environment. They have difficulties interpreting the world around them; they must find a new way to make contact, involving the external world as well as themselves. Seen from a psychological perspective, many participants have lost contact early on with their genuine selves. This might be because they have allowed other people to define their value, which has finally implied that their own self-esteem is primarily based on achievements, such as work output and other external performances. At an existential level, exhaustion syndrome constitutes a type of life crisis (Maslach, 2001). The participants' previous way of living has not enabled them to cope with the stressors they have experienced – they have probably even sought out such stressors in order to show that they can cope.

Medically speaking, constant increases in stress without recovery have devastated the sensitive autonomic nervous system's ability to regulate stress naturally (Währborg, 2003). Successful rehabilitation is based on being able to permanently leave behind one's previous, inadequate stress management patterns and to acquire new strategies that are more appropriate and sustainable. Healing processes are based on intrinsic forces. What therapists can do, with the help of the garden, is to induce health-promoting processes in order to begin the healing our bodies strive for and have the mechanisms to complete. The goal is to heal these injuries, which have been caused by constant flows of the stress hormones adrenaline, noradrenaline and cortisol.

Each participant must first make contact with their surrounding world, involving the person's own thoughts, feelings, senses and muscles. It is important to find places where they feel safe and secure, and to find activities that enable them to make these contacts. The experience of time, the present as well as timelessness, is essential. Thus, the garden or nature setting must have several different kinds of spaces so people have possibilities to start this process.

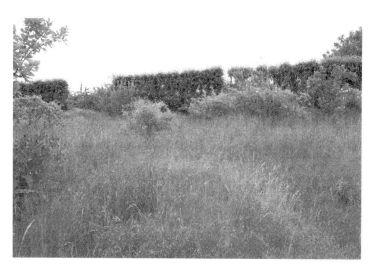

Figure 5.6
Participants regularly take walks in the Meadow. Photograph: Elisabeth von Essen

In the beginning, the participants generally seem lost, astray, and do not want to go far from the staff from whom they seek support. Their activities may consist of managing to come out into the garden, just being there, resting and getting to know it. The first activities involve resting or walking, often together with the therapists, in garden rooms that evoke safety; resting in areas where *Refuge* is the dominant dimension; walking in the Grove and Meadow, and also in the Welcoming Garden.

Despite the fact that the participants are extremely tired when they first arrive, they want to be 'good': they often look for the most work-related places and want to start working and being efficient. The therapists address this by using a very structured scheme for several days in advance, giving targeted/personal suggestions to the participants, so they know exactly what is expected of them. The activities are very simple at first, not intended to be mentally demanding, such as picking fruit together with the therapist. However, this type of activity can be experienced as physically demanding for the participant's body. Some participants struggle just to manage to come to Alnarp. They are experiencing great pain and they are very tired, so picking fruit could still be a demanding activity, both mentally and physically. However, after even just a few days, the participants express palpable relief and liberation, thanks to the peaceful environment that is experienced as having almost no demands, at least no indistinct, trying, and difficult or contradictory demands.

Soon after this phase, the participant is invited to choose their place in the garden, a place that they find is welcoming to them. From now on, the participants put more and more of their reliance on the garden as well as on the staff. An interest starts to grow concerning the different activities in the garden, activities suggested by the staff. The participants choose small garden rooms (Refuge) in the beginning, most often in the Welcoming Garden, and take walks from there and out to the Grove and Meadow. The therapeutic garden invites walks, and both the walks that staff and participants take together and the walks that participants take by themselves have proven to be very important. If the garden had been smaller, these walks would have been difficult to accomplish. In this phase, the walks the participants carry out are very introverted (Tenngart Ivarsson, 2007). They often walk as if in their own world, without participating in their physical and social environment.

Phase 2. Breaking the shell

People experiencing an existential crisis must re-establish communication with their environment as well as build up their self-esteem, self and identity. This involves re-evaluating their situation and finding a new orientation. At this stage, it may be advantageous to try to approach an individual through the physical world, which is somehow directly accessible for communication via all the

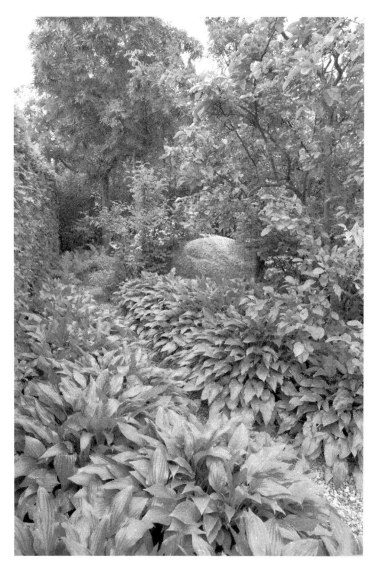

Figure 5.7
A preferred part of
the Welcoming
Garden with a lot
of the quality
refuge.
Photograph:
Elisabeth von
Essen

senses. The nature experience as such is affected by how much of the environment a person is able to take in and by how great their mental powers are.

In this second phase, people participate in several different garden activities. They often change activities several times a day: from being involved in social activities to being on their own, from cultivation to picking fruit and nuts. They still take many walks; however, their walks are certainly more extroverted (Tenngart Ivarsson, 2007). The participants are interested in plants and berries, and in exploring the environment. However, the body is experiencing a great deal of pain, and the participants still become tired. We find that the participant gradually establishes contact with the whole environment, one step at a time. The garden provides different garden rooms for different purposes and moods, and our experiences of the past few years are that this has been significant in every phase, but perhaps especially striking in this phase. Most important is the fact that the garden contains areas for rest and contemplation, as well as for activities and work. Being able to alternate between these extremes has proven to be of great value.

Finding physically challenging activities in a garden is seldom a problem. These can involve everything from digging and compost work to setting stones. Participants often feel that hard physical work in a peaceful environment is liberating and relieves tension. Soothing activities are also easy to create; raking leaves is one good example of such an activity. The calm, sweeping movement has a relaxing, almost meditative effect. People suffering from exhaustion syndrome can practise stress management by, among other things, 'just being' – that is, experiencing nature with all their senses. Some important experiences that can be taken from the garden out into everyday life are stopping work before it is finished, listening when your body tells you it is tired, lowering your ambition levels, reducing the number of obligations you have as well as letting the circumstances of the day determine what you do today.

The activities the participants are to complete must feel meaningful if they and the therapists, working together, are to build up something useful and

Figure 5.8
**Working in the
Traditional Garden
Room.**
Photograph:
Elisabeth von
Essen

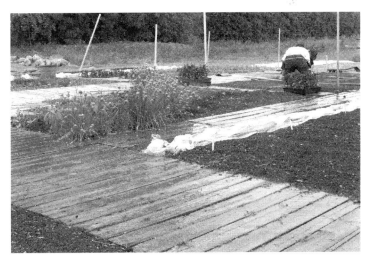

pleasurable. A meaningful activity may be one the person needs to do to manage everyday life, or one that affords joy and a lust for life – this differs from person to person, or from one time to another. Meaningfulness has proven to be of great importance. This is revealed, for example, when therapists are able to use the meaningfulness of an activity to motivate participants suffering from severe pain to carry out movements that they otherwise might hesitate or refuse to carry out. The motivation may lie in the fact that they have built up something together, but may even derive from the individual participant's experience of their illness. For example, therapists can encourage participants to find plants that can be used in teas, ointments and soaps that they can make themselves. Thus, the garden should contain plants that can start this process of curiosity and interest. For instance, this could involve finding herbs that promote sleep and rest or that are good for upset stomachs. This type of reasoning is in line with how participants are encouraged to work with their own health conditions.

After two to three weeks, the fluctuations in stress reactions have diminished substantially. The participants have reached a level of greater mental energy and endurance, and the quality of their sleep is better. We can see a significant change in participants' cognitive functions. They also experience an improvement in their short-term memory and capacity to reflect upon things. Their emotional seclusion diminishes and they become more receptive at the same time. The physical therapist offers a massage, mostly consisting of soft touch, and at this stage the participants regularly describe the result of this massage as an almost shocking awakening, concerning experiences of tensions in the body. The participants express surprise over their new body awareness, reporting that up until now they had not noticed or paid attention to signals from the body. Their self-confidence is increasing regarding their own life history, and an incipient feeling of empathy for their own situation begins to grow. At the same time, we find that their attitudes of guilt and disgrace are diminishing. Concerning their communication with staff and other participants, we notice an increasing versatility in their flow of associations. The participants can talk about their own situation in a humorous way and with self-awareness. We notice that each participant is now more and more reliant, even on other participants. They also express personal desires concerning activities and time spent in the garden, and their activity level is higher.

At the end of this phase, it is clear that participants' hard 'shells' are beginning to soften, which affects the whole body, mentally and physically. This shell was built up when the participant was suffering from severe stress. The shell was protecting them from feelings, as if they had been experiencing a war. This process continues into the next phase.

Figure 5.9
A view of the
labyrinthine paths
in the Welcoming
Garden.
Photograph:
Elisabeth von
Essen

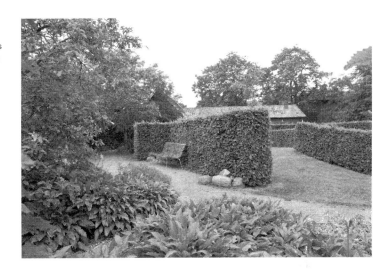

Phase 3. Opening

During the period of rehabilitation, we have observed how participants increase their physical capacity, and improve their underlying mood as well as their ability to concentrate. Through work in the garden, participants' strength gradually increases and they can manage more. During this phase, soft treatment of body awareness is important. Indications from the body can be connected to different affects (primitive emotions like anger, shame, and fear, but also happiness), and can be interpreted in terms of affects. When deep, chronic muscle tension is released, old thinking and behaviour patterns are also dissolved. These old behaviour patterns are a manifestation of the way in which the individual was able to deal with life experiences. Together with activities in the garden – with its soft, sensuous experiences of temperature, scents, sounds and the tactile experiences of plants, soil, water and so on – these affects are increasingly brought to the surface of consciousness.

After four to six weeks, there is a clear reaction in which feelings come pouring out, as when ice thaws. The therapists can certainly feel a sense of irritability in the group. They notice this reaction, and initiate a type of activity that includes finding symbols in the garden. The participants are now in a phase where all senses are involved: impressions from the garden take shape as clear symbols. Violations, infringements, anger towards parents, a spouse, employers and/or dominant brothers or sisters appear. Sorrow over all the years that have been lost in a subdued, secluded and submissive demeanour, and attitudes towards the surrounding world, are expressed. Memories of hard experiences from different times in the participant's life history are awakened and discussed. This occurs most often as a spontaneous need and without pressure from the

139

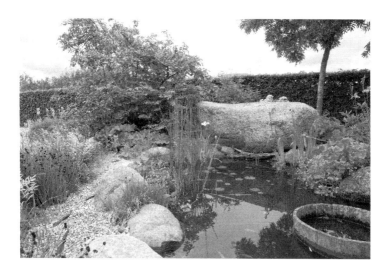

Figure 5.10
The pond in the
Welcoming
Garden has many
symbolic qualities:
stones, water,
flowers, etc.
Photograph:
Elisabeth von
Essen

therapist, and this is often the first time in their life participants tell someone about these experiences. They start to realize and talk about how they have felt, in reality, all these years.

Thus, one important task during this process is to help participants put these new experiences into words. Nature and the garden may here be used on a more symbolic/therapeutic level, such that nature becomes an arena for the person to come into contact with and give shape to their own unique symbolic language. Step by step, more symbolic activities are introduced. At this stage, sowing, picking flowers or working with compost could be activities affecting this process. Sowing a seed and caring for the shoot by watering, applying manure and weeding can cause the participants to consider caring for themselves – to realize that they are worth caring for. Through creative and specific therapeutic methods – for example, art therapy and work with clay inspired by nature – participants are given the opportunity to use their personal symbolic language to visualize events and experiences in their life situations. Nature is full of metaphors and symbols, and these can constitute a link to the unconscious, thereby supporting the healing process. This, in turn, may help people find new strategies for making everyday life more manageable.

The therapist can help to identify an activity or place in the garden that can facilitate participants in their rehabilitation process. This may be anything from handicrafts to conversations that touch upon our innermost places. Many participants now begin to see early patterns in their life history, and start reflecting on why they became sick. Most participants start to concern themselves with their personal matters in an artistic way: they start to arrange plants, write, paint, use clay and so on, and begin to 'thrash things out' with their parents, spouse and others in an artistic way. The participants walk by themselves, trying to find private and positively charged places, where they can be themselves and are their own masters.

Conversational therapy constitutes a supportive, consultative and cognitive/educational approach. At the outset, it is important to provide medical explanations for the varying mental and physical symptoms of exhaustion syndrome. Later, during the conversations in the garden, the individual's unique life and illness histories are tied together, allowing the participant to find some coherence in how and why they became ill. Feelings of abandonment and power-lessness can be toned down and turned into feelings of hope for the future.

In treatment, *time* is an important factor. The participants commu-nicate consciously and unconsciously with phenomena in the garden. A year and its seasons bear witness to the fact that there is a time for everything, which is an important concept. This is often a major adjustment for participants. At work and at home, they have been used to hurrying things along. Now, in the garden, they must yield to nature's own rhythm: taking a pause from one's work does not mean losing time. It is then we exist in time, are present, can see the beauty of nature, the colours, hear the stream ripple, smell the earth and plants, taste the berries and water, and be touched by the moment. We experience things. Sensual moments such as these – when we feel we exist – are moments of recuperation. If things go too fast, we lose our desire – something we must be frugal with.

At the end of this phase, the participants try to say 'No!' in different situations. A newly gained strength can now be found. The participant expresses happiness over the fact that something irrevocable happened as soon as they made contact with their real, genuine, but ill-treated inner ego. This happiness is what the participant wants to keep, no matter what happens in the future.

Phase 4. Growing

During the last two to three weeks, the earlier phase of reactions proceeds to a phase of practice for a new way of perceiving and looking at their life history and situation. Now, the participants start to accept the situation and become reconciled with their life history and their illness. Even the reawakened early traumatic events in childhood are toned down, and during the last weeks these memories have less and less importance in conversations. A participant can accept that, previously in life, they did not have the right resources to manage strain and stress in other ways. The person can see their role in both family and work in a wider perspective, and can understand how different courses of events have originated.

Feelings of guilt continue to diminish and participants' endurance continues to increase. At this stage, when the shell is finally broken, the desire to communicate grows rapidly. This may start a more intense process of communication, where the affects of guilt, shame, anger, fear and so on are mitigated, and the affects of curiosity and happiness are strengthened. This is because the participants can now relate to affects of, for example, guilt and shame, and can accept these feelings. The participants also start to think more and more about their true selves, leaving their old roles, which were perhaps based on good work output. This could be facilitated by performing activities where participants do not have to feel guilty about not having finished every task, which might help them understand that one does not need to be able to manage everything in order to be of value. This phase needs spaces and activities through which individuals can reinforce their basic self-esteem, finding their own needs and a way of looking more optimistically at the future. This phase involves strong efforts to support the true inner self.

At the end of the therapy, participants can take the initiative in starting things and carrying them out; they set about their own, creative projects. At this point, the participants are not as tired as they were at the outset and their bodies are functioning better, and now usually freer from pain. In addition to the mandatory digging and watering, there is also work with various construction projects, allowing participants to do woodwork in the greenhouse and garden. Moreover, they can make use of all the garden crops, thus helping to produce food, firewood and various handicrafts. In all activities, sense experiences such as colours, smells, tastes, balance and the tactile senses are stimulated. For participants with pain, it is important to develop exercises that do not overstrain affected body parts, so that the muscle mass continues to build up properly and the blood circulation to these parts is sufficient. Often, the whole group can share spontaneous reflections and

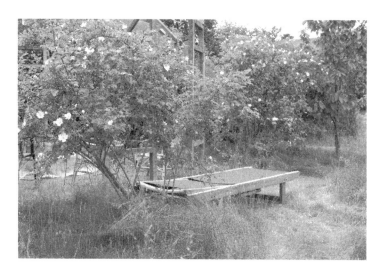

Figure 5.11
A much preferred, more bohemian part of the Wildlife Garden, suitable both for creative work on one's own and for rest. Photograph: Elisabeth von Essen

feelings. Participants report their progress concerning saying 'No!' at home; they practise how to draw the line, and which limits they can accept. They can share with others their inner feelings and even listen to others without feeling burdened. They have acquired a new openness.

During the last weeks, the 'here and now' and the participants' employment come to the forefront in a rather new and different way. Their self-esteem is growing, and together with that comes a new way of seeing their earlier situation on the labour market. Participants start to see a more legitimate, adequate place for themselves in their careers – a personal scope that is beyond dispute. They consider re-entering the labour market, perhaps taking a new bold direction. Their creativity is awakening; they test new ideas and discuss them frequently. Often, thoughts of prestige and status are of less importance than before.

At this moment, the rehabilitation is over, and participants can start to practise their new skills at a workplace. Participants are still allowed ten extra days in the garden, one day a week, as an overlap. As the participants have been sick and have stayed at home for so many years, contact with the work environment may trigger old ingrained reaction patterns. Thus, this overlap is crucial in that the participants are able to return to the garden to get support during the first months to prevent them from falling back into valuing their own identity and self on the basis of performance and efficiency. They must not take a possible failure the 'old' way, but instead look upon it as necessary practice.

Nature-assisted rehabilitation of stress-related mental diseases: a matter of communication

When we started the therapeutic garden in Alnarp, all of us were intent on merging horticultural therapy in a garden setting with restorative experiences in a nature-like area, the goal being to develop a pure nature-assisted therapy. However, after less than two or three months, the therapists saw clear possibilities to integrate pedagogy and traditional occupational therapy, physiotherapy and psychotherapy with this nature-assisted therapy. So, a new model of nature-assisted therapy – the Alnarp model – was developed.

The phases of rehabilitation we observed involved patients' stress reactions decreasing and their power of attention increasing, as was expected according to the ART (Kaplan, 2001) and AAT (Ulrich, 1999) hypotheses. However, they interacted with the garden in other ways not suggested by these hypotheses.

We have found that natural environments, perhaps more than others, seem to activate sensorimotor functions. Moreover, such environments seem to trigger memories through all the senses that are activated there. Some garden rooms speak to us in a familiar way, such that we feel the presence of something that affects our innermost world. We do not simply experience the trees, flowers and gravel roads that are visible. We do not just move through an area containing countless impressions of smells, sounds and sights. A garden or a clearing in the woods cannot merely be described as the sum of all these impressions. Every sensory impression we have – of trees, stones, berries or beaches – occurs in relation to a personal background that is both spatial and temporal. Our experiences are interwoven into our entire life history.

Since time immemorial, people have been forced to find food and water, and shelter from the weather, dangerous animals and enemies. People have been forced to detect how the landscape can afford them enough water, food, shelter and hiding places. The ecological approach to perception claims that we inherently, and through conditioning, look for certain characteristics in our environment that afford us various utilities (Gibson, 1979; Norman, 1999), where pleasure and beauty also may be seen as a kind of utility that offers happiness and the experience of the senses are very important. Thus, we suggest that affordances may play a role in promoting health, and that some affordances are important to all people (for example, water, paths), while other affordances are more private. Some private affordances may even be more or less hidden, from time to time, until they suddenly become apparent at the right moment. These latter affordances seem to be necessary for bringing forth important memories and messages.

Developing a theoretical concept: 'scope of meaning'

In 1991, Grahn suggested that human beings possess a resource he calls *scope of meaning*: an aspect that concerns the self's communication with the external environment, such that the self is extended into the physical space – sometimes more obviously and distinctly, other times less clearly (Grahn, 1991). The meaning of the physical environment can change: it can become vital and clear, strange and chaotic, or be of less importance, depending on the person's own situation and state of mind. Sometimes the external environment even seems to be firmly tied to the individual's ego, to their identity. The scope of meaning may be seen as being made up of all our experiences – bodily/sensory and affective as well as feelings and thoughts – and all our values – how we communicate with the surrounding world in order to function and survive in it. There are people and objects that are defined as bad or good, wholesome or unwholesome, valuable or worthless, dangerous or safe, pleasant or unpleasant. Thus, everything of importance to our functioning in everyday life figures into the scope of meaning (Grahn, 1991, 2005). This concept is partly in line with what have been defined as 'schemes' or 'script' (Stern, 2003; Tomkins, 1995; Bucci, 2007). These 'schemes' concern relations between persons: feelings, activities, memories and roles related to family members, friends and other people, in connection with certain social situations. Moreover, our theory of scope of meaning implies that 'schemes' can change their inherent meaning in part or even completely, depending on the individual's actual situation and state of mind.

The scope of meaning/scope of action theory we are now developing in Alnarp suggests that the surrounding environment communicates with the visitor on many levels: that an environment presents affordances (Norman, 1999; Gibson, 1979) of different intrinsic and perceived worth. These values can sometimes be of huge importance to our ego. An affordance of an environment, Gibson claims, offers us possibilities for different kinds of activities and experiences. Yet, he continues:

> an affordance is neither an objective property nor a subjective property; or it is both if you like. … It is equally a fact of the environment and a fact of behaviour. It is both physical and psychical, yet neither. An affordance points both ways, to the environment and to the observer.
>
> (Gibson, 1979: 129)

We claim that affordances occupy the scope of meaning. Sometimes they can be found for everyone, having clear and shared meanings; in other cases they are more private, and may be concealed until they are suddenly given a lucid meaning.

We usually talk about the self as something that lies deep within us, in our cognitive consciousness. Our physicality, muscles, senses and affects are usually not mentioned. Social context is sometimes included, but rarely physical context. Yet already in infancy, we learn to deal with sensory impressions from our body and surroundings, which we then struggle to master and integrate. In contact with our apparatus of logical thought, these impressions gradually develop to form concepts we use in our personality and emotional intelligence (Ayres, 1983; Goleman, 2004). In order for this to succeed, we must have contact with the surrounding world: communication between the self and the surrounding world is what develops us. This communication is constantly ongoing and is a necessary process, enabling us to develop and maintain our health and identity. This process uses our scope of meaning, including the whole body, sensory-motor function, emotions, cognition, and important parts of the surrounding world – people and objects.

Communication: senses

Communication starts with being aware, with sensing and perceiving our environment. This involves our whole body, and it starts very early, before we are born. Ayres (1983), in her *sensory integration theory*, defines our senses as consisting of vision, hearing, smell, taste, soft touch, temperature, pressure, balance, movement (a 'time/space sense'), muscle position, position of body, vibration, pain, gravitation and visceral sense (sensations from internal organs). However, the single senses are first to be integrated into groups of senses, and then activated and integrated with our whole body including our brain, which is of utmost importance in developing our functional capacities, intelligences and personality.

Ayres (1983) claims that the following senses are basic: soft touch, balance, gravitation, body position and muscle position. Their integration gives us a feeling of being a separate body in space: body awareness. This awareness is of great importance for the feeling of being a self-contained individual. In addition, smell and taste are important. In the clinic she started, she found that the whole place must signal a secure atmosphere, and that the activities must be playful. Otherwise, integration of the senses could not start to develop for her participants, who are children with developmental disabilities.

In the first phases of treatment in our garden, dialogue and reflection seem to occur primarily via bodily contact. Our first goal is to help the participants calm down, feel secure – they are to take frequent breaks. This seems to stimulate their awareness. Several participants have reported how, particularly at the beginning of rehabilitation, they brought mattresses out into the wildest parts of the garden, and how they alternated between sleeping, diving down into the plants or lying on their stomachs, digging their hands down into the earth. One participant told us that she even put her face down into the pure earth, the soil, and that she became very dirty, but felt relieved. Our physiotherapist works with the participant's body awareness, stimulating soft touch through massage, and in our garden the participants practise activities involving balance, body position, gravitation and muscle position. Our findings also show that our participants all improved their body awareness.

Communication: 'emotional tone'

Being aware is one thing, reacting is another. Damasio (2003) defines several types of communication systems. One of the most basic, which can be found in most animals, is the pain and pleasure system. This system deals with withdrawing the organism from unpleasant places and finding more pleasant ones, for example, withdrawing from too hot or cold places to places with a better temperature. A more developed system involves instincts, concerning, for example, hunger, thirst, fight and flight. Both these systems together can be said to concern our *basic instincts of self-preservation* (Damasio, 2003).

More developed than instincts are our emotions (according to Damasio *feeling* is something rather different: a more cognitive, mental representation of an emotion). Like instincts, emotions can be divided into types: Damasio (2003) first mentions basic or categorical affects. Like Tomkins (1995), he classifies them into the following categories: these comprise two positive affects, Enjoyment and Interest; one neutral, Surprise; and six negative, Distress, Fear, Loathing, Anger, Shame and Disgust. All of them can be related to bodily expressions, such as facial expressions and body language. These categorical affects are important in Roger Ulrich's (1993) AAT, which implies that people who are stressed or in a crisis very often react strongly, and negative categorical affects, such as fear, anger or distress, have the upper hand. A person who is very upset and influenced by basic affects interprets the environment in quick holistic images – 'aesthetically' – in terms of being safe or not safe. If they find that the threat is gone, their negative affect will disappear (Ulrich, 1999).

However, other, more developed, types of emotions exist, 'background emotions' (Damasio, 2003; Stern, 2003). While categorical affects are forceful, strong and leave very little scope for other emotions or thoughts, these background types of emotions can be described more in terms of a musical score: emotions grow stronger, then tone down and disappear, sometimes welling up, other times being calmer – like a breeze. Stern (2003) provides examples of how very small infants develop a prelinguistic communication with their parents, for example, being sad or happy together. Expanding on this notion, we consider that this kind of communication can develop in relation to natural elements, such as water, stones or trees. Professor Harold Searles (1960), who studied schizophrenics and how contact with nature appeared to be an important

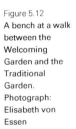

Figure 5.12
A bench at a walk between the Welcoming Garden and the Traditional Garden.
Photograph: Elisabeth von Essen

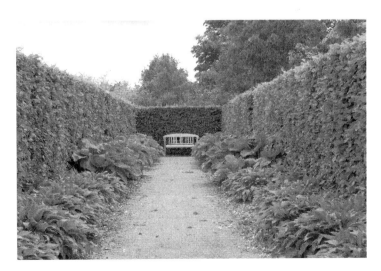

aspect of their well-being, addressed a similar kind of idea. He maintained that we receive signals from nature that are very important, even though we may not consciously perceive them.

In Alnarp, we group all these instincts and emotions together, forming a kind of prelinguistic language we call *emotional tone* (Grahn, 2005; Ottosson and Grahn, 2008). For example, the environment can signal a calm, positive, warm, interesting and secure atmosphere; or a more complex, chilly, precarious or even insecure, threatening and distressing atmosphere.

Marcel Proust, in his *In Search of Lost Time* (Enright ed., 1996), brought up not only the importance of social surroundings to how one perceives security, happiness, threats and so on, but also the importance of physical surroundings. Sensuality, everything from how a Madeleine cookie tastes to how uneven paving stones feel under your foot, all sensory observations are related to:

> the better part of our memories [which] exists outside us, in a blatter of rain, in the smell of an unaired room or of the first crackling brushwood fire in a cold grate: wherever, in short, we happen upon what our mind, having no use for it, had rejected, the last treasure that past has in store, the richest, that which, when all our flow of tears seems to have dried at the source, can make us weep again. Outside us? Within us, rather, but hidden from our eyes in an oblivion more or less prolonged. It is thanks to this oblivion alone that we can from time to time recover the person that we were, place ourselves in relation to things as he was placed, suffer anew because we are no longer ourselves but he, and because he loved what now leaves us indifferent.
>
> (Proust, Enright ed., 1996, vol. 2: 254)

Here, Proust talks about something we would like to define as communication that primarily involves emotional tones. Moreover, these emotional tones connect to some kind of memory, relating to Proust's self, and his innermost scope of meaning – to an affordance that points to his inner self.

However, people can sometimes be 'deaf' or 'blind' concerning this emotional tone; they are unable to detect it. When the Finnish-Swedish poet Edith Södergran became very sick, she had to spend many months in a hospital. Still sick but partly recovered, she finally returned home:

> My childhood's trees stand high in the grass and shake their heads: what has become of you? Rows of pillars stand like reproaches: you are unworthy to walk among us! You are a child and ought to be able to do everything, why are you fettered in the bonds of sickness? You have become a human being, foreign and hateful. When you were a child you conversed long with us, your gaze was wise. Now we want to tell you your life's secret: the key to all

Figure 5.13
Old trees in the
Grove.
Photograph:
Elisabeth von
Essen

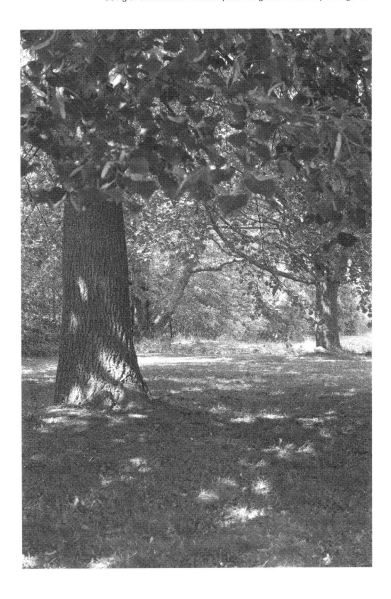

secrets lies in the grass in the raspberry patch. We would knock against your forehead, you sleeping one, we would wake you, dead one, from your sleep.

(Edith Södergran, June 1922, in Södergran, 1992)

Her truly beloved home felt inaccessible. Nevertheless, after several months, the deafness had disappeared:

My childhood's trees stand rejoicing around me: O human! and the grass bids me welcome from foreign lands. I lean my head in the grass: now home at last. Now I shall drink wisdom from the spruces' sap-filled crowns, now I shall drink truth from the withered trunks of the birches, now I shall drink power from the smallest and tenderest grasses: a mighty protector mercifully reaches me his hand.

(Edith Södergran, October 1922, in Södergran, 1992)

And:

November morning. The first flakes fell. Where the waves had written their runic characters in the sand of the riverbed we walked attentively. And the riverbank said to me: Look, this is where you wandered as a child and I am still the same. And the alder that stands by the water is still the same. Say where have you wandered in foreign lands and learnt awkward ways? And what have you gained? Nothing at all. Your feet should tread this field, here is your magic circle from the alders' catkins, certainty comes to you, and the answer to every riddle.

Edith Södergran, November 1922 in Södergran, 1992)

Communication: cognition, Gestalt and depth perception

Perception is often described as the process of achieving cognitive understanding of sensory information (Bell, 1999). If we are to perceive and act appropriately and rapidly in our environment, we cannot pay attention to all information from our senses (Bell, 1999). To avoid chaos when making decisions in our rapid everyday activities, we need to find order and hierarchies. One of the theories of how we discern order from the perceived cues presented to us is *Gestalt* theory, which suggests that separate figures of wholeness – Gestalts – stand out from the rest of the environment (Bell, 1999; Perls, Hefferline and Goodman, 1970).

Ehrenzweig (2000) defines this conscious, rapid type of perception using Gestalts such as 'surface perception'. Sensory information, according to Ehrenzweig (2000), can also be perceived and stored unconsciously as a kind of more undifferentiated information: that is, not Gestalts. He suggests that we detect this information through 'depth perception'. Depth perception is needed to obtain a sense of the 'true world', and it is normally fluently integrated with surface perception. However, Ehrenzweig claims that the separation of depth perception and surface perception (as a result of stress, for example) may cause mental illness. This separation can be mended if we have the possibility and time to make contact with depth perception through unconscious scanning.

Ehrenzweig's 'unconscious scanning' seems to be related to what Stephen and Rachel Kaplan (1989) call 'soft fascination'.

Searles' conception of nature as a link between the conscious and the subconscious is of special relevance in connection with unconscious scanning and soft fascination: contact with nature can contribute substantially to people's recovery from critical situations of various kinds. Signals from nature spark creative processes that are important in the rehabilitation process. This, and being able to master these relationships, says Searles (1960), helps to reduce anxiety and pain, restore our sense of self, improve our perceptions of reality and promote tolerance and understanding (Ottosson and Grahn, 2008; Searles, 1960).

Communication: meaningful activities

After some weeks of therapy, the participants start to open up and reflect. When the participants have started to heal, their interest in the surroundings develops. They start to explore the garden, and to engage in activities. Working with their hands and body makes their interests develop more concretely. An old Swedish proverb says, 'Being alive is wonderful, because then you get to see how things turn out.' Interest in the physical surroundings can be viewed as a fundamental driving force in human beings – the *pursuit of competence* –being able to increase one's physical and mental understanding and compe-tence regarding the environment (Havnesköld and Mothander, 1995). For this driving force to function, it should be accompanied by a positive frame of mind and a positive emotional tone, so that an exchange with the surroundings can emerge that is both pleasurable and marked by curiosity. This playful rela-tionship to the surroundings is said to emerge spontaneously and from birth (Havnesköld and Mothander, 1995).

Here, we relate to physician and psychotherapist professor Poul Bjerre (2004), who talks about how important it is for people in a crisis to enter a positive frame of mind so that they can be influenced by new perspectives and thereby work through the crisis, find a new orientation and grow as individuals. According to Bjerre (2004), in order to be receptive, one must be secure – anger, fear, and so on must not get the upper hand. As we interpret Poul Bjerre, positive affects such as joy and interest/curiosity must have the advantage. Bjerre considers that impressions from certain natural environments as well as from certain works of art or meaningful and creative activities can bring about a long and more lasting positive emotion. The environment and the person attune (Bjerre, 2004), which makes the person more receptive to reorientation. Nature, the special attuning language in nature, functions as a link between the conscious and the unconscious.

Patrik Grahn, Carina Tenngart Ivarsson, Ulrika Stigsdotter and Inga-Lena Bengtsson

Communication: symbol formation, hidden affordances

Through this kind of communication, mainly through the participants' emotional tone, the spatial ambiguities and expressive ambivalences in the garden, generated by their interplay with people's senses, could perhaps imply what Ehrenzweig (2000) has called the 'hidden order', which is 'global, syncretistic, and abstract'. We prefer to interpret this as pre-analytic. A hidden order implies the instability of 'reality constancy' (Frosch, 1966, 1990) as well as unverbalizable perception and preverbal articulation: the use of a language of the senses to convey a holistic sensation – as in, for example, body language.

Each of the rooms in the healing garden, and the rooms together, may be experienced as a whole unto itself, triggering an abstract sense of the existence of an actual message. Thus, what people can hopefully experience in a garden – for all the apparent incommensurateness of the different garden rooms and the more subtle incommensurateness of the parts within each garden room – is an instantaneous sense of unfathomable, unnameable comprehension (a feeling of understanding, a view of the whole, like in a puzzle), a special integrity that is the sign of a transcendental self (Ehrenzweig, 2000; Frosch, 1990; Searles, 1960) – the extent of one's own scope of meaning (Grahn, 1991). Ehrenzweig (2000), like Bjerre (2004), found that the attuning function develops in special environments, and further, that it stimulates the formation of symbols. Successful symbol formation depends on a fusion between the inner and outer worlds, he asserts. Hence, unconscious depth perception can provide us with symbols, thus helping us to restore and deepen our sense of reality by helping us find a hidden order in reality (Ehrenzweig, 2000), or affordances that are initially hidden but become apparent or revealed.

Wilma Bucci has proposed a 'multiple code theory' (Bucci, 2007), maintaining that information derived from our senses is coded and stored in three different ways: *subsymbolic, symbolic imagery* and *symbolic verbal*. Subsymbolic processing operates in somatic, sensory and motor modalities. For instance, it makes the potter able to understand how to treat the clay; the cheese expert able to understand how to treat milk and store cheese; the soccer player able to understand how to treat the ball and the physiotherapist able to understand a participant's inner state. All these knowledge processes occur in specific sensory-somatic modalities rather than in systematic cognitive ways: information is processed via muscles, our inner organs and so on (Bucci, 2007). In contrast to subsymbolic processing, symbols may be images (for example, some kind of picture in a person's mind) or words (for example, verbal interpretations and concepts) (Bucci, 2007).

Figure 5.14
A path to a more
enclosed,
sheltered space in
the Welcoming
Garden.
Photograph:
Elisabeth von
Essen

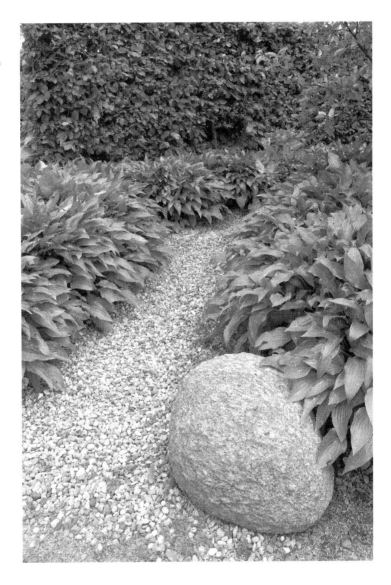

These three systems have different contents and different principles of organizing and storing information in our body and brain. However, they are connected by referential links, with the help of symbolic images, which enable us to symbolize and verbalize our emotional experience and also to understand others (Bucci, 2007). That is, only symbols can transmit messages between our sensorimotor memories and our cognition. Sometimes the three systems have more difficulty connecting, when people do not feel well or are in a crisis. Here, sensations and images from the environment can work as a catalyst, mediating information between the three systems, which is of utmost importance in reha-bilitation and restoration (Bucci, 2007). Although Bucci (2007) does not talk about depth perception or attuning, we interpret this as being in line with her theory: that symbolic images, symbolic activities or painting mediate processes that serve as a referential link between the information coded and stored as subsym-bolic, symbolic imagery and symbolic verbal when the systems are dissociated.

Like Ulrich (1993), Ehrenzweig (2000) mentions 'aesthetic messages' as important and as being found through 'de-differentiation': an all-embracing way of looking that is used by artists to see the parts of a composition as well as the whole simultaneously. According to Ehrenzweig (2000), this is a state of attention to such an extent that it is not retained by conscious memory. Ehrenzweig considers this undifferentiated deep perception to be superior to conscious perception, Gestalts and reasoning. Through this process, one may contact and draw up unconscious aspects of oneself for contemplation. This contemplation, we believe, can occur in garden activities as well as in artistic activities, as Ehrenzweig explains: 'Something like a true conversation takes place between the artist and his own work.' The garden activities, the clay or the painting, by frustrating participants' purely conscious intentions, allow them to contact more submerged parts of their own personality and draw them up for conscious contemplation:

> While the artist struggles with his medium, unknown to himself he wrestles with his unconscious personality revealed by the work of art. Taking back from the work on a conscious level what has been projected into it on an unsubconscious level, is perhaps the most fruitful and painful result of creativity.
>
> (Ehrenzweig, 2000)

Four phases of rehabilitation and the 'scope of meaning/scope of action' theory

We have found that people recover from exhaustion syndrome. Why? The AAT hypothesis (Ulrich, 1993) claims stress reactions should decrease in a restorative setting, suggesting the healing effects of nature are a matter of unconscious processes, affects, located in the oldest, emotion-driven parts of the brain. This can of course be true; however, the theory does not involve cognitive processes, senses other than sight, motor function or the person's life history. The ART hypothesis (Kaplan, 2001) suggests that patients' ability to focus attention should increase. The theory about *directed attention* offers a good explanation for the increase we have found. However, the theory does not involve people's emotions, senses (other than sight) and their life history. According to horticultural therapy, nature and gardens are particularly suitable when the aim is to find meaningful activities that are rewarding (Simson and Straus, 1998; Relf, 1999). However, the theoretical connection to nature is not especially clear.

We believe the 'scope of meaning/scope of action' theory gives a more comprehensive explanation, which can complete or perhaps even include these theories. Yet our participants' life history is essential. In the beginning of rehabilitation, we see participants who are exceptionally tired, many crippled with aches and pains. They are highly stressed, and have severe difficulties concerning body awareness and attention. We suspect that they have appropriated identities according to which they are exceptionally competent people, leaving their true self behind. Their self-esteem is based on achievements, and their self-images tell them they can manage everything. To survive an increasingly desperate situation, they act like soldiers, protecting their false self-image, and becoming increasingly stressed. Stress hormones cause them to stop listening to basic instincts concerning self-preservation, including feeling the warning signals from their own body.

The 'scope of meaning/scope of action' theory suggests that nature-assisted rehabilitation from stress-related mental diseases is a matter of *communication* as regards senses, emotions and cognition. When people feel good, they can cope with and function in most kinds of environments, and may feel that certain environments and persons give them strength and pleasure. Everything fits into their scope of meaning. When people feel weak, the same environments and persons can be perceived as ominous, even intimidating; the scope of meaning changes. It changes completely when people are in a crisis: then, people find it difficult to relate to their surroundings. They seek out what seems secure: what has not changed, what is stable? Certain structures seem to be more permanent, while others can more easily change in meaning. People in crisis seem to be more dependent on the nonhuman environment, on what is communicated by the emotional tone of the nonhuman environment. Moreover, ordinary environments that people perhaps have never noticed before may mean a great deal, in both positive and negative senses.

During a life crisis, communication between the surrounding world and us becomes very difficult; our feelings for objects and people in our scope of meaning change, which in turn changes their cognitive significations and our own scope of action. In such a situation, when one feels almost 'skinless', there seems to be a great need for a physical environment that can help restore individuals, build them up again and even help them develop mentally – here nature acts as a fundamental resource.

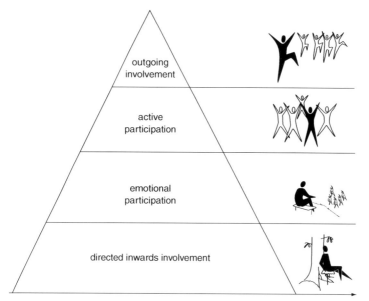

Figure 5.15
Pyramid of executive functions relating to the Scope of Meaning/Scope of Action theory: The lower one is in the pyramid, the greater the need of a supportive non-human environment.

At this point, dialogue and reflection seem to occur in and through the scope of meaning primarily via sensory impressions and emotions, such that the physical environment acts as the counterpart to the dialogue. Very early in childhood, we build a relation, not only to people, but also to our physical surroundings (Frosch, 1990). During childhood, we all go through a developmental phase on the emotional level, in which nature (stones, water, plants, animals) and people communicate with us directly and may gradually be given a more cognitive, symbolic meaning (Searles, 1960; Grahn, 2005; Frosch, 1990).

In situations of crisis, the individual seems to have a need to revert to simpler relations, to simple objects in nature, to the most stable and clear emotional tones (Ottosson and Grahn, 2008). Most complex are our relations to other people, and the simplest relations are those between inanimate objects, such as water, stones and ourselves. Stones and plants are not associated with confusing demands or guilt (Searles, 1960; Ottosson and Grahn, 2008). The experienced nature dimension that has been most important at Alnarp, especially in the beginning of rehabilitation, is Refuge, followed by Nature and Serene. Later, when people start to explore the environment, the dimensions Space and Rich in Species seem to be important, followed by Prospect. When people start searching for symbolic values, the dimension Culture seems to be important. And little by little, the dimension Social becomes important during the rehabilitation program.

For participants in the therapy, we conclude, it is important to:

- Find a garden with many rooms, with demands you can face and handle at a slow pace, from very low-level demands to increasingly advanced levels.
- Find a place where you can feel secure, calm down and be restored, if, for instance, you are deep in thought, irritated or upset.
- Find a place with experienced nature/garden room dimensions – affordances – that you feel you can face and that support your own state of mind.
- Find relaxation in rooms that offer both a more formal and a more bohemian design. Many participants find relief in an area that is far from 'neat', where they can relax.

Figure 5.16
The Wildlife
Garden in Alnarp.
Photograph:
Elisabeth von
Essen

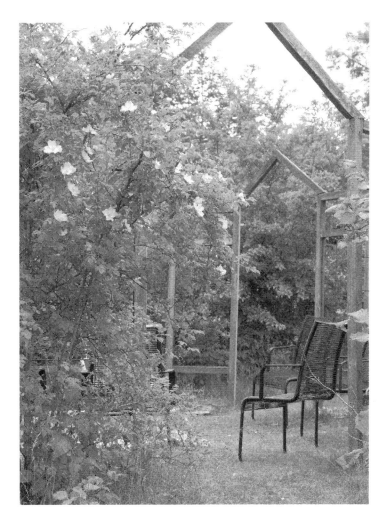

The Alnarp model emphasizes how important it is that the staff, as well as the physical environment, signal security. Rest is necessary, and all the senses require calm stimulation. This, we believe, causes communication to start again between senses, body, emotions and cognition. When the separation between these communication systems is mended, the body can start to work as it should, and gradually the person can start to function. After this has happened, the participants can start to work with more strenuous activities, little by little, including symbolic activities at the end of the therapy. The occupational therapist, the curative educational teacher, the physiotherapist and the psycho-therapist work closely together, and use different affordances in the garden as indispensable tools. Together with affordances in the garden, the therapists can help the participant to function, and to work on and understand their situation.

Developing this theory in an evidence-based health design framework involves different kinds of more applied and basic research. Thus, we continue to improve our garden, from different experiences we have obtained concerning rehabilitation. We have, for example, toned down the display of colours. There are more white and blue flowers, fewer red, yellow and orange, because the participants found it difficult to deal with these intense colours. We have also made more small garden rooms – and there will be even more. There were too few rooms with the dimension of Refuge. We are also busy strengthening the dimension of Nature close to the gate of the garden, so the participants can more easily find their way, walking out to the Grove and the Meadow. We have added more water elements to the garden, and more will come. And in the third phase, when people are trying to find symbols, they lack more malicious ones. One participant brought her mattress to the rubbish heap, which contained old rotting boards. Perhaps she looked upon herself as old lumber? Symbols have become far more important than we could ever have expected. The participants have asked for poisonous and thorny plants, for nettles, thistles and dead trees. So, we will develop a more unpleasant room, perhaps with a Refuge dimension.

In addition, we continue to develop our research, including basic research. For example, in order for rehabilitation to occur, we claim that our activities must be accompanied by a positive emotional tone. At the physiological level, we suspect that oxytocin (a satisfaction and security hormone) secretion begins rather early in the rehabilitation process if accompanied by a positive emotional tone, which stops the mounting stress and high levels of cortisol and catecholamines. This in turn is hypothesized to allow nerve cells to heal, which is followed by an increase in social, concentration and learning abilities. Therefore, we shall start a study including measures of oxytocin and cortisol levels, and neurobiological measurements.

We find all of this to be both important and indeed interesting to develop further. We believe that we are in an early phase of creating knowledge in this field. It has been especially interesting to use action research together with qualitative and quantitative research methods, and we shall continue to use all of these methods. Moreover, involving inputs from many disciplines in the arts and sciences has been stimulating. In the near future, this project will involve researchers from many different disciplines: departments within care and medicine (occupational therapy, physiotherapy, psychotherapy, family medicine, psychiatry, neuroscience, radiology and imaging techniques); departments within gardening and architecture (landscape architecture, horticulture, design) and departments within behaviour sciences (psychology, environmental psychology). This, of course, will develop this area of knowledge further, and involve other ways to explain how people are affected by visiting a therapeutic garden.

References

Aldwin, C. (2007) *Stress, Coping, and Development,* 2nd edn, New York: Guilford.

Atkinson, R. L., Atkinson, R. C., Smith, E. E., Bem, D. J. and Nolen-Hoeksema, S. (1996) *Hilgard's Introduction to Psychology,* Fort Worth, Tex.: Harcourt Brace College.

Ayres, J. (1983) *Sinnenas samspel hos barn* (Sensory integration and the child), Stockholm: Psykologiförlaget.

Barker, R. G. (1968) *Ecological Psychology: Concepts and Methods for Studying the Environment of Human Behavior,* Palo Alto, Calif.: Stanford University Press.

Baum, W. F. (2002) 'From molecular to molar: a paradigm shift in behavior analysis', *Journal of the Experimental Analysis of Behavior,* 78: 95–116.

Bell, S. (1999) *Landscape: Pattern, Perception and Process,* New York: E. & F.N. Spon.

Bjerre, P. (2004) *Död- och förnyelsetankens upprinnelse* (The origin of the idea of death and regeneration), Poul Bjerre-sällskapets årsbok 2003. Grödinge: Poul Bjerre Sällskapet.

Bucci, W. (2007) 'Dissociation from the perspective of multiple code theory', *Contemporary Psychoanalysis,* 43: 305–26.

Damasio, A. R. (2003), *På spaning efter Spinoza – glädje sorg och den kännande hjärnan* (Looking for Spinoza – joy, sorrow and the feeling brain). Stockholm: Natur & Kultur.

Ehrenzweig, A. (2000) *The Hidden Order of Art: A Study on the Psychology of Artistic Imagination,* London: Phoenix.

Frosch, J. (1966) 'A note on reality constancy', in R. M. Loewenstein, L. M. Newman, M. Schur and A. J. M. Solnit (eds), *Psychoanalysis: A General Psychology,* New York: International Universities Press: 349–76.

Frosch, J. (1990) *Psychodynamic Psychiatry: Theory and Practice,* Madison, Wisc.: International University Press.

Gibson, J. J. (1979) *The Ecological Approach to Visual Perception,* Boston, Mass.: Houghton Mifflin.

Goleman, D. (2004) *Emotional Intelligence: Working with Emotional Intelligence,* London: Bloomsbury.

Grahn, P. (1991) *Om parkers betydelse* (On the significance of urban parks), published doctoral thesis, Stad & Land nr 93. Alnarp: Swedish University of Agricultural Sciences.

Grahn, P. (1994) 'Green structures: the importance for health of nature areas and parks', *European Regional Planning,* 56: 89–112 (Council of Europe Press, Strasbourg).

Grahn, P. (1996) 'Wild nature makes children healthy', *Swedish Building Research,* 3 (4): 16–18.

Grahn, P. (2005) 'Om trädgårdsterapi och terapeutiska trädgårdar' (On horticultural therapy and therapeutic gardens), in M. Johansson and M. Küller (eds), *Svensk Miljöpsykologi* (Environmental psychology in Sweden), 245–62, Lund: Studentlitteratur.

Grahn, P. and Stigsdotter, U.K. (2003) 'Landscape Planning and Stress', *Urban Forestry & Urban Greening,* 2: 1–18.

Grahn, P. and Stigsdotter, U.K. (2010). 'The relation between perceived sensory dimensions of urban green space and stress restoration', Landscape and Urban Planning, 94: 264–275.

Grahn, P., Stigsdotter, U.K. and Berggren Bärring, A-M. (2005) 'Human issues: eight experienced qualities in urban green spaces', in *Green Structure and Urban Planning. Final Report*, EC COST Action C11, ESF COST Office, Brussels, pp. 240–8.

Hallsten, L. (2001) 'Utbränning. En processmodell' (Burnout. A model of the process), *Svensk Rehabilitering*, 3: 26–35.

Havnesköld, L. and Mothander, P. R. (1995) *Utvecklingspsykologi. Psykodynamisk teori i nya perspektiv* (Developmental psychology. Psychodynamic theories from a new angle), Stockholm: Liber AB.

Hewson, M. L. (1994) *Horticulture as Therapy*, Guelph, Ontario: Homewood Health Centre.

Kaplan, R. and Kaplan, S. (1989) *The Experience of Nature. A Psychological Perspective*, Cambridge, Mass.: Cambridge University Press.

Kaplan, S. (2001) 'Meditation, restoration, and the management of mental fatigue', *Environment and Behavior*, 33: 480–506.

Kielhofner, G. (1997) *Conceptual Foundations of Occupational Therapy*, Philadelphia: F.A. Davis.

Maslach, C. (2001) *Utbränd. Om omsorgens personliga pris och hur man kan förebygga utbränning* (The truth about burnout. How organizations cause personal stress and what to do about it), Stockholm: Natur & Kultur.

Nordh, H., Grahn, P. and Währborg, P. (2009) 'Meaningful activities in the forest, a way back from exhaustion and long-term sick leave', *Urban Forestry & Urban Greening*, 8: 207–19.

Norman, D.A. (1999) 'Affordances, conventions and design', *Interactions*, 6: 38–43.

Ottosson, J. and Grahn, P. (2008) 'The role of natural settings in crisis rehabilitation. How does the level of crisis influence the response to experiences of nature with regard to measures of rehabilitation?', *Landscape Research*, 33: 51–70.

Parent-Thirion, A., Fernandez Macias, E., Hurley, J. and Vermeylen, G. (2007). *Fourth European Working Conditions Surveys*, Luxembourg: Office for Official Publications of the European Communities.

Perls, F., Hefferline, R. F. and Goodman, P. (1970) *Gestalt Therapy: Excitement and Growth in the Human Personality*, New York: Delta Books.

Proust, M. (1996), *In Search of Lost Time*, vols 1–7, trans. D.J . Enright, London: Vintage.

Relf, D. (1992), 'Human issues in horticulture', *Hort Technology*, 2: 159–71.

Relf, P.D. (1999) 'The role of horticulture in human well-being and quality of life', *Journal of Therapeutic Horticulture*, 10: 10–14.

Searles, H. (1960) *The Nonhuman Environment: In Normal Development and in Schizophrenia*, Madison, Wisc.: International Universities Press.

Simson, S. and Straus, M. C. (1998) *Horticulture as Therapy: Principles and Practice*, New York: Food Products Press.

Socialstyrelsen (2003) *Utmattningssyndrom – Stressrelaterad psykisk ohälsa*, Stockholm: Socialstyrelsen.

Södergran, E. (1992) *Complete Poems*, trans. D. McDuff, Glasgow: Bloodaxe.

Stern, D. (2003) *Spädbarnets interpersonella värld: ett psykoanalytiskt och utvecklingspsykologiskt perspektiv* (The interpersonal world of the the infant: a view from psychoanalysis and developmental psychology), Stockholm: Natur & Kultur.

Stigsdotter, U. A. and Grahn, P. (2003) 'Experiencing a garden: a healing garden for people suffering from burnout diseases', *Journal of Therapeutic Horticulture*, 14: 38–48.

Tenngart Ivarsson, C. (2007) 'Movement in relation to space – different designs support different types of walks in a garden', in *Open Space: People Space 2. Innovative Approaches to Research in Landscape and Health*, ECA conference proceedings, Edinburgh, p. 51.

Tomkins, S. S. (1995) *Exploring Affect*, Cambridge: Cambridge University Press.

Ulrich, R. S. (1984) 'View through a window may influence recovery from surgery', *Science*, 224: 420–1.

Ulrich, R. S. (1993) 'Biophilia, biophobia and natural landscapes', in S. R. Kellert and E. O. Wilson (eds), *The Biophilia Hypothesis*, Washington, D.C.: Island Press.

Ulrich R. S. (1999) 'Effects of gardens on health outcomes: theory and research', in C Cooper Marcus and M. Barnes (eds), *Healing Gardens: Therapeutic Benefits and Design Recommendations*, New York: Wiley.

Währborg, P. (2003) *Stress och den nya ohälsan* (Stress and the new ill-health), Stockholm: Natur & Kultur.

World Health Organization (WHO) (1948) *Preamble to the Constitution of the World Health Organization*, Official Records of the WHO, no. 2, p. 100, New York.

WHO (2008) *Programmes and Projects: Mental Health – Depression*, WHO, available at: <http://www.who.int/mental_health/management/depression/definition/en/> (accessed 24 August 2009).

Part III

Different perspectives on methodology

Chapter 6

Opening space for project pursuit:
affordance, restoration and chills

Brian R. Little

Overview

What methods help us explore person–environment transactions so that we might better explain and enhance human flourishing? The question is a central theme of this book, and is answered at different scales and with alternative foci depending on the authors' fields of inquiry and idiosyncratic personalities. My focus is on Personal Projects Analysis (PPA) (Little, 1983; Little, Salmela-Aro and Phillips, 2007). I start with an overview of the social ecological framework within which the theory and methods of PPA are embedded (Little and Ryan, 1979; Little, 1999a, 2000a). I then explain, selectively, the methodology of PPA, emphasizing how it conjoins assessment of persons and the contexts within which they pursue their projects (Little, 2000b). Next, I explore three emerging issues relevant to our common concerns in this book: how places can provide affordances, restoration and chills to the project pursuer. I conclude with some thoughts about sustainable project pursuit and on the subtleties of opening space for such pursuit.

The social ecology of human flourishing: persons, places and projects

Figure 6.1 provides the elements of a social ecological framework for the study of human well-being and flourishing. The framework examines flourishing (Box F) as a function of personal projects (Box E) and of stable and dynamic personal and contextual attributes (Boxes A, B, C and D).

Brian R. Little

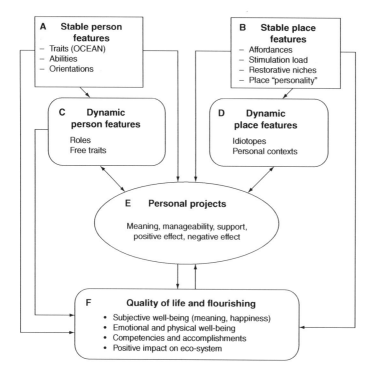

Figure 6 1
A social ecological
framework for
assessing
influences on
human
flourishing.

For present purposes I am substituting 'places' for the more general terms 'contexts' or 'environments', although these more general terms will be used when appropriate. I conceive of human flourishing not only in terms of subjective well-being (including health and happiness) but also as reflecting how people engage with the world adaptively, effectively and creatively. In standard methodological terms, these measures of flourishing comprise our 'outcome' measures or quasi-dependent variables, while measures of the stable and flexible aspects of persons and places, as well as measures of personal projects, are independent or predictor variables. These five blocks of variables have direct, indirect and interactive effects upon human flourishing, partially shown in the directional arrows of Figure 6.1. There is a considerable research literature relating to each of these sources of influence, but a brief and selective overview will help clarify some of the issues to be explored in more detail.

First, relatively fixed traits of personality are reliably associated with different aspects of human flourishing. Five major factors are widely regarded as underlying human personality, captured by the acronym OCEAN (or, in Canada, CANOE): Openness to experience, Conscientiousness, Extraversion, Agreeableness and Neuroticism (for example, John and Srivastava, 1999). These traits are each related to various aspects of human flourishing. For example, extraversion is positively related and neuroticism negatively related to well-being and happiness. Conscientiousness is reliably linked to competence in the work place as well as to health. Agreeableness is associated with the ability to work in groups. Openness to experience is linked to creativity and to the propensity to experience aesthetic chills (McCrae, 2007).

Second, relatively fixed features of environments have been theorized as important to human flourishing. For example, urban density, a relatively fixed feature of one's daily experience, has received considerable attention. The social psychologist Stanley Milgram and the architect Christopher Alexander have each contributed thoughtful, evocative theories about this aspect of urban experience. What is intriguing, however, is that they reach diametrically opposed conclusions about the effects of density on the quality of lives. Milgram (1970) argues that the combination of density and heterogeneity of lifestyles found in cities create a condition of 'information input overload' which, in turn, leads individuals to cope by setting up barriers to such information. Avoiding eye contact, decreasing the length and quality of transactions with others and setting up filters so that certain kinds of individuals are simply not noticed are some of the ways of coping with overload. More perniciously, however, norms of noninvolvement emerge in large cities so that it becomes easier to avoid contact with others.

Alexander (1970) takes a very different view. He argues that human flourishing requires, at each stage of the life cycle, frequent, sustained, intimate, 'warts and all' exchanges with a diversity of other people. Indeed, his design for a city that sustains human contact is explicitly constructed to increase the kind of contact that Milgram and others might regard as noxious overstimulation. I have speculated that Alexanderville and Milgramopolis are actually urban designs made for and by extraverts and introverts, respectively (Little, 1987). That the same features of a place may be interpreted in radically different ways by individuals with differing personality traits illustrates how stable personal features and stable place features can interact to create different conceptions of and possibilities for flourishing.

Third, dynamic features of persons comprise the roles we occupy and 'free traits' which arise out of the personal projects that matter to us. An example of free traits would be the action of an individual who is biogenically introverted (that is, physiologically), but who, in order to advance a core project, behaves in an extraverted fashion (Little, 2000a, 2005, 2008). Similarly, some individuals who score very low on the fixed trait of agreeableness are actually happiest when engaged in activities that involve unpleasant interactions at work (Moskowitz and Côté, 1995). On occasion, however, they may feel constrained to create the illusion of pleasantness when involved in social activities, resulting in free-traited 'pseudo-agreeable' conduct. As we shall see, there are benefits, costs and unintended effects of acting in such a fashion.

Fourth, dynamic features of environments arise from the fact that each of us construes and shapes the environment in an idiosyncratic fashion. The practical implication of this is that attempts to design places that will enhance desired outcomes, such as healthy outdoor venturing, would be frustrated if the designer of those places and spaces assumes that all the potential users construe the environment in the same way. Our idiosyncratic experiences of and preferences for particular places, what we might call our 'idiotopes', are an essential aspect of a broad-based approach to enhancing environmental experience. We have designed some assessment tools for exploring these 'personal contexts' (Little, 1996). One consistent finding in our research has been the importance of relationships with others in the idiosyncratically viewed everyday environment. An environmental design based solely on physical amenities but ignoring the role of social relationships will likely miss the mark.

Finally, personal projects, as shown in Figure 6.1, serve as a transactional conduit through which features of persons and places influence human flourishing. They are the central feature of our social ecological approach to person–environment transactions and human flourishing. We turn now to a more detailed treatment of the significance of personal projects and how we go about assessing them.

Personal projects analysis: What's up? How's it going? Who cares?

Personal projects are *extended sets of personally salient action in context* (Little, 1999b, 2008). They can range from the seemingly simple act of 'putting out the cat' to a complex pursuit such as 'sack Troy', the historical impact of which depends on the precise nature of the verb 'to sack' and whether Troy is an ancient city or an unsuspecting man. Personal projects are units of analysis that simultaneously bring into focus the characteristics of persons and the features of the places within which human action is played out. The theoretical analysis of personal projects developed alongside the creation of new methodological tools for exploring their characteristics and impact (Little, 2000b; Little and Gee, 2007a, 2007b).

It will be helpful to discuss each of the key terms in the definition of personal projects. The *extended* nature of personal projects means that they are inherently temporal, and in this respect they share certain assumptions with time–budget analysis in behavioural geography and other social sciences (for example, Pentland et al., 1999). Their personal saliency requires obtaining accounts by individuals of their idiosyncratic pursuits. This aligns us with those who adopt narrative approaches to the study of people's lives (for example,

McAdams, 1993; Runyan, 1982). The fact that projects are embedded in contexts places our research squarely at the intersection of the study of persons and their environments. We draw both inspiration and guidance from those who design and manage the spaces within which projects are enacted.

Personal projects analysis comprises a suite of assessment modules that, in essence, asks people what they are doing in their lives, how they construe those pursuits, and who or what might facilitate or frustrate such action (Little, 2008).

What's up? The distinctive content and common categories of personal projects

In the first module of PPA, individuals list the current and anticipated personal projects they are pursuing. On average, about fifteen projects are generated, expressed in the idiosyncratic language of the participant.

Simply examining the content of personal projects being pursued by a person is intriguing. Some are commonplace ('losing weight' being the most frequently elicited project); others are idiosyncratic if not singular (for example, 'be a better Druid'). Many different measures can be obtained simply by examining the content of an individual's or group's projects. These include calculating the frequency of major theme areas (for example, recreational, work, health and interpersonal projects), assessing whether they are phrased as 'approach' versus 'avoidance' pursuits, measuring the concentration versus diversity of project domains being pursued, and assessing the level of abstraction at which projects are phrased (for example, 'appreciate the cosmos' versus 'buy kippers') (Little, Salmela-Aro and Phillips, 2007).

It should be emphasized that the attributes of both persons and places need to be taken into account in order to appreciate the viability of a given project. 'Losing weight' is a project that will be facilitated by contexts in which temptations are minimized and diversions from eating abundant. 'Being a better Druid' may be more challenging if the project pursuer is living in a desert rather than a wooded area. The example posed earlier as a 'seemingly simple' act of 'putting out the cat' may not be simple if the cat owner has arthritis, the stairs are badly designed and the cat is unduly feisty. In other words, content alone is not sufficient for understanding the vicissitudes of project pursuit. We need also to look at how each project is construed.

How's it going? The construal of personal projects

After individuals have listed their personal projects in PPA, they rate these projects, or a subset of them, on a set of appraisal scales assessing constructs of theoretical and applied importance. For example, each person rates (from 0–10) each project in terms of its construed degree of stress, importance, controlla-bility, likelihood of completion and visibility to other relevant people. Although we have developed a set of standard appraisal dimensions, we place strong emphasis upon the development of ad hoc or special dimensions of particular relevance to the group or setting under study (Little, 1999b). Once we obtain ratings of a set of projects on a set of appraisal dimensions we can then explore these quantitatively.

PPA appraisal matrices can be examined at the individual level (focusing on intra-individual analysis) as well as at the normative level (focusing on inter-individual analysis). For the former, we examine the correlations between appraisal dimensions across each of the personal projects. For the latter, we take the mean score of each appraisal column in the matrix, creating a vector of scores for each person on each dimension. We can then examine the correlation between appraisal dimensions across individuals, as in traditional research on inter-individual differences. We can also calculate the relation between these project vector scores and measures of the features of persons, places and human flourishing. For some applied purposes, the intra-individual analyses are most important. For more basic research, the inter-individual analyses have been adopted most frequently.

The specific dimensions of personal project appraisal can be reduced to five major factors: project meaning, manageability, support/community, positive affect and negative affect. Project meaning includes such dimensions as how important and self-expressive projects are. Manageability is indexed by such dimensions as perceived control and sense of efficacy experienced in project pursuit. Support/community includes dimensions such as how important relevant other people see the project and how much support is experienced. Positive and negative affects are captured by appraisal dimensions that ask what emotions are experienced when engaged in a project (enjoyment, delight, fear, guilt and so on). Note that positive and negative affect are independent or orthogonal factors, so that some projects may generate both positive and negative affect, or neither.

Each of these five factors has been shown to predict diverse measures of human flourishing. Not surprisingly, the more meaningful, manageable and supported one's projects are construed to be, the more likely it is that one is leading a flourishing life. And similarly with positive and negative affect, which are strong independent predictors of life satisfaction. In this respect, the five factors of personal project appraisals are like the five factors of stable personality traits, in that they have significant and fairly substantial correlates with measures of well-being. There is one key difference, however.

Unlike the relatively fixed features of traits, most personal projects are mutable. They can be reconsidered, reformulated, dropped, expanded, enriched, pared down, handed off to others or re-engaged with passionate intensity. And it is possible to drill down into the content of a person's or group's personal projects to determine which *particular* projects 'carry' the association with measures of well-being and flourishing. We can then examine such projects to see whether they can be made more meaningful, manageable, supported and emotionally satisfying.

From a social policy perspective we can identify targeted issues of concern, such as which projects are the greatest source of stress and challenge for elderly people, or which are the greatest source of enjoyment and self-definition for inner-city teenagers. Such interventions may be done at the individual level in terms of counselling or coaching, or they may be carried out at the community level by improving the nature of the social ecology within which important projects are carried out (for example, Sugiyama and Ward Thompson, 2005).

Who cares? Help, hindrance and emotional support

Another modular option in PPA uses what we called 'open columns' in which, as well as giving numerical ratings on appraisal dimension, individuals also answer open questions such as 'With whom' are you engaged in this project and 'Where' is the primary location in which it is carried out. This allowed us to construct indices related to whether individuals concentrated their project pursuit in one particular location or diverse locations, and whether they pursued projects alone or with others.

Barris (1987) used these indices in her analysis of women at risk for eating disorders. These women were more likely to pursue their projects alone. They also carried out their projects in a more limited range of environmental settings than women without eating disorders, and were particularly likely to engage in projects at home. One consequence of such an inward-focused project style is the decreased likelihood that one will gain support from others for projects that matter.

A consistent finding in our research programme has been that the support of others in our projects is a key factor in predicting aspects of flourishing. Whether it is looking at indicators of successful childbirth (McKeen, 1984) or the bottom line of new entrepreneurs (Dowden, 2004), the support of a partner is a critical factor. Such support can be material help, emotional encouragement or more likely a combination of these. But it should also be noted that the person who is our major source of help is also frequently the major source of hindrance in our project pursuits (Ruehlman and Wolchik, 1988). One of the PPA assessment modules, the joint cross-impact matrix, explicitly allows us to explore how couples appraise whether their projects are facilitated or frustrated by the projects of the partner. Hwang (2004) has shown that an excellent predictor of relationship success is simply the number of shared projects that romantically involved couples are pursuing together.

The development of social technologies, such as instant messaging and the emergence of a young and vigorous twittering class, raise fascinating questions about how we provide support for each other's projects. Are these devices likely to provide the same kind of support as the direct contact espoused by Alexander? Is a timely text message saying 'Fantastic' as effective as a hug in helping advance our core projects when we need reassurance?

Three emerging themes: affordance, restoration and chills

Three themes that have emerged in our research programme will highlight some of the subtleties of person–environment transactions and point to some rather different ways of approaching the design of environments for human flourishing.

Affordance: shaping project pursuit

The concept of affordance, developed originally by Gibson (1979) in the field of perception, has become one of the most basic and important concepts in the social sciences (Heft, 1997). Affordance is that feature of an environment or place that will facilitate or afford action. The concept is inherently relational – a place that says 'Come on down' for one creature may be a 'Do not enter' zone for another.

The social ecology of project pursuit is, in part, an exploration of the affordances that will allow an individual to pursue projects (Sugiyama and Ward Thompson, 2005; Wallenius, 1999). Some projects, such as 'Bite my tongue more' can be carried out almost anywhere, while others, such as 'Climb to the highest point in the Maldives' are best carried out on a particular archipelago in the Indian Ocean. When difficulties in pursuing a project arise, three possibilities ensue. We can change the person, the place or the project.

A poignant example of how affordances are influenced by the interplay of person, place and project is given by Karl Weick in his account of the forest fire in 1949 at Mann Gulch in Montana (Weick, 1999). The fire was out of control, but despite explicit instructions to do so, most of the firefighters would not drop their heavy equipment. They were locked into the project of 'Fight the fire.' Their inability to switch projects from 'fire fighting' to 'saving ourselves' had tragic consequences, and thirteen died.

Our own research suggests that the affordance of situations in project pursuit is rather different for men and women. Men preferred work environments that did not impede the progress of their projects. For women, this was not a core concern. Rather, they were particularly happy in work environments providing the opportunity for connections with others (Phillips, Little and Goodine, 1997).

Restoration: fixed traits, free traits and places fit to live in

The study of restorative environments has been a major area of research in environmental psychology (Hartig, 2007; Kaplan, 1995). Typically, restorative environments are assumed to be salutary for most people, with relatively little attention paid to individual differences in what would constitute a restorative environment. I wish to propose a rather different approach by discussing first the notion of person–environment 'fit', and then getting into the more nuanced aspects of free traits and restoration.

Person–environment fit, fixed traits and restorative processes

Individuals' well-being will be enhanced to the extent that daily pursuits are carried out in places that 'fit' with their relatively stable traits – their needs, orientations and dispositions. For example, extraverted individuals have a biogenic (that is, physiological) need for stimulating and exciting environments in contrast to introverts. For extraverts, environments that are quiet, calm and slow-paced may actually extract a toll, and the density and intensity of going downtown would be restorative. Similarly, individuals high in openness to experience seek out places that offer numerous and diverse choices for exploration, whereas their more closed neighbours may find the plenitude of possibilities rather disconcerting.

So we can suggest that if there is a lack of fit between individuals' natural propensities and the places they live in, costs will be incurred and restoration will be required. But the exact nature of those restorative settings will show substantial individual differences. 'Hell', said one famous French existentialist introvert, 'is other people.' After frenetic and protracted exchanges with the denizens of left-bank Paris, escaping to a bare room with time to drink slowly and reflect deeply will be heavenly for Jean-Paul and other introverts (existentialist or not).

One of the most creative examples of exploring the 'fit' between people and places is recent research examining how cities and regions can themselves be regarded as having personalities, based on the concentration of individuals of differing personalities living in those places (Florida, 2008; Rentfrow, Gosling and Potter, 2008). These researchers have literally mapped how different cities and regions of the United States show strong patterns of concentrated personality characteristics. The West Coast is high in openness to experience, parts of the Eastern seaboard high in neuroticism, and the Midwest, radiating out from Chicago, is the epicentre of extraversion. Interestingly, and I suspect surprisingly to most, North Dakota, at the state level, has both the highest average scores on extraversion and agreeableness. It is also dead last on openness to experience. Given the salutary effect of living in places that are concordant with one's personality, or at least visiting them for restorative purposes, we might recommend that highly extraverted and agreeable people move to Fargo. But only if they are closed to the idea.

Free traits, acting out of character and restorative niches

Although conflict between fixed traits and the environments we inhabit may generate stress that requires alternative forms of restoration, a more complicated form of restorative need occurs when individuals engage in free-traited action. Free traits, as mentioned above, are patterns of conduct that resemble the big five factors of fixed traits, but are, in fact, strategic enactments intended to advance a core personal project. Here, the notion of restoration becomes particularly important.

When introverted individuals are faced with an environment that is too stimulating, the most efficient strategy will be to find different environments that are less stimulating. However, that introvert may have a core project that requires acting out of character. Because of values that are central to them and projects with which they identify deeply they act as extraverts, or more accurately as 'pseudo-extraverts'. In so doing they both enter into and also create the environment that they are least able to tolerate at a biogenic level. They may not realize the conflict between their biogenic needs and their personal projects until they have reached the edge of burnout. Then, a restorative niche consistent with their first nature is not simply a pleasant adaptive option. It becomes a health necessity (Little, 2008; Little and Joseph, 2007).

It is under these circumstances where it becomes clear that the various aspects of human flourishing listed in Figure 6.1 may conflict. The successful pursuit of a core personal project may bring us an exceptional sense of personal meaning. It may also provide a valued good for others we care about. But it might also bring us to our knees. That diverse forms of the human good may themselves conflict is one of the unfortunate but perhaps inevitable consequences of the complexity and contingency of human lives.

Chills: prudence and piloerections

I hope to have made clear that project pursuit is a vital aspect of human flourishing, and places that provide affordances and restorations for such pursuit deserve our study and support. However, there is something incomplete about this view of flourishing. Let me address this by restating our conclusions so far in this way: to enhance human flourishing, individuals need to be agents who identify core projects that they then pursue passionately. How could there be anything wrong with such a notion?

There are two problems. First, investing in core projects and shaping one's life around them will almost inevitably lead a person into territory where aspirations are frustrated and life plans are upset. The fewer and the more passionately held the projects, the more damaging is likely to be the effect of frustrated project pursuit. If I could paraphrase and (even worse) anglicize Rabbie Burns, we need to accept that for both mice and moms things can go astray, leaving both with grief and pain for intimated joy.

Although this is a problem, it can be circumvented by the virtue of prudence, which involves the judicious balancing of projects and flexibility of pursuit so that one is not vulnerable to losing everything to the nasty intrusions of a particular Thursday morning. Indeed, adoption of a philosophy of life in which one does not invest too heavily in one's personal pursuits is a respectable and ancient approach to living well, particularly as taught by the Hellenistic schools of Stoic and Skeptic philosophy (Nussbaum, 1994). Being aware of environmental affordances and of one's own strengths and weaknesses provides protection from the vicissitudes of life. This means that we might indeed, with self-regulatory and social ecological intelligence, muddle through our lives, and with luck, achieve much more.

The second problem, however, is more fundamental. What if the whole notion of taking control of our lives and shaping them so as to achieve our articulated goals is foundationally flawed? Larmore (1999) has made an eloquent case for precisely this view in his critique of theories of justice based on individuals pursuing and achieving a rational life plan:

> The good life is not, I have argued, the life lived in accord with a rational plan. It is the life lived with a sense of our dual nature as active and passive beings, bent on achieving the goals we espouse, but also liable to be surprised by forms of good we never anticipated. A life lived in the light of this more complex ideal can accommodate, it can even welcome, the way in which an unexpected good may challenge our existing projects.
>
> (Larmore, 1999:111)

In other words, interrupted plans may not bring the joy we originally anticipated, but as long as we are not too wee and timorous, they may alert us to new delights and stimulate new projects that take us to different places in our lives. Who, we might ask, are the people most likely to create such space in their lives? I believe it is those individuals who are most open to experience, one of the relatively fixed traits of personality. Although openness is associated with creativity, it is not strongly linked to most of the measures of well-being and flourishing with which we have been concerned. However, there is one area that has been shown to be uniquely associated with openness to experience: the proclivity to experience aesthetic chills (McCrae, 2007).

Hairy creatures experience a particular kind of chill – piloerections (literally hair standing up). For the relatively hairless, goosebumps also serve as an indicator of chills (I am focusing only on positive chills, not those indicative of fear or dread). What causes goosebumps? I propose that chills, like affordances and restorations, are inherently *relational* – they are a finely orchestrated exchange between a receptive person and something estimable external to that person.

I have been doing some exploratory studies on the various domains in which people report experiencing chills. Music and nature are frequently mentioned, but viewing exceptional achievements can also give us chills. I recently read that Lord Black of Cross Harbour found reading Winston Churchill's speeches gave him 'giant goosebumps'. Again, there are considerable individual differences to be found. The stunning view from a mountaintop may bring chills of awe to some. For others it is the fact that they beat everyone else to the top that brings on the high fives and the positive chills. Peak experiences and pilo-erections can arise from competitive as well as contemplative ascent.

I believe that the tendency to experience chills tells us something important about the intricate relations between persons, projects and places. Recall that we need not only receptive people but forces external to us for aesthetic chills to occur. It is difficult, if not impossible, to *command* chills. Rather they need to be experienced when we are in that passive mode that Larmore prescribed as central to the human good. They sweep over us, surprise us and bring us unanticipated delight. When our projects have gone stale, might chills serve as an invitation to explore new domains? And might not these chill-induced explorations create new project pursuits that may subsequently bring deep meaning and pleasure in our lives? I suspect this is so, but at this point these are simply speculative ruminations.

Sustainability: opening inner and outer space

I have saved to the last our central theoretical proposition about personal projects and human flourishing. It is this: *human flourishing is enhanced to the extent that individuals are engaged in the sustainable pursuit of core personal projects.* Core projects are those that are central to an individual's identity and which would be relinquished only with a sense of deep loss. For such projects to be sustainable the major sources of influence depicted in Figure 6.1 need to be taken into account. Being in places that will facilitate project pursuit is important, and if the relatively fixed features of our environments do not provide the necessary affordance, restorative niches and chill-inducing experiences, we can modify them or move elsewhere. Of course this presupposes that one has the power and the resources to modify and move. As this is not the case for many, planners and designers often serve to mobilize and facilitate needed change.

Sustainable pursuit also requires that one's relatively stable traits are conducive to pursuing core projects. Although he can always leave Paris, it is difficult for Jean-Paul to leave Jean-Paul. However, just as we can change the relatively flexible features of our personal contexts, we can also engage in free traits, which temporarily override our fixed traits in the service of advancing our projects. But as we have seen, protractedly acting out of character, even for a project that is deeply resonant, can take a toll. Ensuring that restorative niches are available may mitigate the costs of doing that which runs against our nature but matters dearly to us.

Earlier I suggested that passionate project pursuit might be insufficient for enhancing the quality of lives. The reason for this was that sustainability could be compromised if passionate project pursuit is not balanced by prudential considerations. The project pursuer may be at risk because passionate pursuit can exhaust us. If we are doggedly pursuing our projects, ignoring distractions and pushing very hard against our social ecology, there is another risk. Our social ecologies may themselves be fragile, and continued pursuit of our core projects within them may no longer be feasible. Both self-regulation and skills in managing our social ecologies are required for sustainable project pursuit.

It seems reasonable to suggest that a balance between passion and prudence is best for enhancing human flourishing. Passion creates the energy to persevere even when you and your best friends are ready to call it quits. Prudence helps us avoid getting gobsmacked.

Finally, we need to consider the situation where a person no longer seems able to identify core projects, where whatever has served as an impellent to action in the past seems no longer worth pursuing. Here is where openness can have a powerful effect on human flourishing. And here is where living in chill-inducing places is salutary. Being open, of course, means that you can be both stirred and shaken by fortuity. Flourishing requires both courage and luck: courage to drop projects that have gone stale and risking something new, and luck to be in places rich with possibilities. Both inner and outer spaces need opening.

Concluding practical speculations

My major goal in this chapter has been to demonstrate both how and why to assess the personal projects that link persons with places. From the felicitous design of cities to the restorative effects of outdoor spaces, environmental design can play a key role in inviting new project pursuit, in facilitating current projects, and in providing diverse forms of restorative experience. In concluding, I wish to speculate on four practical implications of this line of argument for those whose role is the actual creation of such environments.

Brian R. Little

First, it is possible to use the current personal projects of a group of individuals as a basis for examining their link to modifiable aspects of the environment. Two creative examples of this have been undertaken in Edinburgh. The OPENspace research centre at Edinburgh College of Art has developed a rigorous research programme that explores, in part, how outdoor environments support the personal projects of older individuals. They have found some preliminary evidence that such support is linked to the quality of lives of those individuals (Sugiyama and Ward Thompson, 2005). Also in Edinburgh, there has been some innovative use of conjoint analysis of personal projects to explore the most useful therapeutic interventions with individuals with low-level visibility problems such as macular degeneration (Aspinall, 2005). For a woman whose core project was the creation of dinner parties, the greatest utility was found to be in redesigning her cooking facilities with larger dials. In her case, vision difficulties precluded much by way of improvement in outdoor activities, but it is entirely possible that therapeutic interventions based on an analysis of core projects can lead to modifications of access to and movement through the outdoor environment.

Second, environmental designers could take into account not only a person's ongoing projects but also those personal projects that are desired by individuals but which have been put on hold, perhaps forever, because of the lack of environmental affordance. One way in which this can be explored is by using the priming function in personal projects (see Little and Gee, 2007a). This involves asking individuals, after they have finished generating their list of personal projects, to step back and think of additional projects that they would value pursuing but that they are not actively pursuing, for whatever reason. This list of desired projects will, I suspect, reveal possible pursuits that might be taken off the shelf by reshaping of the affordance structure of the daily physical environment. A 'get fit' project, long put on hold, might be brought into the daily flow of personal activity for an individual by the provision of accessible bicycle paths nearby.

Third, given the exceptional advances in simulation technology that allows individuals to actually see possible changes in their local landscape, it would be intriguing to see how such simulated changes could generate new personal projects or activity preferences that may not have occurred to the resident. In such an approach, environmental modification would be based on evidence of the perceived salutary effect of these 'possible places'. This process could be used to detect changes likely to increase the affordance not only of current projects, but also of those that have been shelved and those that have been newly instigated by awareness of new affordances and places that beckon.

Fourth, the design of restorative environments, amply demonstrated in this volume, takes a somewhat different form when considering personal projects and free traits. Although there may well be environments that are restorative to all people, particularly natural landscapes, individual differences in personality will frustrate attempts to provide a 'one niche fits all' strategy for restoration.

What kind of environment would provide a restorative retreat for individuals whose first nature is neurotic, closed, introverted, disagreeable and disorganized? As a psychologist I am relieved not to have to conjure up an answer to that question! However, it is not a frivolous one. The best-laid schemes of landscape designers may go 'agley' precisely because a particular client group is primarily comprised of individuals whose personalities and projects are perplexing. The only solution to such a dilemma is for dialogue between designers and clients, precisely the kind of dialogue and interchange that is the driving force behind this volume. Opening inner and outer space will require both openness to the complexity of human personalities and inwardness with the notion that the optimal design of places is inherently contestable.

References

Alexander, C. (1970) 'The city as a mechanism for sustaining human contact', in W. Ewald (ed.), *Environment for Man*, Bloomington, Ind.: Indiana University Press.

Aspinall, P. (2005) 'On quality of life' (unpublished manuscript), School of the Built Environment, Heriot-Watt University, Edinburgh, Scotland.

Barris, R. (1987) 'Relationships between eating behaviors and person/environment interactions in college women', *Occupational Therapy*, 7: 273–88.

Dowden, C. E. (2004) 'Managing to be 'free': personality, personal projects and well-being in entrepreneurs' (unpublished doctoral dissertation), Carleton University, Ottawa, ON, Canada.

Florida, R. (2008) *Who's Your City? How the Creative Economy is Making Where to Live the Most Important Decision of your Life*, Toronto: Random House Canada.

Gibson, J. J. (1979) *The Ecological Approach to Visual Perception*, Boston, Mass.: Houghton-Mifflin.

Hartig, T. (2007) 'Three steps to understanding restorative environments as health resources', in C. Ward Thompson and P. Travlou (eds), *Open Space: People Space*, London: Taylor & Francis.

Heft, H. (1997) 'Affordances and the body: an intentional analysis of Gibson's ecological approach to visual perception', *Journal for the Theory of Social Behaviour*, 19: 1–30.

Hwang, A. A. (2004) 'Yours, mine, ours: the role of joint personal projects in close relationships' (unpublished doctoral dissertation), Harvard University, Cambridge, Mass.

John, O. P. and Srivastava, S. (1999) 'The big five trait taxonomy: history, measurement, and theoretical perspectives', in L.A. Pervin and O. P. John (eds), *Handbook of Personality: Theory and Research*, 2nd edn, 102–39, New York: Guilford.

Kaplan, S. (1995) 'The restorative benefits of nature: toward an integrative framework', *Journal of Environmental Psychology*, 15: 169–82.

Larmore, C. (1999) 'The idea of a life plan', in E. E. Paul, F. Miller Jr. and J. Paul (eds), *Human Flourishing*, 96–112, New York: Cambridge University Press.

Little, B. R. (1983) 'Personal projects: a rationale and method for investigation', *Environment and Behavior*, 15: 273–309.

Little, B. R. (1987) 'Personality and the environment', in D. Stokols and I. Altman (eds), *Handbook of Environmental Psychology*, New York: Wiley.

Little, B. R. (1996) 'Free traits, personal projects and idio-tapes: three tiers for personality psychology', *Psychological Inquiry*, 7: 340–4.

Little, B. R. (1999a) 'Personal projects and social ecology: themes and variations across the life span', in J. Brandtstadter and R. M. Lerner (eds), *Action and Self-Development: Theory and Research Through the Life Span*, Thousand Oaks, Calif.: Sage.

Little, B. R. (1999b) 'Personality and motivation: personal action and the conative evolution', in L. A. Pervin and O. P. John (eds), *Handbook of Personality: Theory and Research*, 2nd edn, New York: Guilford.

Brian R. Little

Little, B. R. (2000a) 'Free traits and personal contexts: expanding a social ecological model of well-being', in W. B. Walsh, K. H. Craik and R. Price (eds), *Person Environment Psychology*, 2nd edn, New York: Guilford, 87–116.

Little, B. R. (2000b) 'Persons, contexts and personal projects: assumptive themes of a methodological transactionalism', in S. Wapner, J. Demick, T. Yamamoto and H. Minami (eds), *Theoretical Perspectives in Environment–Behavior Research*, 79–88, New York: Plenum.

Little, B. R. (2005) 'Personality science and personal projects: six impossible things before breakfast', *Journal of Research in Personality*, 39: 4–21.

Little, B. R. (2008) 'Personal projects and free traits: personality and motivation reconsidered', *Social and Personality Psychology Compass*, 2: 1235–54.

Little, B. R. and Gee, T. L. (2007a) 'The methodology of personal projects analysis: four modules and a funnel', in B. R. Little, K. Salmela-Aro and S. D. Phillips (eds), *Personal Project Pursuit: Goals, Action and Human Flourishing*, Mahwah, N.H.: Lawrence Erlbaum Associates, 51–93.

Little, B. R. and Gee, T. L. (2007b) 'Personal projects analysis', in N. Salkind (ed.), *Encyclopedia of Measurement and Statistics*, Thousand Oaks, Calif.: Sage.

Little, B. R. and Joseph, M. F. (2007) 'Personal projects and free traits: mutable selves and well beings', in B. R. Little, K. Salmela-Aro and S. D. Phillips (eds), *Personal Project Pursuit: Goals, Action and Human Flourishing*, Mahwah, N.J.: Lawrence Erlbaum Associates, 375–400.

Little, B. R. and Ryan, T. J. (1979) 'A social ecological model of development', in K. Ishwaran (ed.), *Childhood and Adolescence in Canada*, Toronto: McGraw-Hill Ryerson, 273–301.

Little, B. R., Salmela-Aro, K. and Phillips, S. D. (2007) *Personal Project Pursuit: Goals, Action and Human Flourishing*, Mahwah, N.J.: Lawrence Erlbaum Associates.

McAdams, D. P. (1993) *The Stories We Live by: Personal Myths and the Making of the Self*, New York: William Morrow.

McCrae, R. R. (2007) 'Aesthetic chills as a universal marker of openness to experience', *Motivation and Emotion*, 31: 5–11.

McKeen, N. A. (1984) 'The personal projects of pregnant women', unpublished bachelor's thesis, Carleton University, Ottawa, ON, Canada.

Milgram, S. (1970) 'The experience of living in cities', *Science*, 167: 1461–68.

Moskowitz, D. S. and Côté, S. (1995) 'Do interpersonal traits predict affect? A comparison of three models', *Journal of Personality and Social Psychology*, 69: 915–24.

Nussbaum, M. (1994) *The Therapy of Desire: Theory and Practice in Hellenistic Ethics*, Princeton, N.J.: Princeton University Press.

Pentland, W. E., Harvey, A. S., Lawton, M. P. and McColl, M. A. (1999) *Time Use in the Social Sciences*, New York: Kluwer Academic/Plenum.

Phillips, S. D., Little, B. R. and Goodine, L. A. (1977) 'Reconsidering gender and public administration: five steps beyond conventional research', *Canadian Journal of Public Administration*, 40: 563–81.

Rentfrow, P. J., Gosling, S. D. and Potter, J. (2008) 'A theory of the emergence, persistence, and expression of geographic variation in psychological characteristics', *Perspectives on Psychological Science*, 3: 339–69.

Ruehlman, L. and Wolchik, S. (1988) 'Personal goals and interpersonal support and hindrance as factors in psychological distress and well-being', *Journal of Personality and Social Psychology*, 55: 293–301.

Runyan, W. M. (1982) *Life Histories and Psychobiography*, New York: Oxford University Press.

Sugiyama, T. and Ward Thompson, C. (2005) 'Environmental support for outdoor activities and older people's quality of life', *Journal of Housing for the Elderly*, 19: 169–87.

Wallenius, M. (1999) 'Personal projects in everyday places: perceived supportiveness of the environment and psychological well-being', *Journal of Environmental Psychology*, 19: 131–43.

Weick, K. E. (1999) 'That's moving: theories that matter', *Journal of Management Inquiry*, 8: 134–42.

Chapter 7

On environmental preference:
applying conjoint analysis to visiting parks and buying houses

Peter Aspinall

The contribution of the environment to health, well-being and quality of life is a central theme in this book. The relationship itself and the terms involved are complex, and have different meanings and definitions in different situations. For example, 'quality of life' when used in situations involving visually impaired people has a very narrow definition. It is the degree to which a person's vision loss impacts on their ability to carry out a series of daily tasks that they need or wish to do – for example, reading newspapers, negotiating steps, crossing roads and preparing food. This is appropriate for the immediate medical concerns of those involved (that is, ophthalmologists and optometrists) and, furthermore, from the perspective of environmental support for these activities, an application of basic lighting design principles (that is, maximising visual contrast and minimising glare) can produce real benefits.

On the other hand, broader definitions of quality of life within social science (for example, Higgs et al., 2003) involve discussion and assessment around concepts such as autonomy, self-esteem, sense of control, stress reduction and satisfaction. The role of environmental support for these facets of quality of life is much less clear. Within OPENspace we are exploring personal project analysis (see Little, Chapter 6, this volume) as a way of developing a better understanding of the environment/quality of life relationship, and our early evidence looks promising. However, whatever the situation or context, most definitions of quality of life and well-being invariably subsume the notion of individual freedom and choice. Understanding people's choices and preferences is therefore essential to caring for them and supporting their quality of life.

The aim of this chapter is to demonstrate a particular methodological approach for investigating people's preferences and priorities. The family of methods is known as conjoint analysis, and the selected examples to demonstrate its use are from the natural and built environment – visiting parks and buying houses.

Before I embark on the details of conjoint analysis it is important to give a wider perspective to the psychology of preference, choice and decision making. This perspective raises issues relevant to all research attempts to assess preference and choice. Its implementation has progressed in parallel with the emergence of conjoint methodologies. As will be shown in the next section, some of these issues (for example, coping with context effects) have been central to the development of conjoint analysis.

General introduction

Any methodology directed at understanding people's choices or preferences needs to take account of a simple truth: it is that all our perceptions are, of their nature, both relative and selective. Information is not perceived, remembered or interpreted in isolation, but in the light of past experience and the context in which it occurs. In other words, there is no such thing as context-free judgement or decision making. In any situation, we only attend to a fraction of the available information, and our perceptions and judgements are influenced by the physiological, cognitive or motivational context in which the information is provided (Plous, 1993). For example, many studies have shown that expectations strongly influence perception. When people are shown five playing cards and asked if there is anything strange about them, many people fail to notice that one card is a black three of hearts (Bruner and Postman, 1949). Or again, subjects who thought they had been given a gin and tonic showed smaller increases in heart rate in a social situation than subjects who thought they had been given a tonic alone, even when the tonic contained alcohol (Wilson and Abrams, 1977). From the behavioural perspective, similarly misleading information resulted in greater risks in overtaking when driving (McMillen, Smith and Wells-Parker, 1989).

Perception is also influenced not only by what people expect to see but also by what they want to see – that is motivational factors, which include their hopes, desires and emotional attachments. For example, people watching the same event (such as two sets of supporters watching a football match) might simply be interpreting the event in a different way and forming different attitudes to it. However, studies suggest a more radical explanation (Hastorf and Cantril, 1954). It is argued that, such is their emotional attachment to different teams, supporters are not seeing the same event at all but actually seeing different events unfold. The inevitable conclusion is that, from the simplest of tasks to complex settings, an explicit or implicit context is invariably present to shape our choices or behaviour. In a research situation, if the researcher does not provide a context then one will invariably be assumed by participating subjects. It follows therefore that in Figure 7.1, the general question about liking a landscape (as is sometimes used in research) is quite ambiguous and might elicit quite different answers from many different respondent perspectives. If this is the research intention, then fine, but it presents a researcher with real difficulty in drawing inferences from the responses.

When judging or deciding some basic context, dependent effects have been identified (Plous, 1993). These include contrast (how a prior experience changes the judgement of a subsequent one –for example, when an estate agent shows potential buyers an overpriced or rundown property before the home under serious consideration); primacy (first impressions or informational cues are given greater importance); and recency (the last informational cues are more easily remembered and accessed). These three effects are concerned with how a stimulus or piece of information can have a differential effect depending on its presentational order in a sequence of information. However, the 'halo effect' is not dependent on order of presentation, but about how positive or negative information in one area spreads to another. For example, in one study, essays were rated higher in quality when attributed to a physically attractive author rather than an average or unattractive one (Landy and Sigall, 1974). Indeed, it was apparent to Thorndyke (1920) that competent professionals were unable to treat an individual as a 'compound of separate qualities and to assign a magnitude to each of these independent of the others'. Of course, there are limits to the influence of context effects, but they are important in decision making and may even be underestimated in experimental studies with respect to daily situations (Hershey and Schoemaker, 1980).

Figure 7.1
Ambiguities in
responding to a
landscape
preference study.

How much do you like this landscape?

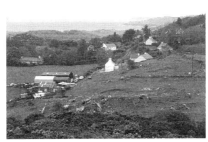

Response depends on
anticipated behaviours

e.g. as a place

- To live in

- For a holiday

- For a walk with friends

- To retire

- To grow up

Each question elicits a different response.

In early research on people's preference's and choices, there was considerable interest in what it meant to act rationally. A classical theoretical account of this, which involved maximising utility (value or worth), was developed by Neumann and Morgenstern (1947). This was not intended to describe how people actually behaved, but how they should behave if they wished to act rationally. However, problems with rational models of decision making soon arose. First, several internal paradoxes undermining their basic assumptions emerged. For example one, the Allais paradox (1953), showed that when people were in a state of uncertainty where large sums of money were concerned, a rational choice did not follow from normative predictions – perhaps something today's bankers might revisit! And in addition, an enormous amount of psychological evidence was accumulating (which could not be dismissed as irrational) describing how people actually perceived alternative courses of action in making choices. One particular example of this was experimental evidence of preference reversals and intransitivity (Plous, 1993). For example, in a rational decision it is assumed that a decision maker who prefers Outcome A to Outcome B, and Outcome B to Outcome C, should prefer Outcome A to Outcome C. However, in a series of cleverly designed situations, Tversky (1969) showed that a third of subjects behaved intransitively (that is, they did not follow this logic) and two-thirds of these consistently so – reliable intransitivity! In addition, preference reversals were not just a laboratory oddity. Lichtenstein and Slovic (1971) replicated their experimental results in a casino in Las Vegas on forty-four gamblers and professional dealers. Preference reversals were robust. When people are asked to choose between two bets, they oscillated in paying particular attention to either the likelihood of winning or to the size of the potential payoff.

This kind of evidence led to the notion of 'framing' effects in decision-making, which were highlighted in further innovative work by Tversky and Kahneman (1981). For these authors, a decision frame is 'the decision makers' conception of the acts, outcomes, and contingencies associated with a particular choice'. The frame was seen to be partly controlled by the way a problem was formulated, and partly controlled by the norms, habits and characteristics of the decision maker.

Perhaps the most famous example of framing is Tversky and Kahemann's (1981) 'Asian disease problem'. Medical doctors were presented with a situation in which it was imagined that an outbreak of an Asian disease was likely to kill 600 people in the United States. In one representation of the problem, a possible programme of action was said to result in either 200 people being saved or that there was a one in three chance 600 would be saved. In a second representation of the problem, equivalent outcomes of the programme were used in stating that either 400 people would die or there was a two in three chance 600 would die. Results showed doctors to be risk averse in choosing the first option in the first presentation, and risk seeking in being more prepared to gamble in choosing the second option of the second presentation. Changing the frame of reference from 'lives saved' to 'lives lost' flipped the choice of preferred programme. Furthermore, decision makers had framed both their perception of choices and the outcomes of those choices. Tversky and Kahnemann also showed how, in a range of daily situations from buying theatre tickets to missing a flight, outcomes were evaluated against a reference frame of gains and losses. Their subsequent development of 'prospect theory' (Kahneman and Tversky, 1979) is still the most widely accepted account of this effect in decision making. Prospect theory redefined classical accounts of utility (value or worth) to account for these experimental findings on attitudes to gains and losses.

These are some of the findings on how people respond in a choice situation. This literature on people's perceptions and choices is both informative and entertaining. It cuts across both the selective nature of perception and decision making, and forms a background to methodological approaches to exploring choice behaviour. It is apparent that, in studying preferences and choices, psychological factors play a major role, as does the presentational context of the choice situation. This background provides the context for the origins and development of conjoint analysis within academic psychology and economics. In addition to the factors already discussed, there are other psychological matters which, while not under the control of a researcher, are relevant to any decisional situation. These are biases related to the way information is processed – heuristic short-cuts, anchoring effects, a response to randomness, and responses to high and low probabilities touched on earlier. Awareness of these (for example, see Plous, 1993) will also be of benefit, as the key issue for research methodology is to either understand or minimise the potential impact of these effects.

Background to conjoint analysis

A paper by Luce and Tukey in the *Journal of Mathematical Psychology* in 1964 was the beginning of conjoint measurement. Central to its development, and echoing Thorndyke's remark in 1920, was the premise that a person's preference for an object cannot be expressed reliably by combining the ratings or weights of its various separate components. Instead, in a conjoint analysis, a decompositional approach is taken, in which people's ratings of an object's components are deduced from their overall evaluations of the whole object. This seems to be more realistic and closer to how people make decisions in everyday situations, and what's more, it works. This has been conjoint's obvious attraction to marketing science, where there is a very clear and simple validity check: does it predict consumer behaviour? As Orme comments, despite its assumptions, imperfections and leaps of faith, conjoint analysis works well in practice and still 'trumps' other methods (Orme, 2005).

Early academic developments in conjoint came to the attention of Green and Rao who, in 1971, published an historic article on conjoint measurement in the *Journal of Marketing Research*. By the 1980s the use of conjoint analysis was spreading, but mainly among researchers and academics with statistical backgrounds and computer programming skills. However, another influential case study (Goldberg, Green and Wind, 1984) was a successful application of conjoint to help Marriott design its new courtyard hotels, and when commercial software became available in 1985, the breakthrough to its wider application occurred. Early software was Adaptive Conjoint Analysis (ACA, see Orme, 1996), which included 'what-if?' market simulators. Once a set of preferences had been established, researchers or business managers could explore market acceptance in a simulated competitive environment.

Adaptive conjoint was the most widely used method until 1993, when discrete choice software became available (Choice-based Conjoint or CBC: see Orme, 1996). A second important development in favour of CBC was the application of hierarchical Bayesian (HB) methods, from which estimates of utility at an individual level could be derived from discrete choice models. With individual-level data, problems resulting from aggregation of data (such as the IIA or blue bus, red bus problem[1]) were solved. Another key development was the application of latent class models, which enabled groups of individuals with homogeneous preferences to be identified. Over the last ten years academics have explored HB-related methods to develop:

- more complex models of preference in which earlier assumptions that the value of a product is equal to the sum of the value of its parts have been relaxed
- partial profile methods in which choice-based conjoint can be used in a situation of many attributes, although any one respondent only sees a subset of attribute combinations
- recently, new software which combines aspects of adaptive and choice-based conjoint to overcome problems of noncompensation in decision making – that is, situations where an individual refuses to trade on one or more attributes under consideration.

Finally, as a general summary of how conjoint analysis addresses a number of the issues raised:

- The context is designed to be as close as possible to that which would naturally occur in a real decisional situation.
- The participant is always presented with a relative choice in which two or more profiles (for example, of objects, or elements of situations) are compared across several characteristics or attributes.

- Each relevant element in a choice situation is placed in a variety of different contexts; individual elements are not artificially isolated for assessment but compared together.
- By using a series of different contexts for each choice task, framing effects associated with context bias are minimised.

In the examples that follow, a full CBC application and a partial profile CBC application are used, as well as an ACA application. The examples highlight different ways of dealing with more complex multiple attribute choice situations.

First-time house buyers and their preferences (full CBC using text and images)

Context

In a study for the Joseph Rowntree Foundation (Leishman et al., 2004) the central research question concerned first-time house buyers and their priorities and preferences in buying a house. It seemed that there had been relatively little research into house buyers' needs, preferences and trade-offs, and therefore the extent to which new-build housing met people's needs. The reason for this was that studies of preference among moving households had tended to be dominated by the 'big picture' factors such as price, location and property size related to needs such as more bedrooms or a garden for the children, being in the right school catchment area or wanting a smaller more manageable home when nearing retirement. There was therefore little fine-grained information available to distinguish between what made one (similar) house preferable to another. In addition, satisfaction studies among recent movers raised the concern of post hoc rationalisation. Having just made the biggest financial commitment that most households make in their lifetime, few would wish to admit that their chosen house was less than ideal.

Methodology

The study set out to examine house buyers' needs by analysing the physical, locational and quality characteristics of housing actually constructed by house builders. Four hundred participants were involved – 200 based in Edinburgh and 200 in Glasgow. Of particular interest to the Rowntree Foundation (and the government) was the question of what would be needed to persuade buyers to live in higher-density inner city areas and thus help to minimise urban sprawl. The study focused on those who had recently bought new-build housing or flats, although some participants were prospective purchasers of new-build housing. Prior to running a conjoint study we carried out:

- a review of literature and existing housing preference studies
- a series of six focus groups with recent buyers of new houses, drawn from across the two cities, to capture experience across the price range of new-build housing
- a series of interviews with 16 people – prospective buyers responded to a leaflet left in show homes, while actual new-build buyers were recruited by sampling a range of estates (in terms of builders and prices).

The outcome of this initial work suggested eight main housing attributes would be particularly relevant to include in a conjoint analysis. These were:

- price: six different price bands were used
- location: city centre, near city centre, suburban, out of town
- neighbourhood: five types which varied in terms of density, amenities, and transportation links
- property type: six types ranging from detached, semi-detached to several flat types
- public room layout: six different room options and allocations
- bedroom layout: five different options in terms of number of rooms, size and layout.
- front garden: none, small, or large
- back garden: none small or large.

Although the conjoint software for a full-profile CBC analysis allows for up to ten attributes, the research group was of the view that eight attributes would be too much information for a participant to take in at one time. However, we wished to take advantage of the greater robustness of choice-based conjoint as opposed to adaptive conjoint. We decided to overcome the excessive list of attributes by splitting them into a format similar to that used by estate agents, which is a mix of images and text. This is in line with the spirit of conjoint, which is to use as realistic a context as possible for preference and choice. The first three attributes above were presented by text, and the other five shown in the form of facades and plans of houses.[2]

A series of posters was prepared, each of which contained an image and a description of two houses side by side. In presenting the choices to partici-pants, they were asked, 'In your recent (or current) situation of wanting to buy a house, which of these two would you prefer to buy?' We could have added a third option of 'neither' on each poster, but opted to use a forced, paired-choice presentation which seemed a realistic choice for respondents to make.

Findings

The focus groups revealed interesting insights into the range of factors that people considered important concerning locational and neighbourhood factors. However, the analysis based on the choice-based conjoint survey data produced far more detailed and insightful findings. The data was analysed using the Sawtooth CBC software (Orme, 1996). This produced average measures of relative importance, and through the Hierarchical Bayesian module, generated individual measures of relative importance across all levels of all attributes for each participant. This individual data set on importances was then subjected to latent class analysis to see whether there were subgroups of individuals with differing sets of preference and relative importances. The analysis indicated that the 400 respondents fell into four different identifiable preference groups. The sociodemographic characteristics of these groups were then explored to produce the profiles shown in Table 7.1.

It should be remembered that the four groups in Table 7.1 have been identified from a group of new-build house and flat buyers, so that the groups relate to a particular subset of buyers rather than all house buyers of both new and secondhand houses. The ways in which the groups prioritised the eight attributes is shown in Figure 7.2.

Figure 7.2 summarises the strength of preference for the eight attributes for each of the consumer groups using 'cobweb' diagrams. The diagrams are scaled so that the inner octagon represents a score of 12.5 and the outer octagon represents 25. Since there are eight attributes, any point lying on the inner octagon is equivalent to (that is, not more or less than) proportionate importance. Attributes that are further from the centre point are more important than attributes that are closer to this point.

Table 7.1 Characteristics of the four consumer groups identified.

	Consumer group	Characteristics
Group 1	'DINKYs' (double income, no kids yet)	Predominantly younger single households and couples.
Group 2	'Neo-DINKYs'	As group 1 but a slightly higher prevalence of couples and non-professional occupations.
Group 3	'Middle-SEG (socio-economic group) families'	Slightly older buyers, over half of whom have children.
Group 4	'Higher-SEG families'	As group 3 but with a higher prevalence of single person households and a greater predominance of professional occupations.

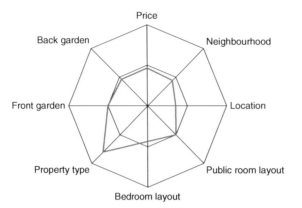

Figure 7.2a
Summary of
preferences for
DINKYs.

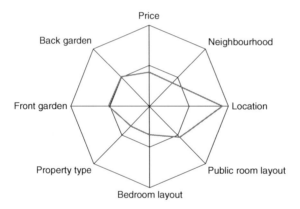

Figure 7.2b
Summary of
preferences for
neo-DINKYs.

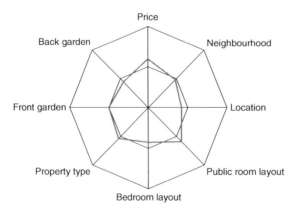

Figure 7.2c
Summary of
preferences for
middle-SEG
families.

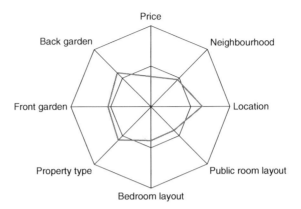

Figure 7.2d
Summary of
preferences for
higher-SEG
families.

Details on the groups in Table 7.1 are as follows.

- **DINKYs ('double income, no kids yet' participants)**. The diagrams show that property type is the single most important attribute to DINKYs, while location is the least important factor. DINKYs are likely to be drawn to new-build housing sites that feature the property types and public room options that appeal to them. This really means flats with above-average external space, or detached houses with functional public room layouts (large living rooms, small kitchens and utility rooms). The revealed preferences of the DINKYs are similar to those articulated by younger city dwellers in the quali-tative stage of the CASPAR (City-centre Apartments for Single People at Affordable Rents) project (Oakes and McKee, 1997). These younger people also sought to live in a safe area, convenient for local amenities and public transport. However, most of the participants were employed in the city, and although they enjoyed the anonymity of the city, they also valued being close to open spaces where it was possible to 'escape from work'. Although the interiors of the properties were considered more important than the facades, the participants nonetheless valued traditional buildings and conver-sions more highly than new-build apartments. Their major concerns included sound insulation and having good space and light. In new-build flats, balconies were considered to be desirable and a large main room was seen as a priority. The picture that emerges is that property design and specifi-cation factors are of particular importance to such households.
- **Neo DINKYs** – the revealed preferences of the neo-DINKYs are a stark contrast. These buyers rate location as the most important attribute by a considerable margin, and consequently will be drawn to particular locations (out of town being particularly preferred) rather than property types. These locational preferences were found to be difficult to overcome in trade-offs

against other attributes. For example, even though the provision of better public rooms and garden characteristics were considered next most important, they could not compensate for location in the decisional process of these buyers.

- **Middle SEGs (socioeconomic groups)** – in the third group, the Middle SEG families are attracted to housing options that are in their preferred price bracket. However, as Figure 7.2 shows, public room layout and property characteristics are only marginally less important than price. The analysis suggests that this group's preference for suburban locations and low-density neighbourhoods can be overcome through the provision of preferred public room options or property types in alternative locations, provided these are marketed at the right price. Buyers in this group have a strong aversion to flats. In theory it would be possible to compensate for failure to achieve preferred location (suburbs) through the provision of similar priced low-density housing in centrally located low-density neighbourhoods. However, there are obvious difficulties in actually providing such a combination.
- **Higher SEGs (socioeconomic groups)** – finally, the Higher SEG families are attracted to location, garden characteristics and property types as shown in Figure 7.2. Internal property characteristics and price are relatively unimportant factors to these buyers, although detached housing is generally preferred to higher-density property types. Buyers in this group have a strong preference for out of town locations.

In summary, there are many proponents of the view that the three most important attributes to house buyers are 'location, location, location'. The conjoint findings outlined here on a subgroup of first-time buyers show this is not the case. Two of the consumer identified groups did consider location as the most important attribute of housing, although for only one group was location the dominant factor (neo-DINKYs). The analysis shows how property type, specification, layout and garden features play different roles for the four identified groups.

From the conjoint perspective, the analysis revealed combinations of priorities in differently identified groups of buyers which were not expected and which had not previously been reported. As a footnote to the method, a comparison was made between the attributes that were presented in visual form and those presented by text. Little evidence is available on this, although Dijkstra, van Leeuwen and Timmermans (2003) consider that pictorial representations contribute to the degree of realism of the evaluation task. However, they suffer from difficulties in producing images that accurately reflect particular combinations of attributes assigned to each option, and in determining whether such attributes have been noticed by respondents in coming to a decision. In addition, respondents' decisions may be overly influenced by lighting, composition, people featured in the images and so on, which may have comparatively low priority in real-life decision making (Laing et al., 2008). Results on attribute comparisons are shown in Table 7.2. While across the four groups there is an even split of text to visual importance, it is interesting that the average importance of visual attributes is significantly higher than that for those represented by text.

As a postscript to the Joseph Rowntree Study, we in OPENspace are currently undertaking a European study (PLUREL) which also involves housing preference. This study is based on the idea that different factors affected by land use change (for example, green space, air quality) combine in different ways to increase or decrease the quality of life for people living in a particular place. However, each of the factors involved in making a place attractive is of course valued differently by the different types of people likely to live or move there. Each may play a different role, therefore, in configuring how attractive a place is for living. The factors chosen, which emerged from an extensive review, included house or flat suitability, public access to green spaces, air quality, public transport, noise pollution, perceptions of safety and security, convenience of shopping facilities and household-waste collection (Bell and Zuin, 2008).

Among the types of conjoint analysis available, adaptive conjoint analysis was chosen for this study, as it provides a respondent-friendly interview process and accommodates a greater number of attributes than other types of conjoint analysis. The term 'adaptive' refers to the fact that the computer-administered interview is customised for each respondent; at each step, previous answers are used to decide which question to ask next, in order to obtain the most information about the respondent's preferences. Adaptive conjoint analysis

Table 7.2 Visual and text-based attributes.

Use of images
Study on housing preference for Joseph Rowntree Foundation (Leishman, Aspinall, Munro, 2004).

12 attribute conjoint paired comparison task using
a) text (e.g. cost, local amenities)
b) images (e.g. garden size, number of bedrooms)
c) 4 different group preferences

	visual	**text**
• All respondents	10.605	4.652
• Group pref 1	3.206	3.391
• Group pref 2	6.273	3.060
• Group pref 3	30.985	9.617
• Group pref 4	1.957	2.540
• Images - House type/no of rooms/room configuration/garden size		

is being used to measure the perceived importance of the quality of life indicators relating to the attractiveness of an area as a place to live, as outlined above, and to incorporate them into the impact assessment process. This will allow researchers to map out the perceived quality of hypothetical living environments resulting from forecasted land-use scenarios. For example, the analysis will be used to examine how people's preferences and perceived affordances (see Heft, Chapter 1 in this book) relating to land use are affected by membership of different groups and segments in the population, such as older people and groups of immigrants.

Visiting neighbourhood open space: older people's preferences

In this second example, a similar methodological problem presented itself. The number of potential attributes seen to be relevant in answering the research question – which features of open space are important in influencing preferences for neighbourhood open space? – was large. In the housing study, we resolved the problem of large attribute numbers by a mix of visual and text presentations (although there was little prior evidence on the consequence of this). In this study, the alternative chosen methodology was to stick with text but use a choice-based conjoint partial profile design (explained below).

Context

Neighbourhood outdoor spaces such as parks can contribute positively to people's health and quality of life status, as is reviewed in de Vries' chapter (3) in this book. Increasing the use of the local outdoor environment would seem therefore a good way of promoting older people's health and well-being, but what features of open spaces are likely to influence an older person's choice over whether to go outdoors and where to go? Some general evidence is available. For example, a study in the United Kingdom has shown that older people's walking patterns are associated with a space's attractiveness, facilities (such as café or toilets), lack of nuisance, and the quality of paths to such spaces (Sugiyama and Ward Thompson, 2008). A US study has found that higher density of green space in urban areas, which is equivalent to better access to parks, is conducive to walking by older adults (Li et al., 2005). In addition, path connectedness has been positively linked to instrumental and recreational walking in retirement community campuses (Joseph and Zimring, 2007). Finally, safety and pleasantness in local open spaces have been associated with life satisfaction in the United Kingdom (Sugiyama, Ward Thompson and Alves, 2009).

However, from studies to date it is not clear how people prioritise features of the environment that might have a bearing on their preferences and possible actions. Nor is it clear whether there are identifiable subgroups of older people with significantly different preferences between outdoor open spaces. Addressing the issue of facilitating and encouraging older people's outdoor activity is of practical importance for those involved in designing and managing open spaces. It is especially relevant in a planning context where resources to invest in the environment may be strongly constrained. This is ideal territory for conjoint analysis.

This study was undertaken as part of a wider EPSRC Consortium project entitled I'DGO (Inclusive Design for Getting Outdoors), which explored aspects of the outdoor environment – its planning and design – that have an impact on older people's quality of life and use of outdoor spaces. More detail is available in Alves and colleagues (2008); and Aspinall and colleagues (2010).

Methodology

There were two stages in preparing the content of the conjoint questionnaire, similar to the structure of the housing choice study. In the first stage, eight focus group interviews were carried out with people aged 65 and older across urban, suburban and rural settings in Britain. The focus groups explored what aspects of the outdoor environment were relevant to older people's outdoor activities, health and quality of life. A review of literature and a content analysis of the focus group interviews generated a number of environmental attributes potentially relevant to older people's preference for outdoor open spaces. Fifteen attributes were finally selected for inclusion in the CBC questionnaire. They included eight attributes relating to the environment and travel options en route to a local park, such as distance to the park, pavement quality, presence of trees and seats along footpaths, and levels of traffic. In addition there were seven attributes related to the environment within a local park, such as the density of trees and plants; the availability of facilities such as cafés and toilets; the presence of seats, water features, car parks or things to watch; levels of maintenance and nuisance. Each of the selected attributes had between two and four levels. The full list of attributes and levels is shown in Table 7.3.

In this case we did not use images as in the housing study but written descriptions of the parks. Both alternatives have their merits, but here it was for three reasons which relate to the unique and specific characteristics of an image. First, this uniqueness would negate the variability of season, weather, atmosphere and vegetation state, which is part of our experience of the outdoor environment and affects preference. Second, text profiles of parks allowed greater flexibility in generalisation so that participants could relate the information provided to their local park. Third, a text presentation provides clarity on what aspects of the environment are to be considered.

Peter Aspinall

Table 7.3 The fifteen attributes and their levels.

1   Distance:
    - 0–5 minutes walk;
    - 5–10 minutes walk;
    - 10–15 minutes walk; and
    - 15 minutes or more.
2   Pavement existence:
    - pavement all the way;
    - pavement part of the way; and
    - no pavement.
3   Pavement quality:
    - high quality pavement; and
    - low quality pavement.
4   Tree along footpath:
    - tree-lined paths; and
    - no trees along path.
5   Seats en route:
    - some seats en route; and
    - no seats on route.
6   Traffic:
    - light traffic en route;
    - medium traffic ; and
    - heavy traffic.
7   Tree/plants:
    - dense trees/plants;
    - many trees/plants;
    - some trees/plants; and
    - no trees/plants.
8   Facility:
    - café/toilets;
    - toilets; and
    - no special facility.
9   Seats:
    - many seats in the park; and
    - few seats in the park.
10 Things to watch:
    - good views;
    - wildlife;
    - other's activities; and
    - nothing special to watch.

11 Maintenance:
- well maintained; and
- not well maintained.

12 Nuisance:
- youngsters hanging around;
- dog fouling;
- signs of vandalism; and
- no particular nuisance.

13 Water feature:
- some water feature; and
- no water feature.

14 Public transport:
- easy access to public transport; and
- no easy access to public transport.

15 Car park:
- car park nearby; and
- no car park.

The second stage involved the conjoint tasks themselves. A paired comparison task was chosen because it is the simplest format for a choice-based conjoint design and was considered appropriate for older respondents. In addition, the number of attributes shown in each comparison task was limited to four (out of the available fifteen),[3] again to reduce the burden of memorising and comparing the options. An example of a typical paired comparison task used in the questionnaire is shown in Figure 7.3. For each task, participants were asked to compare the two hypothetical parks and to choose the one they would prefer as their local open space (assuming that these parks are equal in all other respects).

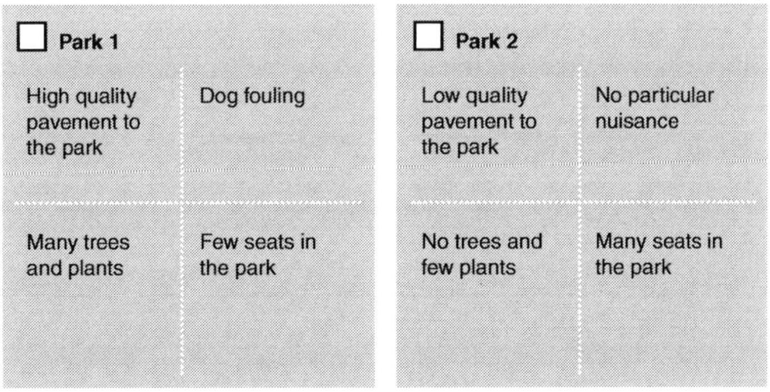

Figure 7.3
Example of the paired comparison conjoint task.

☐ **Park 1**		☐ **Park 2**	
High quality pavement to the park	Dog fouling	Low quality pavement to the park	No particular nuisance
Many trees and plants	Few seats in the park	No trees and few plants	Many seats in the park

The fifteen versions of the CBC questionnaire generated, each containing eleven paired comparison tasks, showed a design efficiency of over 95 per cent. Three 'holdout' tasks, involving predetermined scenarios, were added in the final questionnaire to give a total of fourteen comparison tasks. The 'holdout' questions were used for an internal validity check: that is, the actual preferences of participants on these tasks are compared with those predicted by the conjoint software from the eleven nonholdout tasks.

The demographic variables noted were age, gender, living arrangement (own home or shelter/care home), household composition (living alone or not), postcode (from which living in an urban or rural area was derived), and distance in minutes it took to get to the local park (by foot, car or public transport). Levels of hearing, vision and mobility impairment for participants were also identified. The choice-based conjoint questionnaire was mailed directly to 1,860 older people in twenty local authorities across Britain (seventeen from England, two from Scotland and one from Wales) in 2005. These locations were chosen considering population distribution, geographic location, residential density, type of industry, level of social deprivation (according to the national Index of Multiple Deprivation) and the balance of urban to rural areas, in an attempt to cover a diverse yet reasonably representative range of areas across Britain.

Findings

A total of 237 usable questionnaires were obtained by survey. Table 7.4 shows the characteristics of the sample. Participants' ages ranged from 60 to 97 (mean = 74.7; SD = 7.9), and just over half (52 per cent) were women. Most participants lived at home (90 per cent), rather than in sheltered or care accommodation, and had no difficulty in seeing (90.2 per cent). However, some participants had difficulty in hearing (23.3 per cent) and in getting around (29.3 per cent) Many participants visited local parks on a weekly basis (49.8 per cent). The majority could reach their local park on foot (61.6 per cent), and the average travel time to reach the park was 12.7 minutes.

Results from the holdout tasks showed internal validity at 85 per cent. This suggests that the conjoint model is robust in predicting choices. The conjoint model was run with and without interaction effects. The latter did not significantly improve the fit of the main effects model.

(i) Relative importance of environmental attributes

The first main summary from the analysis is the average relative importances across the whole sample. Figure 7.4 shows the rank order of utilities, with confidence limits, for the fifteen attributes. The attribute 'nuisance' (youngsters

Table 7.4 Characteristics of participants.

Characteristics	n (%)
Age	
60–74	116 (49.6)
75+	118 (50.4)
Gender	
Men	111 (47.4)
Women	123 (52.6)
Living arrangement	
Home	207 (90.0)
Shelter/Care	23 (10.0)
Living alone or not	
Alone	84 (36.1)
With someone	149 (63.9)
Difficulty seeing	
Not difficult	184 (90.2)
Difficult	18 (8.8)
Very difficult	2 (1.0)
Difficulty hearing	
Not difficult	165 (76.7)
Difficult	41 (19.1)
Very difficult	9 (4.2)
Difficulty moving	
Not difficult	155 (70.8)
Difficult	54 (24.7)
Very difficult	10 (4.6)
Distance to local park (in travel minutes)	Mean: 12.7 Median: 10.0 Std Deviation 7.9
Means to go to local park	
Foot	138 (61.6)
Car	79 (35.3)
Public transport	7 (3.1)
Frequency of visits to local parks	
Less than once a week	112 (49.8)
Once a week	65 (28.9)
Twice a week or more	22 (9.8)

Missing cases: Age (3); Living arrangement (7); Living alone or not (4); Difficulty—Seeing (33), Hearing (22), and Moving (18); Distance to local park (11); Means to go to local park (13); Frequency of visits per week (12)

Peter Aspinall

hanging around, dog fouling, signs of vandalism, and no particular nuisance) was the most important, followed by 'facilities' and 'trees/plants'. 'Traffic' and 'things to watch' assumed the fourth and fifth rankings. The least important attribute in the relative context of alternative attributes was 'distance' (analysed as 0–5, 5–10, 10–15, and 15+ minutes' walk). An important aspect of conjoint analysis arises from this apparently counterintuitive finding on distance. This does not imply that distance in general is an unimportant variable. Rather, it is that the range of distances presented in this study (from zero to fifteen minutes as the longest journey time) is seen as relatively unimportant, when compared to the ranges presented for the other attributes. An increase in the distance range would almost certainly increase its relative importance. This emphasises the importance of careful consideration of the levels to include when planning a conjoint study.

(ii) Differences within and between attributes

An example of the influence of levels within attributes is shown in Figure 7.5 for the top two attributes. In Figure 7.5 the levels of an attribute are shown on the x axis and the relative importances (utilities or part-worths) are shown on the y axis. Higher positive utilities indicate higher relative importances, with each graph centred on a mean of zero. In the case of the nuisance variable the highest importance understandably is for 'no nuisance'. The worst value that nuisance can take is 'signs of vandalism'. 'Dog fouling' is less bad, and the least nuisance considered is 'youngsters hanging around'. For the facilities variable the least preferred situation is the absence of both a café and a toilet. Providing

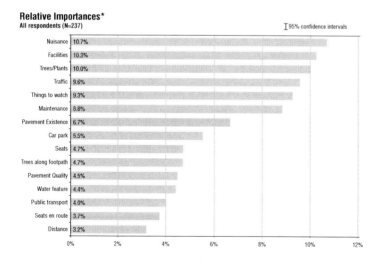

Figure 7.4 Relative importance in rank order of the fifteen attributes.

200

a toilet makes a significant difference, while the best situation is the presence of both. These findings are to be expected and are not surprising. It is the following inference which can be made from the differences in these relative importances that is interesting. If we consider levels within an attribute, the difference between two levels indicates the relative importance of the change between the levels. In other words, because the difference between 'no nuisance' and 'signs of vandalism' is larger than that between 'no nuisance' and 'youngsters hanging around ($t = 20.1$, $p<0.01$), then removing signs of vandalism is seen as more important than preventing youngsters hanging around. Or again by comparing relevant differences, Figure 7.5 shows that providing a toilet in a park currently without one is seen as more important than adding a café to a park that already has a toilet.

A similar comparison can be made between attributes. For example, which environmental change do people consider more important – adding a toilet to a park without one, or reducing traffic intensity from medium to light? Figure 7.6 shows the evidence: adding a toilet is by far the more important. Or how do signs of vandalism compare with traffic reduction from heavy to medium? Figure 7.7 shows that vandalism is the more important.

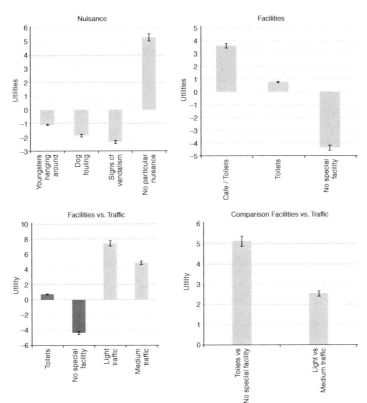

Figure 7.5
Relative
importances
within levels of an
attribute.

Figure 7.6
Relative
importance
between
attributes.

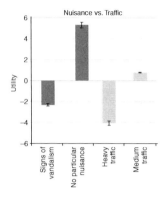 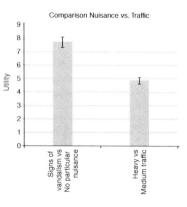

Figure 7.7
Relative
importance
between
attributes.

The analysis is enabling us to make quantitative comparisons between different levels of a nominal scale.

(iii) Subgroups with different preferences: redundancy analysis

Subgroups within the respondents have been explored using redundancy analysis (Stewart and Love, 1968; Legendre and Anderson, 1999). This is a kind of principal component analysis in reverse. What it does is to map the demographic characteristics of people within the same spatial structure which contains their preferences. Greater distance from the origin reflects more importance, while spatial proximity reflects links between characteristics of people and their preferences (Legendre and Legendre, 1998; Ter Braak and Smilauer, 2002). The diagram in Figure 7.8 shows the variation in importance scores that can be accounted for by individual characteristics.

In the diagram, respondents' characteristics are represented by diamonds, and park attributes by squares. A series of multivariate F tests based on Monte Carlo permutations are shown in Figure 7.8, in which the two significant individual characteristics are seen to be whether someone lives alone or with someone, and the degree of difficulty they have in getting around. The results suggest that participants who differed in these characteristics were significantly different in the way they prioritised the environmental attributes. These individual factors form two main orthogonal axes through the origin of the diagram in Figure 7.8, one from bottom left (living with someone) to top right (living alone); and one from top left (difficulty getting around) to bottom right. Notice that the top left corresponds to the older age group and the bottom right the younger age group. The diagram shows that those with difficulty getting around place a relatively

Figure 7.8
Redundancy
analysis with
demographic
variables and park
attributes.

Redundancy Analysis (RDA)

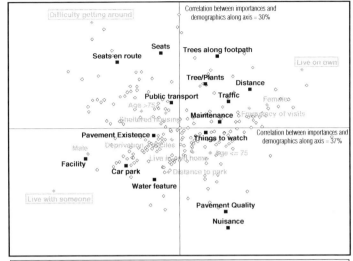

Redundancy Analysis
RDA is Principal Components Analysis (PCA) with explanatory variables. A linear regression analysis is performed between the two sets of variables. The chart produced displays only the variation in the importance scores that can be explained by the demographic variables. The chart represents the respondents as locations (white diamonds) and the importances (black) and the demographics (light grey) as directions radiating out from the centre of the chart. RDA is able to show the relative differences between respondents unlike MDPref which shows respondents actual preferences.

What the chart shows
The chart shows that people who have greater difficulty getting around, place a relatively greater importance on the provision of seats both at the park and en route. They would appear to be willing to trade pavement quality and less nuisance in order to have more seats. Those respondents who live with someone place a relatively higher importance on the provision of facilities and a car park. Those respondents who live alone place a relatively higher importance on the distance to the park and whether there are trees planted along the footpath.

Significance tests (Multivariate F based on Monte Carlo Permutations)

Attribute	F	P
Live on own / with someone	3.57	0.001
Difficulty getting around	3.37	0.002
Frequency of visits	1.35	0.199
Gender	0.91	0.504
Live in own home / sheltered housing	0.91	0.506
Deprivation - deciles	0.86	0.536
Distance to park	0.73	0.678
Age	0.16	0.999

greater importance on the provision of seats both at the park and en route. They would appear to be willing to trade pavement quality and increased nuisance in order to have more seats. Those respondents who live with someone place a relatively higher importance on the provision of facilities and a car park. Those who live alone place a relatively high importance on the distance to the park, and the presence of trees and plants both along the footpath and at the park (for further details and discussion, see Aspinall et al., 2010).

A detailed breakdown of the impact of living state and degree of mobility on importance shows that if you live alone and have no mobility problems, then 'nuisance' is most important, with 'facilities' being relatively unimportant. On the other hand if you either live with someone or have a mobility problem, then 'facilities' is the most important or jointly most important attribute. More generally, the results are also valuable in illustrating the importance of trees and plants for all groups, but especially for those living alone and with mobility impairment. It confirms the value of the natural environment and aesthetic experience by comparison with concerns over nuisance or practical issues such as traffic or facilities.

(iv) Preference share using 'what if' simulations

A simple extension of the comparison of differences between attributes illustrated in section (ii) (above) enables us to make comparisons across several attributes and levels that make up the profile of a particular park. This analysis forms the 'market' simulator, used to convert utility data into share of preference data, which is more practically useful. The simulator allows the

Simulator   Break by | Who live with x difficulty getting about ▼ |

	Park 1 ☑	Park 2 ☑	Park 3 ☑
Distance	5–10 min walk ▼	5–10 min walk ▼	15 min or more ▼
Pavement Existence	Pavement all the way ▼	Pavement part of the way ▼	Pavement part of the way ▼
Pavement Quality	Low quality pavement ▼	Low quality pavement ▼	High quality pavement ▼
Trees along footpath	No trees along paths ▼	Tree-lined paths ▼	No trees along paths ▼
Seats en route	No seats en route ▼	No seats en route ▼	Some seats en route ▼
Traffic	Light traffic ▼	Light traffic ▼	Heavy traffic ▼
Trees / Plants	No trees / few plants ▼	Many trees / plants ▼	Some trees / plants ▼
Facilities	Cafe / Toilets ▼	No special facility ▼	Toilets ▼
Seats	Few seats in the park ▼	Few seats in the park ▼	Few seats in the park ▼
Things to watch	Other's activities ▼	Wildlife ▼	Good views ▼
Maintenance	Well maintained ▼	Well maintained ▼	Well maintained ▼
Nuisance	Youngsters hanging around ▼	Youngsters hanging around ▼	Youngsters hanging around ▼
Water feature	Some water features ▼	Some water features ▼	Some water features ▼
Public transport	Easy access by public transport ▼	Easy access by public transport ▼	Easy access by public transport ▼
Car park	Car park nearby ▼	No car park ▼	Car park nearby ▼
All respondents (n=237)	30%	33%	37%
Live alone & not difficult (n=53)	25%	50%	25%
Live alone & difficult (n=24)	20%	44%	36%
Live with someone & not difficult (n=100)	35%	27%	39%

Figure 7.9
A 'What If?' simulator for a comparison of three parks.

researcher to run 'what if' scenarios in which alternative permutations of the full set of attributes can be compared for share of preference. This is illustrated in Figure 7.9 for three hypothetical parks. In the example chosen the share of preference is given below the simulator for the total sample and for three of the significant subgroups identified by redundancy analysis – that is, those living alone, with someone and with or without mobility difficulties.

For the total sample the combination of attribute levels in the profile of Park 3 receives the highest preference share at 37 per cent. However, for those living alone the highest preference is for Park 2 at 50 per cent. For those living with someone preference matches that for the total sample (that is, for Park 3) with a slightly higher share at 39 per cent. Note that some attributes have been set at the same level across all parks (for example, youngsters hanging around, some water features, and easy access) so they do not influence preference share.

In the dynamic model available from the software, any combination of attribute levels can be compared towards predicting choice and this can be modified by any segmentation of the data by demographics.

(v) Sensitivity analysis

Finally, sensitivity analysis is illustrated in Figure 7.10. Here the information recorded in the profile of Park 1 in the simulator is used as a reference level to explore the potential by which any attribute that increases or decreases in level may influence the share of preference. This analysis might offer the most practical solutions to those faced with planning change to an existing park and anticipating their consequences.

Figure 7.10
Sensitivity
analysis
(preference share
for scenario 1).

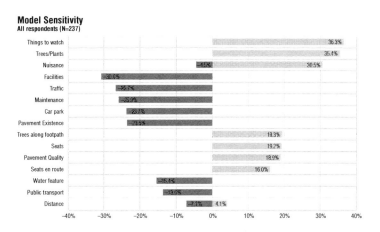

The diagram shows horizontal bars to the right or left of a vertical line. Those to the left represent levels of an attribute that are present in the profile of Park 1 and that are positively viewed by respondents – the farther to the left, the more positive the perception. In contrast horizontal bars to the right represent levels of attributes that are not present in Park 1 but have the potential to bring about positive change – again, the farther to the right the greater the potential benefit. The longest bar to the left is facilities, and corresponds in the Profile of Park 1 in Figure 7.9 to the presence of both a café and toilets. Given this is the level associated with the highest existing preference (and given in this hypothetical context the only change allowed is within the existing levels of an attribute – so excluding, say, a second toilet) the only change available would result in a negative relative change to facilities and a corresponding reduction to the length of the horizontal bar to the left. One of the longest bars to the right in Figure 7.10 is 'trees and plants'. In Figure 7.9, Park 1 is set at 'no trees and few plants', which is the lowest level for this attribute. Any change to this attribute is going to be positive. In addition because this is one of the longest horizontal lines, adding trees and plants would be one practical move to bring most improvement to Park 1's rating.

Sensitivity analysis therefore gives a picture of an existing situation and indicates which attribute will be most effective to bring about the greatest positive change. It might also be used to find the minimum changes required to attain a certain level of preference, or to discover how trade-offs between attributes allow an existing level of preference to be maintained in changing circumstances.

Concluding observations

Conjoint analysis has the advantage, as Orme (2005) puts it, that it 'works' in anticipating priorities and consumer behaviour. Its central idea is that choices presented in a natural context, which are then disaggregated to understand the contribution of their components, offer a better way of predicting choices in real-life situations than those where an aggregation of components is used. In this way, conjoint always presents each component in a choice task in a varying context of other components so that typical biases inherent in the relative nature of perception and choice are minimised. It must be emphasised, of course, that conjoint importances (that is, utilities or part-worths) are always dependent on and relative to the set of components considered. Adding a new attribute can change the structure, particularly if it interacts with those present.

As a consequence of its practical success, the popularity of conjoint analysis has now spread into many different areas. However, the degree to which it will translate into these other areas is a more open question. As mentioned at the beginning, in the OPENspace research group one of our central interests is the environmental contribution to quality of life. We are aware that within medicine, NICE UK (2004) has recommended that researchers move to discrete choice methods (for example, conjoint analysis) for quality of life assessment. However, evidence in ophthalmology (Aspinall et al., 2007, 2008) has provided puzzling results. While this evidence shows that conjoint results are robust to order and presentational effects, and are also replicable and have good internal validity, the results from Hierarchical Bayesian generated individual utility measures correlate poorly with standard quality of life measures obtained from conventional questionnaires – and this is in a field where definitions of quality of life are strict and apparently unambiguous. However, a recent finding within the OPENspace research group if replicated may help resolve this. A study on people's attitudes to and priorities for the area in which they lived used both conventional attitudinal questionnaires and an adaptive conjoint analysis questionnaire (OPENspace, 2009). Predictors of satisfaction ratings were strongest from other evaluative ratings and weakest from the conjoint measures. On the other hand, predictors of people's actions (that is, where they go to and how frequently they go) were strongest from the conjoint measures. Is it the case therefore that the conjoint measures of relative importance are more closely linked with behaviour rather than attitudes? If correct this would be a constructive solution because otherwise fundamental questions of methodology and external validity are raised, for which at present there is no clear explanation.

The two examples chosen here shared the same methodological problem – that the numbers of attributes relevant to preference were greater than that recommended for choice tasks in a full profile text-based conjoint. In other words, the number of presented attributes must take account of the informational limits to which a person can attend. To address this, two approaches were taken. One was to mix text and image and to present several attributes in pictorial form; the second was to use a partial profile design, in which only limited sets of attributes are presented together in any one choice task. While the partial profile approach already has credibility, the comparative presentational impact of either visual or text-based information on utilities has received less attention and requires more research.

The housing study focused on a particular group of first-time buyers. Conjoint analysis identified more subtle profiles of four different subgroups of buyers than had previously occurred. Here the benefit of Hierarchical Bayesian, followed by latent class, analysis was demonstrated. The neighbourhood open space study set out to identify environmental factors that preferentially facilitated or inhibited outdoor visits to neighbourhood open space by older people. It showed what these characteristics might be for the British context, using a small but diverse sample representing a range of living contexts. The exploration of subgroup differences in priorities revealed two main factors. The results suggest that whether or not an older person lives alone is a key influence on priorities in relation to a local park and access to it, as is the degree to which people's mobility is impaired.

In this study a fuller range of conjoint outputs was demonstrated, including trade-offs between attributes, park profile comparisons, sensitivity analysis and redundancy analysis. These offer not only research data but also decisional management tools for planners and designers concerned with effective environmental change towards access and use. Here is a practical basis for linking environmental manipulation to one of the themes of this book – improvements in exercise, health and quality of life. Within the context of research-informed practice, these type of outputs involving dynamic modelling and scenario building may in the longer term be the most important and useful of all.

Acknowledgements

The author would like to thank The Joseph Rowntree Foundation and EPSRC through the IDGO Consortium for financial support. In addition thanks are due to Chris Leishman (then Heriot Watt University) and Roger Brice and Adrian Vickers (Adelphi Research Group Bollington) for their contribution to analysis and graphic presentation.

Notes

1 This is where the introduction of a new attribute takes a disproportionate share from the existing ones – for example, suppose, in a transport choice situation, a blue bus is added to a set of attributes already containing a red bus. Two similar options of this sort may provide misleading evidence for the more general question of preference for buses as a form of transport.

2 The combinations of attributes and levels present in any paired comparison task were generated by the Sawtooth software program <www.sawtoothsoftware.com/download/techpap/admtech.pdf>. Several sets of paired comparison tasks were generated which were then screened for a balance of 'degree of difficulty' (that is, we wanted two very easy choices with the rest at gradations of difficulty) and for practical anomalies (that is, we rejected obvious impractical combinations such as the largest house at the lowest price). The software also calculated a design efficiency measure related to the number of paired comparisons necessary and the number of versions of the questionnaire needed.

3 As in the housing study, the number of comparison tasks for each participant and the number of different versions of the questionnaire were determined from a measure of the 'design efficiency' of the analysis. Design efficiency, which is computed using the Sawtooth software program <www.sawtoothsoftware.com/download/techpap/admtech.pdf>, refers to the accuracy of the estimated measure, obtained from the number of comparison tasks relative to the number of questionnaire versions, attributes and levels.

References

Allais, P. (1953) 'The behaviour of rational man in risk situations: a critique of the axioms and postulates of the American School', *Econometrica*, 21: 503–46.

Alves, S., Aspinall, P. A., Ward Thompson, C., Sugiyama, T., Brice, R. and Vickers, A. (2008) 'Preferences of older people for environmental attributes of local parks', *Facilities*, 26 (11/12): 433–53.

Aspinall, P. A., Johnson, Z. K., Azuara-Blanco, A., Montarzino, A., Brice, R. and Vickers, A. (2008) 'Evaluation of quality of life and priorities of patients with glaucoma', *Investigative Ophthalmology and Visual Science*, 49: 1907–15.

Aspinall, P. A., Hill, A. R., Dhillon, B., Armbrecht, A. M., Nelson, P., Lumsden, C., Farini-Hudson, E., Brice, R., Vickers, A. and Buchholz, P. (2007) 'Quality of life and relative importance: a comparison of time trade-off and conjoint analysis methods in patients with age-related macular degeneration', *British Journal of Ophthalmology*, 91 (6): 766–72.

Aspinall P. A., Ward-Thompson C., Alves S., Sugiyama T., Brice, R. and Vickers, A. (2010) 'Preference and relative importance for environmental attributes of neighbourhood open space in older people', *Environment and Planning B* (in press).

Bell, S. and Zuin, A. (2008) Social and Quality of Life indicators: selection of indicators and development of conjoint study. PLUREL Milestone numbers 4.3.5 and 4.3.10, December 2008. Sustainability Impact Assessment Module no. 4.

Bruner, J. and Postman, L. (1949) 'On the perception of incongruity: a paradigm', *Journal of Personality*, 18: 206, 223.

Dijkstra, J., van Leeuwen, J. and Timmermans, H. (2003) 'Evaluating design alternatives using conjoint experiments in virtual reality', *Environment and Planning B: Planning and Design*, 30: 357–67.

Goldberg S., Green P. and Wind, Y. (1984) 'Conjoint analysis of price premiums for hotel amenities', *Journal of Business*, 57 (1), pt 2.

Green, P. and Rao, V. (1971) 'Conjoint measurement for quantifying judgemental data', *Journal of Marketing Research*, 8 (3): 355–63.

Hastorf, A. and Cantrill, H. (1954) 'They saw a game: a case study', *Journal of Abnormal and Social Psychology*, 49: 129–34.

Hershey, J. and Schoemaker, P. (1980) 'Risk taking and problem context in the domain of losses: an expected utility analysis', *Journal of Risk and Insurance*, 47: 111–32.

Higgs, P., Hyde, M., Wiggins, R. and Blane, D. (2003) 'Researching quality of life in early old age: the importance of the sociological dimension', *Social Policy and Administration*, 37 (3): 239–52.

Joseph, A. and Zimring, C. (2007) 'Where active older adults walk: understanding the factors related to path choice for walking among active retirement community residents', *Environment and Behavior*, 39 (1): 75–105.

Kahneman, D. and Tversky, A. (1979) 'Prospect theory: an analysis of decision under risk', *Econometrica*, 47: 263–91.

Laing, R., Davies, A.-M., Miller, D. Conniff, A. Scott. S. and Morrice, J. (2008) 'The application of visual environmental economics in the study of public preference and urban greenspace', *Environment and Planning B: Planning and Design*, advance online publication, doi:10.1068/b33140.

Landy, D. and Sigall, H. (1974) 'Beauty is talent: task evaluation as a function of the performers' physical attractiveness', *Journal of Personality and Social Psychology*, 29: 299–304.

Legendre, P. and Anderson, M. J. (1999) 'Distance based redundancy analysis testing multispecies responses in multifactorial ecological experiments', *Ecological Monographs*, 69 (1): 1–24.

Legendre, P. and Legendre, L. (1998) *Numerical Ecology*, 2nd edn, Amsterdam: Elsevier Science: 579–93.

Leishman, C., Aspinall, P. A., Munro, M. and Warren, F. (2004) *Preference for New Build Houses*, York: Joseph Rowntree Foundation.

Li, F. Z., Fisher, K. J., Bauman, A., Ory, M. G., Chodzko-Zajko,W. and Harmer, P. (2005) 'Neighborhood influences on physical activity in middle-aged and older adults: A multilevel perspective', *Journal of Aging and Physical Activity*, 13: 87–114.

Lichtenstein, S. and Slovic, P. (1971) 'Reversals of preference between bids and choices in gambling decisions', *Journal of Experimental Psychology*, 89: 46–55.

Luce, R. and Tukey, J. (1964) 'Simultaneous conjoint measurement: a new type of fundamental measurement', *Journal of Mathematical Psychology*, 1 (1): 1–27.

McMillen, D., Smith, S. and Wells-Parker, E. (1989) 'The effects of alcohol, expectancy and sensation seeking on driving risk taking', *Addictive Behaviour*, 14: 477–83.

National Institute for Health and Clinical Excellence (NICE) (2004) *Guide to the Methods of Technology Appraisal.* Report April 2004 (Section 5.5: Valuing health effects, p. 24), London: Department of Health.

Neumann, J. von and Morgenstern, O. (1947) *Theory of Games and Economic Behaviour*, Princeton, N.J.: Princeton University Press.

Oakes ,C. and McKee, E. (1997) *The Market for a New Private Rented Sector* (Housing Research Findings, 214), York: Joseph Rowntree Foundation.

Orme, B. (1996) *Which Conjoint Method Should I Use?*, Sawtooth Technical Papers, Sawtooth Solutions.

Orme, B. (2005) *The CBC/HB system for hierarchical Bayes estimation, Version 4*, Sawtooth Technical Papers, Sawtooth Solutions.

OPENspace (2009) *Not so Green and Pleasant? Final Report, Part B, Understanding the Impact of Quality of Urban Green Space on Well-being*, unpublished report for Commission for Architecture and the Built Environment (CABE), Edinburgh: OPENspace research centre.

Plous, S. (1993) *The Psychology of Judgement and Decision Making*, New York: McGraw-Hill.

Stewart, D. and Love, W. (1968) 'A general canonical correlation index', *Psychological Bulletin*, 70 (3): 160–3.

Sugiyama, T. and Ward Thompson, C. (2008) 'Associations between characteristics of neighbourhood open space and older people's walking', *Urban Forestry and Urban Greening*, 7 (1): 41–51.

Sugiyama, T., Ward Thompson, C. and Alves, S. (2009) 'Associations between neighbourhood open space attributes and quality of life for older people in Britain', *Environment and Behavior*, 41 (1): 3–21.

Ter Braak, C. J. F. and Smilauer, P. (2002) *CANOCO Reference Manual and CanoDraw for Windows User's Guide*, Version 4.5, Ithaca, N.Y.: Microcomputer Power.

Thorndyke, E. (1920) 'A constant error in psychological ratings', *Journal of Applied Psychology*, 4: 25–9.

Tversky, A. (1969) 'Intransitivity of preferences', *Psychological Review*, 76: 31–48.

Tversky, A. and Kahneman, D. (1981) 'The framing of decisions and the psychology of choice', *Science*, 211: 453–8.

Wilson, R. and Abrams, D. (1977) 'Effects of alcohol on social anxiety and physiological arousal: cognitive versus pharmacological processes', *Cognition Research and Therapy*, 1: 195–210.

Part IV

Applications in practice: spatial structure, landscape design and landscape use

Chapter 8

Feeling good and feeling safe in the landscape:
a 'syntactic' approach

Ruth Conroy Dalton and Julienne Hanson

Introduction

Space syntax is a theory and set of tools and techniques for the analysis of spatial configurations. It was developed at University College London (UCL) in the late 1970s, as an approach to understanding human spatial organisation, and to help architects, planners and urban designers to simulate the likely social consequences of their projects at the design stage. The fundamental proposition of space syntax is that a building or place can be broken down into spatial components, so that an analysis of the interrelations of all the components will yield information about the pattern of space that is meaningful and functionally relevant. Over the past 30 years, space syntax has been applied successfully to resolve problems as diverse as master planning entire cities or revealing the imprint of culture in domestic settings.

One important finding from syntactic studies of urban environments is that syntactic measures of spatial 'integration' (the closeness of each spatial element to all others) are normally a strong predictor of space occupancy and movement, and this has proved critical in designing well-used places. Space syntax has also been used to study modern town precincts and residential areas, to show how the natural and expected relation between spatial integration and pedestrian movement can be disrupted by dysfunctional design and layout. However, it has rarely been applied to the looser spatial arrangements found in landscape architecture, where prospects and vistas are shaped more generously and at a larger scale than in townscape, and where, unlike the built environment, the spatial boundaries of living landscapes not only change in transparency or opacity with the course of the seasons, but are also less well delineated.

With this in mind, this chapter explores the opportunities and challenges in taking a syntactic approach to the spatial analysis of landscape. To
the extent that people avoid walking through landscapes in which they feel
apprehensive, understanding the spatial characteristics of such environments
should enable landscape designers to create vital landscapes that support
healthy lifestyles and avoid those conditions where people may feel insecure.
This chapter will therefore focus on how the tools and techniques of space
syntax can be adapted to understand the circumstances under which people
feel motivated to explore their local landscape, and the spatial factors that
may deter people from incorporating walking into their personal strategy for
healthy living.

How space syntax works

Space syntax is built on three classes of spatial unit, each associated with a
distinct and different representation; axial lines, convex spaces and visual
fields (isovists): see Figure 8.1. Movement is essentially a linear activity,
whereas social interaction is best supported by a convex space in which all
points can see all others. Finally, from any point in space it is possible to
construct a 360-degree visual field that describes the area and the boundary
that can be directly seen from that location. Following Benedikt (1979), space
syntax normally uses the term *isovist* (related terms from landscape studies/
geography would be *vista* and *viewshed*, discussed in detail by Conroy-Dalton
and Bafna, 2003) to refer to these irregularly shaped slices through the environment. Space syntax proposes that as people move through the complex
patterns of space that are typical of buildings or cities, they build up an
enduring picture of the pattern of space as a whole. Each of these representations therefore describes some aspect of how people use and experience
space practically, retrieve information from and understand space analytically,
or generate space creatively through architectural and urban design. A central
proposition of space syntax is that there is a link between the representations
of space that are adopted and those aspects of functionality that are laid open
to investigation.

However, the syntactic (space syntax) approach to architectural and
urban space is concerned not just with the properties of individual spaces, but
with the relationships between the many spaces that make up the spatial
layout of a building or a city. Space syntax uses the term *configuration* to refer
to the way in which each space in a layout contributes to how all the spaces in
the system affect one another. A fundamental notion of space syntax is that the
layout of a network of spaces appears to be different when seen from different
locations in the system.

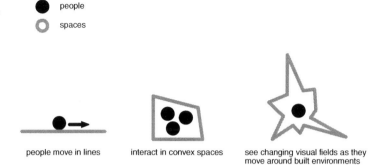

Figure 8.1
The social logic of
axial and convex
spaces and
isovists.

people

spaces

people move in lines   interact in convex spaces   see changing visual fields as they
move around built environments

This can be illustrated by drawing a *justified access graph* from
different spaces in a layout, as shown in Figure 8.2. The graphs drawn from space
5 (left) and space 10 (right) look quite different, but they are actually the same
graph looked at from different points of view. Although different, each graph
gives an accurate picture of what the whole layout looks like from that particular
space, and thus each graph expresses a real property of the layout.

The shape of the graphs from each space can then be used to assign
numerical values to each space.[1] The syntactic, graph-theoretic measure of *integration*, for example, calculates the extent to which it is necessary to pass
through other spaces to go from each space to all others. This will be high or low
according to whether the graph is shallow, as on the left, or deep, as on the right.
To the degree that the graph from a space is shallow, it will be relatively accessible to all others in the system and therefore integrated; to the degree that it is
deep, most of the other spaces in the system will be relatively inaccessible and
so the location is termed segregated.

Space syntax utilises several such configurational measures, the most
important of which is integration, to analyse the spatial patterns that are created
by buildings and cities. Systems of axial lines, convex spaces and isovists can all
be analysed in the same relational way, depending on the topic under investigation. For large systems, space syntax utilises computer modelling using

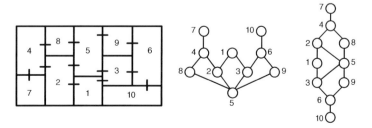

Figure 8.2
Configuration -
access graphs
from different
spaces in a
system.

215

DepthMap[2] software to compute the relations between each space and all other spaces, calculate the integration value of each and colour each element according to its degree of integration, where red indicates the most integrated spaces, through the colour spectrum to blue, which identifies the most segregated spaces of all. A greyscale version indicates maximum integration by black, with dark to pale grey representing increasing degrees of segregation.

Since space syntax was first developed, numerous studies from all parts of the world have shown how social and cultural patterns are imprinted in spatial layouts, and how spatial layouts affect the functioning of buildings and cities. One of the most important and robust relationships in urban systems is that between the degree of integration of a street (axial line) and the amount of pedestrian movement carried by that street; all other things being equal, the more integrated the street the busier it will be, and the more segregated it is the quieter it will be (Hillier, 1996, 2001; Hillier et al., 1987, 1993; Hillier and Iida, 2005).

Other studies have used space syntax to describe and quantify the characteristics of different complex public buildings such as museums (Tzortzi, 2004; Peponis et al., 2004), university campuses (Greene and Penn, 1997), laboratories (Hillier et al., 1985), offices (Penn, 1994; Penn, Desyllas and Vaughan, 1999; Schnädelbach et al., 2006) hospitals (Haq and Girotto, 2003), shopping malls (Batty, 2004) and similar settings where way finding may be a significant issue. Space syntax has been used to study the relationship between spatial layouts and social affects such as crime (Hillier and Shu, 2000; Hillier, 2004), traffic flow (Penn et al., 1998; Conroy Dalton, 2007) and the like, and in design applications in architecture, urban design, planning, transport studies and interior design (Hillier et al., 1991).

The syntactic analysis of landscapes

Practical applications of space syntax to landscape studies tend to be directed towards promoting the use of green routes and public parks in urban areas through people-aware design. For example, in 2003 Space Syntax Limited, a commercial spin-off company from the university-based research group at UCL, was commissioned by Thames Chase Community Forest to study the use of two Greenways on the outskirts of London. Greenways are:

> a car free component of a network for non-motorised use, connecting people to facilities and open spaces in and around towns, cities and the countryside, for shared use by people of all abilities on foot, bike or horseback, for commuting, play or leisure.
>
> (Countryside Agency, 1998)

The study analysed local travel patterns on and around the Greenways, and gathered information about the needs and motivations of walkers, in order to suggest ways to improve levels of use, especially for short trips. The key spatial factors that seemed to influence the observed levels of activity on the Greenways were integration, visibility and co-presence (Rose, 2003). The report's recommendations were therefore that to maximise their potential as transport corridors, Greenways should be well integrated with pre-existing pedestrian movement patterns and local street networks, good visibility should be maintained to nearby streets to make people feel safer, and well-used routes should also be well maintained.

Similarly, a detailed observation study of the use of a local Thameside park in the heart of London adjacent to the iconic Greater London Authority building, the headquarters of London's mayor (Savic and Rose, 2003), found that while routes at the perimeter of the park were well used, those in the heart of the park were less busy. Because public spaces are more likely to be used where there are already people walking and cycling nearby, this report stressed the importance of locating city parks at strategic points in the urban grid, drawing movement from the surrounding streets into the park from several directions by fitting the routes through the park into the natural movement patterns of the area, and ensuring that good visibility is maintained between the park and its surroundings by minimising dense and tall foliage, especially at the entrances. It also recommended that adequate seating, lighting and high-quality planting should be provided to encourage passers-by to sit down, and that provision should be made for commercial and community facilities that can maintain a more permanent presence and informally 'police' the park.

Studies of a similar nature have been carried out in several parts of the world (Baser, 2007; Grajewski and Psarra, 2001; Guler, 2007; Makhzoumi et al., 2005; Papargyropoulou, 2006). A common theme in many of these studies is the relationship between visibility (what can be seen), accessibility (where people can go) and observed use and movement (where people actually are, considered in terms of static occupancy of space as well as through-movement). An intriguing insight (Papargyropoulou, 2006) is that the spatial configuration of a parkland setting may be unique in respect of the freedom of choice that it offers its users in terms of where to go, what to look at and who else is co-present with the observer in the visual field.

A second strand of work is rather more theoretical, in that it seeks to understand and quantify the unique properties of landscape as distinct from urban space. For example, Makhzoumi and Zako (1999) have drawn attention to the difficulty of defining landscape elements. Elements such as orchards, fields, woodland and buildings have clear physical boundaries and can readily be distin-guished, but others such as maquis (scrub) may be both extensive and amor-phous. Makhzoumi and Zako resolved this problem by first defining the boundaries of all the clear elements in the landscape, then treating the maquis as the 'connective tissue' of the landscape, analogous to the streets of a town, which was then analysed using conventional syntactic methods.[3] The results were interpreted using Appleton's (1975) concepts of prospect and refuge. Davies, Mora and Peebles (2006) have also drawn attention to the amorphous nature of large open green spaces with large amounts of vegetation, where conventional isovist measures such as the area/perimeter ratio (Benedikt, 1979) may become difficult to calculate, yielding distorted and unrealistic results when compared with those for urban space.

The issue of visibility has been extensively explored in the field of geoinformation science (GISci) through *viewshed* analysis.[4] This concept has generated an extensive technical literature, which concentrates mainly on mapping the properties of individual viewsheds as opposed to showing how viewsheds with different properties relate systematically to one another in landscapes with different appearances and characteristics. However, Turner and colleagues (2001) have proposed a method for utilising a set of isovists laid out in a spatial environment (architects' houses and art galleries were used to demonstrate the approach) on a 1 m square regular grid in order to generate a graph that captured the mutual visibility between locations, or *visibility graph*. In a subsequent paper, O'Sullivan and Turner (2001) applied the approach to landscape, and suggested that it may provide tools for quantifying the perceptual characteristics of landscape, such as the extent to which an observer in a landscape setting perceives themselves 'inside' or surrounded by the landscape, thus pointing towards the possibility of quantifying concepts like those of prospect and refuge, referred to earlier. In similar vein, Llobera (2003) has suggested that these kinds of visual analysis, which he terms 'visualscapes', may be capable of giving a rigorous, mathematical definition of an object's visual prominence or visual exposure in a landscape.

In this respect, interesting work is being done to develop an algorithm to express the probability that a target object really can be seen from a given location in the landscape, a factor termed 'probabilistic visibility' (Skov-Petersen and Snizek, 2007a, 2007b). Building upon an earlier study of the landscape of Queensland (Preston, 2002), the authors propose that when analysing visibility in small-scale landscapes using visual fields (whether isovists or viewsheds), factors such as the ruggedness of the terrain, the presence of ground-level planting and even the weather and light conditions might interfere with visual contact. They have therefore proposed a measure of 'visibility decay' which takes account of the physical distance between the viewer and the target, the relative transparency of the environment and the viewing angle (concepts frequently employed in computer graphics in order to render natural scenes realistically: Rokita, 1993). These ideas were tested empirically in a field study located in a beech forest setting. This revealed that other features that may need to be taken into account include the exposure time of the target, whether it is moving or stationary and its appearance.

Drawing on the developments outlined above, and previous experience of employing space syntax to analyse a wide range of settings from people's homes (Hanson, 1998) to virtual environments (Conroy Dalton, 2001, 2002), the remainder of this chapter uses the new town of Milton Keynes as a vehicle to examine the potential of space syntax theories and methods to explore people's experiences of walking in landscaped settings. Access to parks and natural landscapes is believed to promote walking as a form of healthy, natural exercise that is accessible to the majority of the population. As Burgess, Harrison and Limb describe, people report:

> a profound sense of personal satisfaction ... gained from experiencing the sensuous pleasures of being outside in open spaces: enjoying the changing seasons, feeling the sun, the wind or the rain, being able to walk, run or just sit down and enjoy the view.
>
> (Burgess et al., 1988: 460)

To that end, many towns and cities, including Milton Keynes, have developed walking strategies to encourage local residents to walk more, and so reduce their chances of succumbing to a range of chronic health conditions such as obesity or heart disease, as well as maintain good mental health. Aspects of the landscape that are of particular interest here are not only functional in respect of how people move through the landscape, but also cognitive, relating to how they feel about it. The relationship between spatial configuration and space occupancy and movement is well understood, so the test for space syntax analysis is whether it is possible to develop representations that pin down the relationship between the more functional properties of movement and co-presence, and the experiential spatial attributes that lead people to feel good and feel safe in the landscape.

Milton Keynes

Milton Keynes is the most recent and radical of the English New Towns. It is located 45 miles north of London and was originally planned to cover 8,900 hectares (22,000 acres) of the north Buckinghamshire countryside.[5] It was conceived of as a low-density development with a planned capacity of 250,000.[6] From its inception in 1967, the town adopted an innovative approach to master planning, by layering a 1 kilometre square grid of high speed roads, local distributor roads, cycleways and bridleways, pedestrian routes, linear parks and a variety of local play spaces, in order to create attractive, safe, car-free and healthy landscapes within reach of everyone's home. The planning concept was for 'environmental areas' each occupying a grid square and forming a semi-autonomous community, built in a variety of architectural styles and centred on a primary school, local retail centre and community facilities. The landscape design concept was of a 'forest city', and to that end, 20 per cent of the designated area of the town was allocated to creating a citywide parkland landscape (Walker, 1994). A comprehensive network of footpaths and cycleways threads through the grid squares to link them to the town's varied facilities and amenities, but this is completely separate from the high-speed vehicular grid roads. The town actively seeks to encourage walking and cycling, so pedestrian and cycle links between the grid squares are achieved by either bridges or underpasses.

Footpaths in Milton Keynes are mostly short links within housing estates; there are no footpaths between estates, and for longer journeys pedestrians have to use the cycleways (known locally as Redways, due to their use of distinctive coloured tarmac). These have become synonymous with perceived low personal security. Fear of crime is a barrier to walking, though only 1 per cent of all reported crime in Milton Keynes takes place on the Redways (MKC, 2003). Nevertheless, more people report feeling unsafe walking alone in Milton Keynes than in any other part of the entire region (Milton Keynes Council and Thames Valley Police, 1998). Amongst the contributory factors are the abundant and dense vegetation which lines many routes and contributes to poor visibility, poor lighting (especially at night) and the narrowness and isolation of many routes, which means that it is impossible to take evasive action if a person who appears to be acting suspiciously is encountered while walking or cycling (Franklin, 1999). Another reason may be that '[m]ost Redways have been constructed as a maze of largely indirect local paths' (MKC, 1998) rather than as direct routes linking desirable destinations. Underpasses and bridges contribute to the meandering, maze-like effect. Small wonder, then, that the town's Director of Public Health has highlighted obesity as a growing threat to health, adding that because the town has been designed to facilitate car use, there is a need to promote higher levels of physical activity within the local population (Hicks, 2007).

The spatial structure of Milton Keynes

The master planning of Milton Keynes has led to a very distinctive axial structure in respect of its urban grid (see Figure 8.3). The most integrated (black) line, running southeast to northwest towards the left side of the map, is that of Watling Street, originally a Roman road and now the A5. Integration picks out the mesh of supergrid roads in darker grey tones, while irrespective of their geometric position in the town grid, the local roads are almost all pale grey (segregated). The shopping centre can immediately be identified as a local intensification of mid-grey

Figure 8.3
Axial map of
Milton Keynes.

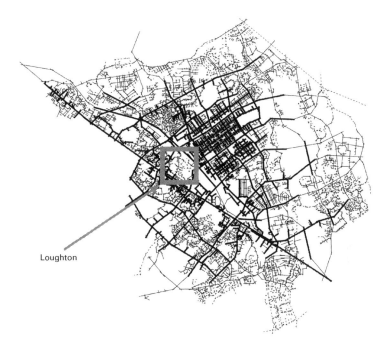

Loughton

lines at the geometric centre of the map. Put simply, integration favours the high-speed roads where there is no provision for pedestrians or cyclists; the local environments where people might walk are uniformly segregated and inaccessible.

The polarization between cars and pedestrians can be further illustrated by homing in on one of the grid squares, Loughton, to study in more detail the pattern of local roads, pedestrian paths and Redways, in relation to the local landscape and streetscape. The village of Loughton dates back to at least the *Domesday Book* and is one of the most desirable of Milton Keynes' neighbourhoods. As Figure 8.3 shows, Loughton is strategically located between the station end of the shopping centre and the A5. It lies immediately to the east of the most integrated road in the new town's supergrid, and most of the local roads within the grid square itself are reasonably well integrated. The station is about ten minutes walk away and the town centre can be accessed by the Redways in 15–20 minutes.

Figure 8.4 is an aerial photograph of Loughton. The grid square contains about 1,000 dwellings, both old and new, and the areas of new housing are interspersed with large green spaces that include the playing fields of the local middle school and primary school, the village green, a section of Loughton Valley Linear Park, several pony paddocks, allotments and an equestrian centre.

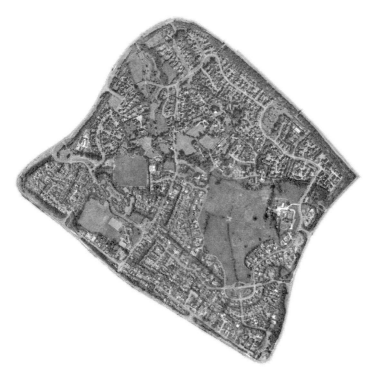

Figure 8.4
Aerial photograph
of the grid square
containing the
original village of
Loughton and the
Loughton Valley
Linear Park
(© 2009 Google -
Map data © 2009
Tele Atlas).

At the heart of the village is a thirteenth-century church, which stands at the top of a slight hill that rises above the flood plain of Loughton Brook. The older houses are scattered parallel to Loughton Brook along the Bradwell Road, which before the arrival of the new town used to connect Watling Street and Loughton village to the neighbouring village of Bradwell.

Loughton ought to be an attractive environment in which to walk, and its low density notwithstanding, its location and degree of integration should support reasonable levels of pedestrian activity, yet as Figure 8.5 shows, it is a complex and multilayered environment that even residents of many years find difficult to comprehend.[7] Levels of pedestrian activity are generally low, and despite their beauty and high amenity, Loughton's parks are empty for most of the time. The village environment therefore offers a challenging test bed in which to extend space syntax analysis by exploring issues that relate to feelings of safety, security and well-being as well as functional activity patterns in land-scaped settings.

Figure 8.5
The network of
vehicular roads
(A), pedestrian
footpaths (B),
cycle ways (C),
social trails (D)
and bridle paths
(E) in Loughton.
Image F is the
space syntax
'integration'
pattern of the
combined
network.

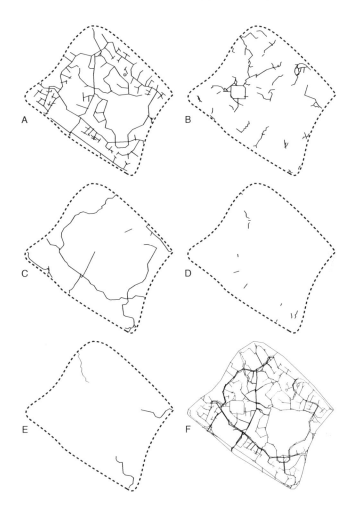

Spatial analysis

The question that this chapter set out to explore was whether the kinds of
objective, configuration-based analyses typically employed by space syntax
researchers can be brought to bear on the problem of representing and understanding the role of the natural landscape, particularly with reference to pedestrian movement. In this final section, we shall attempt to demonstrate how
certain space syntax techniques may begin to be adapted or extended in order to
address this problem, as well as to outline a strategy for future research. It is
proposed that there are, broadly, three ways in which space syntax methods may
be applied to the study of natural landscapes. These can be characterized as:

- 'assigning attributes to spatial units' (or the nodes in the graph-based representation)
- 'assigning attributes to the relationships between spatial units' (or the edges in the graph)
- the use of multilayered graphs.

Some of the goals of these tactics are to be able to account for the seasonal variation found in the natural landscape, the imprecise nature of natural boundaries and the multiplicity of types of path and/or use. Each of these approaches is briefly described below.

Assigning attributes to spatial units

As discussed in an earlier section of this chapter, there are three kinds of spatial representation or unit that are typically employed in breaking up a continuous spatial setting into discrete chunks amenable to quantitative, graph-based analysis: axial line, convex space and isovist. One method of enriching these spatial descriptors is to assign values or attributes to them, depending upon the specific research question. For example, it has long been recognised that the attribute termed 'constitution', or the degree to which a space is interfaced by doors and/or windows (providing natural surveillance), plays a significant role not only in the perception of crime but also in recorded instances of it (Hillier and Shu, 2000).

Using the grid square of Loughton as an example, the constitution of a space (an intrinsic property of a space) can be combined with its integration value (a configuration property). It is then possible to classify Loughton's paths through the village and its landscape according to how 'integrated and consti-tuted' (I+C), 'integrated and unconstituted' (I+U), segregated and constituted (S+C), or segregated and unconstituted (S+U) each is, in order to test the hypothesis that this may begin to provide an index for perceived safety when walking outdoors (Figure 8.6). Of course, the degree to which a space is over-looked may itself vary, depending upon the time of year. Seasonal variation might mean that a temporary abundance of foliage could have the effect of obscuring views that would be present at other times of year, and a method to allow for such variation is discussed in the next section of the paper.

Another method of assigning a nonconfigurational attribute to a space is by the use of a weighted network graph. In this case each space, or node in the graph, is given a weight according to its position on a spectrum of predefined values. For example, a space could be characterized by the composition of its bounding vertical surfaces. Within a dense urban environment, a significant proportion of a spatial boundary could be expected to be 'hard' brick or masonry vertical surfaces; conversely, in the natural landscape, a spatial boundary could be (fuzzily) delineated

Figure 8.6
Four illustrative
routes in Loughton
that are: integrated
and constituted'
(I+C), integrated
and unconstituted
(I+U), segregated
and unconstituted
(S+U) and
segregated and
constituted (S+C),
respectively.

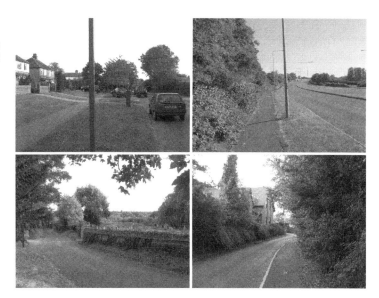

by vegetation. Boundaries could therefore be classified as consisting of relative proportions of, for example, building face, solid brick or masonry wall, decorative pierced
block wall or screen wall, continuous fence, visually pervious fencing, railings, culti-
vated hedge, semi-cultivated hedge/shrubbery, trees and so on. Depending upon the
relative proportion of 'hard' to 'soft' surfaces, a corresponding value could be assigned
to the corresponding node in the network graph. As with the previous example, which
combined the values of constitution and integration, these surface attributes could be
considered in isolation or combined with other configurational values.

The act of considering the type of surface boundary of, for example, a
convex space or isovist, is not new. Benedikt (1979) discussed the difference
between the real-world perimeter of an isovist (that section of an isovist's
perimeter formed by a material surface) versus those sections of an isovist's
perimeter formed by an occluding radial (a line of sight that links the corner of an
occluding surface to its termination point at another surface, located at a distance
beyond the first point). His measure of 'occlusivity' was intended to capture the
ratio between these two types of surface perimeter. Equally, Zako, in her study
of London housing estates (Zako and Hanson, 2009), classified sections of a
housing estate's boundary according to similar hard-to-soft categories.

Assigning attributes to the relationships between spatial units

After demonstrating how intrinsic and configurational properties might be
combined, it is suggested that one method to permit a greater sensitivity to the

effect of the changing seasons upon our perception of space might be to assign a weight to the edges of a network graph. In conventional space syntax analysis, the edges between two nodes in a graph represent the relationship between those two corresponding spaces. Usually this relationship is a binary one: two spaces are either connected, meaning that there is a condition of mutual visibility and permeability between them, or they are not. However, if we consider the natural landscape, it may well be that two locations that are visible from each other might only be so in the winter, and not so in the spring or summer (Figure 8.7).

So, for example, if two spaces are mutually visible/accessible all year round, this might be expressed as an edge-weight of 4, as opposed to a pair of

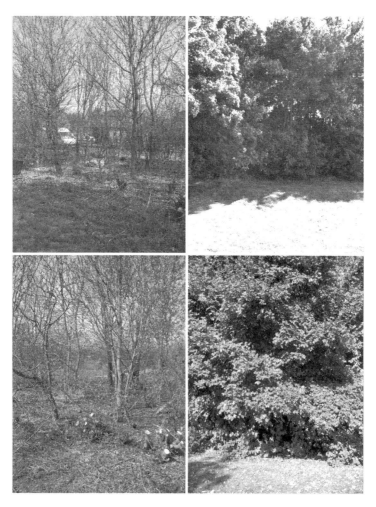

Figure 8.7
The view between a residential lane and an adjacent park in winter and summer. In winter the houses and the park are visible to one another, in summer the view both ways is completely obscured by foliage.

spaces being mutually visible only in winter, which might be expressed as a weight of only 1 (with the weights of 2 and 3 corresponding to the numbers of seasons during which such a relationship is present). In this way a *weighted graph* could be created in which the 'strength' of an edge corresponds to the relative permanence of the spatial relationship. Peponis and colleagues (2004) employed such a method in their study of science exhibitions. In this case, the mutual visibility between separate exhibits was expressed on a scale of 0 to 3 depending upon the perceptual clarity of the visual link. A weighted, spatial network graph was then formed, permitting further configurational analyses. This can be seen as being a way of augmenting or extending commonly used space syntax techniques to add a richer layer of information, pertaining to the experience of being within a natural environment.

Multilayered graphs

In the grid-square of Loughton we have chosen to represent a number of different kinds of paths (Figure 8.5 and Figure 8.8), these being the vehicular, pedestrian, cycle and bridle paths as well as more informal 'social trails' (undesignated paths often evidenced as an eroded track providing a spatial short-cut). One method that can be employed to understand how these different kinds of paths function together is to treat them as separate but layered graphs that happen to intersect at specific, identified points in space. Again, this is taking typical 'tried and tested' space syntax techniques of representation and analysis, and modifying them to be able to address the specific issues that may arise in the natural landscape. The different network graphs from our example area of Loughton can thus be combined to give an overall impression of how these different uses coexist, and the effect that each may have upon the other. This employs a technique described by Dalton (2007). Imagine that each distinct graph from Figure 8.5 becomes a layer in a larger graph, and that these layers are connected at certain points: for example, where a bridle path crosses over a road.

Figure 8.8
Left:
the network of vehicular roads, pedestrian footpaths, cycle ways, social trails and bridle paths in Loughton, showing points of possible transition between layers.
Right:
the underlying graph network, showing how different layered subgraphs (differentiated by colour) may be connected at strategic points to form a larger graph.

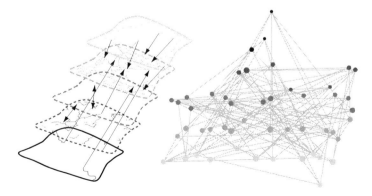

Typically in space syntax analyses, these two lines would either be considered to be linked, or be held to be 'unlinked' depending upon the criteria applied. In the case of multilayered graphs, each layer (for example, the footpath layer and the car layer) could remain as distinct graphs that intersect at specific locations represented by *directed* links. In the case of the footpath and the car layers, the link would 'point' from the footpath to the car layer, indicating that a person could walk along a road but a car would be unable to walk upon a footpath. These inequalities could be coded into every possible pair of layers, to produce an overall layered graph. Of course, these techniques could be combined with those described above to produced layered and *weighted graphs* if appropriate.

Discussion

This chapter has begun to make some tentative suggestions as to how the family of techniques and methods employed in space syntax analysis, commonly applied to buildings and urban environments, might begin to be both extended and modified in order to begin to quantify the experience of being in and moving through the natural landscape. Some of the properties previously described that may discourage walking – isolated routes, lack of connectivity, poor visibility, and maze-like layouts – are tractable to syntactic analysis. The next step is to pilot the modified and extended 'syntactic' representations and measures described above, to see whether any accord with people's reported experiences.[8] It is clear that the way forward should include a synthesis of three types of expertise: an ability to quantify natural spaces objectively (the contribution of space syntax), environmental/cognitive psychology methods of, for example, verbal protocols and other forms of self-reporting in order to attempt to elicit the types of affordances provided by the natural landscape, and knowledge of the landscape itself, providing structured methods of classification and evaluation. This chapter, therefore, ends with a plea for future, interdisciplinary collaboration, as this will provide the best opportunity to understand the reasons why people are reluctant to make full use of the available, natural environment, and hence feel both good and safe in the landscape.

Notes

1 For a full explanation of the mathematical derivation of the measures, see Hillier and Hanson (1984).
2 Developed by Alasdair Turner, UCL Depthmap is a computer program that performs visibility analysis on architectural and urban systems. It takes input in the form of a plan of the system, and is able to construct a map of 'visually integrated' locations within it. It was first written for the Silicon Graphics IRIX operating system as a simple isovist processing program in 1998.

Since then it has gone through several metamorphoses to reach the current version 4, for the Windows platform. It is designed to run on Windows 2000 and XP operating systems.

3 In this case, a combination of convex analysis, all-line axial maps and isovists.

4 Unlike the usual syntactic interpretation of an isovist, a viewshed need not be spatially continuous.

5 In 2004, the government announced plans to expand the town's designated area to the west and east, in order to raise the population to 300,000 by 2031.

6 At the 2001 census, the population of the urban area stood at just over 184,000.

7 Hanson has lived in Loughton for 18 years; Conroy Dalton for five years.

8 Offering an interpretation for these spatial attributes of landscape is, however, likely to prove challenging; to a fit and active youth a bush may simply present itself as an attractive landscape feature, but a frail older woman may be more wary and avoid the same bush in case it conceals a mugger.

References

Appleton, J. (1975) *The Experience of Landscape*, London: Wiley.

Audit Commission (2006) *Corporate Assessment: Milton Keynes Council,* London: Audit Commission.

Baser, B. (2007) 'A new landscape design strategy for creating continuous, perceptible and productive urban green: a case study of Kadikoy, Istanbul', proceedings of the Sixth International Space Syntax Symposium, 11–14 June 2007.

Batty, M. (2003) 'Agent-based pedestrian modelling', CASA Working Paper no. 61. London: Centre for Advanced Spatial Analysis (UCL).

Benedikt, M. (1979) 'To take hold of space; isovists and isovist fields', *Environment and Planning B*, 6: 47–65.

Burgess, J., Harrison, C. M. and Limb, M. (1988) 'People, parks and the urban green: a study of popular meanings and values for open spaces in the city', *Urban Studies*, 25 (6): 455–73.

Conroy Dalton, R. (2001) 'Spatial navigation in immersive virtual environments', doctoral thesis, University College London.

Conroy Dalton, R. (2002) 'Is spatial intelligibility critical to the design of largescale virtual environments?' *International Journal of Design Computing*, 4.

Conroy Dalton, R. (2007) 'Social exclusion and transportation in Peachtree City, Georgia', *Progress in Planning*, 67 (4).

Conroy Dalton, R. and Bafna, S. (2003) 'The syntactical image of the city: a reciprocal definition of spatial elements and spatial syntaxes', paper presented at the Fourth International Space Syntax Symposium, 17–19 June 2003, London.

Countryside Agency (1998) *The Greenways Handbook*, London: Natural England.

Dalton, N. (2007) Personal communication [email].

Davies, C., Mora, R. and Peebles, D. (2006) *Isovists for Orientation: Can Space Syntax Help us to Predict Directional Confusion?* London: Ordnance Survey.

Franklin J. (1999) 'Two decades of the Redway cycle paths in Milton Keynes', *Traffic Engineering and Control*, July/August 1999.

Gibson, J. J. (1979) *The Ecological Approach to Visual Perception*, Boston, Mass.: Houghton Mifflin.

Grajewski, T. and Psarra, S. (2001) *The Evaluation of Park Layouts and their Impact on the Patterns of Use and Movement: Warley Woods: A Case Study*, Reading: Urban Parks Forum.

Greene, M. and Penn, A. (1997) 'Socio-spatial analysis of four university campuses: the implications of spatial configuration on creation and transmission of knowledge', paper presented at the Space Syntax First International Symposium, London, April 1997.

Guler, G. (2007) 'Measuring the effects of the bridges on Istanbul's green system using space syntax and GIS tools', paper presented at Le Notre Conference, Belgrade, 10–14 October 2007.

Hanson, J. (1998) *Decoding Homes and Houses*, Cambridge: Cambridge University Press.

Haq, S. and Girotto, S. (2003) 'Ability and intelligibility; wayfinding and environmental cognition in the designed environment', Proceedings of the Fourth International Space Syntax Symposium, London, June 2003.

Hicks, N. (2007) *Blueprint for the Health of Milton Keynes: Director of Public Health's Annual Report*, Milton Keynes Primary Care Trust, 19 April.

Hillier, B. (1996) 'Cities as movement economies', *Urban Design International*, 1 (1): 41–60.

Hillier, B. (2001) 'A theory of the city as object: or, how spatial laws mediate the social construction of urban space', Proceedings of the Third International Space Syntax Symposium, Atlanta, Georgia, USA, 7–11 May 2001.

Hillier, B. (2004) 'Can streets be made safe?', *Urban Design International*, 9: 31–45.

Hillier, B. and Hanson, J. (1984) *The Social Logic of Space*, Cambridge: Cambridge University Press.

Hillier, B. and Iida, S. (2005) 'Network and psychological effects in urban movement', in A. G. Cohn and D. M. Mark, (eds), *Spatial Information Theory: COSIT 2005*, Lecture Notes in Computer Science no. 3693, 475-490, Berlin: Springer-Verlag.

Hillier, B. and Shu, S. (2000) 'Crime and urban layout: the need for evidence', in: S. Ballantyne, V. MacLaren and K. Pease (eds), *Secure Foundations: Key Issues in Crime Prevention, Crime Reduction and Community Safety*, London: Institute for Public Policy Research.

Hillier, B., Penn, A., Grajewski, T., Burdett, R. and Musgrove, J. (1985) 'Space standards and configuration in research laboratories', technical report, Bartlett School of Architecture and Planning, University College London.

Hillier, B., Penn, A., Grajewski, T. and Jianming, X. (1991) 'Brindleyplace, Birmingham: the UCL study of the potential of the site and the Farrell masterplan', discussion paper, University College London.

Hillier, B., Penn, A., Hanson, J., Grajewski, T. and Xu, J. (1993) 'Natural movement: or, configuration and attraction in urban pedestrian movement', *Environment and Planning B*, 20 (1): 29–66.

Hillier, B., Burdett, R., Peponis, J. and Penn, A. (1987) 'Creating life: or, does architecture determine anything?', *Architecture and Comportement/Architecture and Behaviour*, 3 (3): 233–50.

Llobera, M. (2003) 'Extending GIS-based visual analysis: the concept of "visualscapes"', *International Journal of Geographical Information Science*, 17 (1): 25–48.

Makhzoumi, J. and Zako, R. (1999) 'Investigating the spatial pattern of Mediterranean rural landscapes', poster presented at the Second International Space Syntax Symposium, Brasilia, 29 March–2 April 1999.

Makhzoumi, J., Zako, R., Zougheib, D. and Mabsout, S. (2005) 'Aligning campus sustainability and historic landscapes preservation', poster presented at the Fifth International Space Syntax Symposium, Delft, Netherlands.

Milton Keynes Council (1998) *Milton Keynes Redways and Leisure Routes: An Information Sheet*, Milton Keynes: Milton Keynes Council.

Milton Keynes Council (2003) *Milton Keynes Walking Strategy*, Milton Keynes: Milton Keynes Council.

Milton Keynes Council and Thames Valley Police (1998) *Milton Keynes Crime and Community Safety Partnership Audit Report*, Milton Keynes: Milton Keynes Council and Thames Valley Police.

Norman, D. (1988) *The Design of Everyday Things*, London: MIT Press.

O'Sullivan, D. and Turner, A. (2001) 'Visibility graphs and landscape visibility analysis', *International Journal of Geographical Information Science*, 15 (3): 221–37.

Papargyropoulou, P. (2006) 'Park interpretations: an exploration of the spatial properties and urban performance of Regent's Park, London and Pedion Areos Park, Athens', M.Sc. thesis, University College London.

Penn, A. (1994) 'Space for innovation: effects of spatial configuration on social and knowledge generation', *Proceedings of the First Workshop for Cooperation between Japan and the UK on SOFT Science & Technology*, STA, Osaka, Japan, 126–8.

Penn, A., Desyllas, J. and Vaughan, L. (1999) 'The space of innovation: interaction and communication in the work environment', *Environment and Planning B: Planning and Design*, 26 (2): 193–218.

Penn, A., Hillier, B., Banister, D. and Xu, J. (1998) 'Configurational modelling of urban movement networks', *Environment and Planning B: Planning and Design*, 25: 59–84.

Penning-Rowsell, E. and Burgess, J. (1997) 'River landscapes: changing the concrete overcoat?', *Landscape Research*, 22 (1): 5–11.

Peponis, J., Conroy Dalton, R., Wineman, J. and Dalton, N. (2004) 'Measuring the effects of layout upon visitors' spatial behaviors in open plan exhibition settings', *Environment and Planning B: Planning and Design*, 31: 453–73.

Preston, R. (2002) *Visual Exposure of the Landscapes in the Bremer River Catchment and the Middle Brisbane River Catchment*, available at: <http://www.epa.qld.gov.au/publications/p00872.html> (accessed 3 August 2009).

Rokita, P. (1993) 'Fast generation of depth of field effects in computer graphics', *Computer and Graphics*, 17 (5): 505–624.

Rose, A. (2003) *Greenways: Walking at the Urban Fringe*, London: Space Syntax Limited.

Savic, B. and Rose, A. (2003) *Potter's Field Park: A Report on Existing Patterns of Space Use and Spatial Potentials*, London: Space Syntax Limited.

Schnädelbach, H., Penn, A., Steadman, P., Benford, S., Koleva, B. and Rodden, T. (2006) 'Moving office: inhabiting a dynamic building', in *Proceedings of the 20th Anniversary Conference on Computer Supported Cooperative Work (CSCW)*, Banff, Canada: ACM Press.

Skov-Petersen, H. and Snizek, B. (2007a) 'Probability of visual encounters', in R. H. Gimblett and H. Skov-Peteresen (eds), *Monitoring, Simulation and Management of Visitor Landscapes*, Tucson, Az.: University of Arizona Press.

Skov-Petersen, H. and Snizek, B. (2007b) 'To see or not to see: assessment of probabilistic visibility', paper presented at Tenth AGILE Conference, Aalborg, Denmark, 8–11 April 2007.

Synott, M. (2006) Personal communication [email].

Turner, A., Doxa, M., O'Sullivan, D. and Penn, A. (2001) 'From isovists to visibility graphs: a methodology for the analysis of architectural space', *Environment and Planning B*, 28: 103–21.

Tzortzi, K. (2004) 'Building and exhibition layout: Sainsbury Wing compared with Castelvecchio', *Architectural Research Quarterly*, 8 (2): 128–40.

Walker, D. (1994) 'Introduction', in *Architectural Design Profile No. 111, New Towns*, London: Academy Group.

Zako, R. and Hanson, J. (2009) 'Housing in the twentieth-century city', in R. Cooper, G. Evans and C. Boyko (eds), *Designing Sustainable Cities*, London: Wiley Blackwell.

Chapter 9

Landscape quality and quality of life

Catharine Ward Thompson

Introduction

Commonsense tells us that the quality of the landscape in which we lead our lives makes a difference to the quality of the lived experience. Indeed, how could it be otherwise? Yet there remain many unanswered questions as to what kind of environment might offer maximum benefit for people's quality of life, given the increasingly urbanised nature of society and its ageing demographic structure. Although health is only a part of what makes for quality of life, the World Health Organization (WHO) definition of health's broad embrace, including 'complete physical, mental and social well-being' (WHO, 1946), suggests it is a central component, and therefore of key interest in understanding links between landscape and quality of life.

If we consider the era after the Second World War, it is only very recently that the potential public health benefits of access to landscapes such as parks, riversides or woodlands and similar green or semi-natural open space have been given serious attention, despite the fact that such considerations were the focus of the first public park movement more than 150 years ago (Ward Thompson, 2005; Worpole, 2007). Now that the health benefits of green space are again in the spotlight, there is a new demand for evidence on how the quantity and quality of green space might actually make a measurable difference to health outcomes. If we can understand better how people experience the landscape of everyday life, and how they experience green or natural landscapes in particular, this might illuminate an understanding of the relationship between landscape, health and quality of life, and contribute to better decision making on management of the environment.

The scale at which the landscape is considered is clearly important here, and such questions can be explored at many levels, from the whole urban environment and its green infrastructure to the details of garden or street design immediately outside someone's home. This chapter explores some of the issues at the local and neighbourhood level, drawing on recent and ongoing work at OPENspace research centre in Edinburgh, where we have been investigating different ways of understanding people's engagement with the landscape in attempts to provide evidence in support of good policy and practice. We are interested in how planning and design of outdoor environments might offer an enhanced quality of life for people, and in researching how much difference this might make in practice to people's health and well-being.

As we attempt to address different aspects of such questions, we also seek to understand the mechanisms and patterns behind relationships between health or quality of life and the availability of different kinds of green and outdoor environments. This throws up many challenges, and suggests the need for better theoretical frameworks as well as practical tools with which to research them. In this chapter, I explore some of the conceptual and practical challenges we face as a research community, and offer examples of recent work that has attempted to address them.

Landscape and health challenges: the environment as 'the patient'

For those concerned with public health, the appeal in researching how to identify and develop salutogenic environments (that is, environments that support healthy behaviours and responses) is that these may have more permanent and population-wide effects than other forms of public health interventions targeted at individuals (for example, as explored by Saelens et al., 2003; see also Bull, Giles-Corti and Wood, Chapter 4, this volume). However, the methods conventionally used in health research are not necessarily well suited to exploring the environment, particularly when we want to research the influence of specific outdoor places rather than make generalisations at national level. A key here is the perspective taken on the target or object of research investigation by different disciplines. Medical research will focus on the person as the 'patient', the locus around which interventions are determined. For example, if someone has difficulty getting out and about because of visual or mobility impairment, the medical and therapy specialists will focus on what can be done to improve the individual's capabilities and give them assistance in negotiating a range of outdoor environments. By contrast, environmental planners and designers focus on the physical environment as 'the patient' or the target of interventions: how can one adapt a particular environment, with all its idiosyncrasies, to serve people with a range of abilities and needs? And although landscape designers will usually have human well-being as a primary aim of their interventions, this may be just one of a range of concerns, sitting alongside biodiversity, hydrological systems management, carbon footprints and so on, as other measures of healthy landscapes.

While this difference may seem obvious it is not trivial, and can add to the challenge in developing the research agenda around environment and health. Randomised controlled trials have been developed as the best way to determine the effectiveness and value of interventions aimed at the individual. However, at a conceptual level, above and beyond any practical considerations, they are not the ideal tool for evaluating the influence of environment on health. They are based on the principle (admittedly not always easy to achieve in practice) that all but one factor can be held constant across a group of individuals, and that a single targeted change likely to influence health can consistently be applied to (or withheld from) each person. But the environment, particularly the outdoor environment, is multi-faceted and resistant to control in all kinds of ways. Setting aside important considerations of the social environment, the physical environment reflects major differences such as patterns of climate and weather but also the variations in development over different timescales, geological, biogeographical and historical, which are impossible to hold uniform when considering how one place might influence the health of one group of people compared with another.

When we consider the outdoors, most people's everyday living environments cannot be marshalled into categories that vary only in one or two aspects of the environment. Indeed, it is precisely this variation in season, time and at all scales of place that is a defining characteristic of the outdoor environment and can offer pleasure and interest, or discomfort and avoidance. It makes even longitudinal approaches, which can overcome many of the difficulties in studying the influence of landscape on health, subject to challenge at times. How do we manage this, then, in researching where best to intervene to improve health?

The answers, not surprisingly, are complex. One answer must be to look at specific places and to explore in depth what people experience when leading their everyday lives in such places. This requires qualitative approaches, sensitive methods to record the experience, and careful interpretation to tease out any relationship between landscape and well-being, especially if the researcher is to get a sense of what are likely to be several different mechanisms at work simultaneously. But in order to be able to generalise about salutogenic landscapes in any meaningful way, we also need to gather data systematically across a number of people and places, and to be able to test how robustly findings stand up when compared in this way. This is not new conceptually, of course, but of practical concern is the question of just how much data on the environment, and on individuals' experience of that environment, needs to be collected. Can we distinguish between aspects of the environment that matter and those that do not?

At present, researchers are attempting to include an ever-widening array of potentially relevant environmental factors in their data collection because we are not yet confident in our understanding of environment–human health relationships. Despite the analytical advantages that geographic information systems (GIS) now offer, such technology and computing power encourage us to collect and compile ever more data; yet this can be hugely time-consuming, especially if much of it must be newly collected in the field. The 'walkability' audit tools developed in various parts of the world to measure aspects of the urban street environment relevant to supporting people's walking behaviours are a case in point (see Pikora et al., 2002; De Bourdeaudhuij et al., 2005; Pikora et al., 2006; Bull et al., Chapter 4, this volume, and Millington et al., under review), where a vast effort in data collection often reveals how little we can be confident about in understanding what encourages people to walk. If we are to be efficient in our research, any insight or evidence that will help target data collection more effectively is to be welcomed.

Certain analytical options, such as multilevel modelling, recently being used by researchers to manage better the complexities of environmental data (for example, Maas et al., 2008; Burton et al., 2009), offer ways out of some of the difficulties described above. They are valuable in recognising the different scales at which the environment may have an influence, mirroring the multiple scales at which landscape planners, designers and managers have to work. I do not want to focus on such statistical techniques here, however, but rather on some other challenges in the basis for our approach to environmental research and its practical consequences for the environmental design professions.

The ecological approach and its multiple meanings

Just as the adjective 'sustainable' has had much of its meaning leached out through a myriad of interpretations, valuable though the underlying concept is, so also with the word 'ecological'. The view from different professional disciplines reveals quite different perspectives on what an ecological approach might mean. For many biologists and not a few landscape ecologists, the global environment is at the heart of any ecological approach, and a biocentric rather than anthropocentric view places humankind as just one among many species whose continuing existence relies on the health and equilibrium of the biosphere (Thompson, 2000). Here, the environment really is 'the patient', the focus of efforts to manage or intervene for better health and quality of life on the planet (see the Convention on Biological Diversity, 1993). Of course, the health of the planet is important for the health of humans, individually and collectively, but the emphasis for many environmental and conservation scientists is on the wider spectrum of biodi-versity and at a point on the scale quite distant from that of direct human concerns (see, for example, Margulis, 2000).

At the other end of the scale, with a clearly anthropocentric perspective, sits Bronfenbrenner's human ecology theory, drawing on the work of Vygotsky and others (Bronfenbrenner, 1979, 2005), where the individual human is the focus, 'the patient', around which nested ecological systems are located. Such ecological models have been taken up by researchers in a variety of ways, from the ecological psychology of Gibson and others (see Gibson 1979; Heft, Chapter 1, this volume), with its emphasis on the reciprocal relationship between perceiver and environment, to the socio-ecological models of behaviour change that underlie recent work on physical activity and health (see Bauer, 2003; Bull et al, Chapter 4, this volume) and emphasise the individual, societal and environmental context in which human behaviour takes place.

While these different perspectives require us to be careful, especially in landscape research, about just which perspective informs the 'ecological approach' being taken when one is described or promoted, they also offer some opportunities to think creatively. Landscape architects work within a framework where, implicitly or explicitly, the usual assumption is that environmental design is for human comfort and for biogeographical health at whatever scale the envir-onment is being considered. Mediation between approaches to ecology is a necessity and yet the ecological models available tend to sit in disciplinary silos. I believe there is an opportunity for landscape researchers to develop new models or approaches that bridge or transcend such divides, as a recent expert group have suggested (James et al., 2009).

For landscape planners and designers, one of the most useful, prac-tical outcomes of research on ecology from the biological sciences perspective has been the conceptual models produced by Forman and colleagues for the kinds of landscape patterns necessary to support different groups of animal species – concepts such as the landscape mosaic of patch, corridor and matrix – which offer a basis for making planning decisions that minimise habitat loss (Forman, 1995; Dramstad, Olson and Forman, 1996). However, *Homo sapiens* is not one of the species conventionally included in this model, other than as a destroyer or disrupter of other species' habitats, so the concepts serve the interests of biodiversity but not directly of human well-being. We need to develop models that take such ideas as Forman's and interpret them for human habitat, identifying the patterns of green and open space, in particular, that optimise quality of life and help humans flourish. Researchers are beginning to amass the arguments and the evidence that will help provide the basis for such models (Kaplan, Kaplan and Ryan, 1998; Ward Thompson, 2002; Handley et al., 2003; Sugiyama et al., 2008) but there is much still to be done to provide practicable guidance for environmental planning and design.

Environmental support for individuals' needs and desires

Research in environmental design, as outlined above, is likely to be focused on needs from and responses to the environment that are common across most of the population. How can one environment best enhance well-being for the diversity of people who spend time within it? If we take the Forman approach, the primary focus would be on biological needs – those aspects of the environment that serve our most fundamental requirements for survival and well-being at an instinctive level – and indeed it would be an enormously valuable contribution to landscape planning if our understanding of fundamental needs for engagement with the natural environment were better understood. Researchers such as Kaplan and Kaplan (1989), Kellert and Wilson with their biophilia hypothesis (1993), Hartig (2007) and Grahn and colleagues (Chapter 5, this volume) continue to make important contributions towards this goal.

Yet, if we are to understand what qualities of the environment are important to people's quality of life, we need to acknowledge the diversity as well as the commonality that exists in people's capabilities, experience, desires and needs. We need to understand the cultural, the social and the individual influences on what people seek, perceive and experience in the landscape around them, as Bronfenbrenner's approach to human ecology suggests. This is a challenge for landscape designers. Can one environment really serve this diversity? Is universal design really possible at all scales? And if there are conflicts, how can one identify and address them in design terms? The conventional approach in landscape planning and design has been to look for factors in the environment that matter to most people, or to one or more defined groups of people, and to address those factors with little regard for their relative importance (see, for example, the guidance by Project for Public Spaces: PPS, 2009). Yet, although many factors may be considered important (and often are) by respondents to conventional questionnaires on aspects of landscape and green space preference, some factors may weigh much more heavily in practice than others. The virtues of techniques such as conjoint analysis are that they can explore relative importance in a meaningful way, and help identify subgroups within a population for whom there are different priorities (see Aspinall, Chapter 7, this volume). Such techniques offer considerable practical benefits for planners in helping prioritise expenditure on the environment in the most effective way.

Recent research by OPENspace on older people's engagement with outdoor environments as part of the I'DGO project (Inclusive Design for Getting Outdoors – a collaboration with the Universities of Salford and Oxford Brookes) highlighted the necessity of considering environmental design from diverse user perspectives. As we focus more closely on the individual, it becomes apparent how different qualities and elements in the environment may be a matter of indif-ference (for example, certain colours if someone is visually impaired) or very important (for example, proximity of an accessible toilet if someone has a weak bladder). Our approach at OPENspace begins with a recognition of people's trans-actional relationship with place (Canter, 1985; Myers and Ward Thompson, 2003; Ward Thompson and Myers, 2004): that is, that people and their environment are part of a dynamic, interactive system where each reciprocally affects the other.

In exploring older people's access outdoors, where participants' life circumstances and abilities varied widely, it became apparent that there was considerable diversity in aspirations and requirements for getting outdoors. Equally, people limited their expectations of being able to use and enjoy the wider environment of streets and open spaces according to recent experience they had of such places. Bearing this in mind, we developed an approach that focused alternately on the environment and on the individual, recognising that, for any one person, the two are intimately linked, as the concept of affordance suggests (Heft, Chapter 1, this volume).

Initially we explored the notion of 'environmental supportiveness' as a way of conceptualising the relationship between the outdoor environment and an individual person's activities (Sugiyama and Ward Thompson, 2007c) (see Figure 9.1).

We developed two instruments to measure the quality of the envir-onment relevant to older people's outdoor activity, on the premise that environ-ments that make chosen outdoor activities easy and enjoyable are contributing to

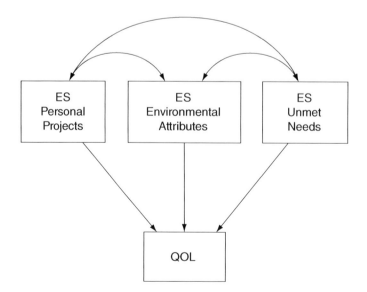

Figure 9.1 Quality of Life (QoL) predicted by Three Different Types of Environmental Support (ES) (from Sugiyama and Ward Thompson 2007c).

a better quality of life. One approach took a common set of environmental characteristics, identified as likely to be important from previous investigations, and
asked for individual responses to these; the other focused on each individual's
particular and unique demands for environmental support. For this latter, we
used Little's personal projects (1983 and Chapter 6, this volume) as a methodological approach, founded on Kelly's (1955) personal construct theory. In contrast
with normative ways of measuring the quality of the environment, where criteria
are fixed and are assumed to be salient to all, this idiographic method makes it
possible to assess environmental supportiveness based on individuals' personal
projects – the things they plan or would like to do – and a relevant setting within
which such projects or activities would be undertaken. It offers a unique way of
investigating how well individuals' needs, desires and aspirations are supported
or frustrated by their environment and how well people cope with the environment in which they find themselves (Sugiyama and Ward Thompson, 2007a).

Some typical personal projects that involve going outdoors for our
older participants included:

- 'playing with my grandchildren'
- 'cleaning the car once a week'
- 'going shopping'
- 'gardening'.

However, we also elicited less usual projects from some people:

- 'practising putting [for golf] in my garden'
- 'being the school [road] crossing patrol'
- 'being the "appropriate adult" in police station interviews' [for when a
juvenile or mentally vulnerable person has been detained in police custody].

Clearly the kind of environment needed to support some of these projects (for
example, playing with grandchildren, or practising putting) is quite different than
for others (for instance, getting to the police station) but the environment can
potentially make any of them easy and pleasant, or difficult and frustrating.

Ongoing analysis of results from this exploratory work helps us understand better the difference that landscape design can make to a variety of idiosyncratic demands from the environment, while choice-based conjoint analysis
(one variant of the conjoint family of methods – see Aspinall, Chapter 7, this
volume) has helped us to understand what aspects of a local park make most
difference to older people as a group, and how differing priorities distinguish
between subgroups within this population (Alves et al., 2008; Aspinall et al.,
2010, in press). In this sample of participants from the I'DGO project, those who
live with someone else but have difficulty getting around consider facilities such

as toilets and a café to have greater importance than nuisances such as vandalism or dog fouling. By contrast, for those who live alone and have no mobility difficulties, nuisances are the most important factor and facilities less so. In both cases, trees and plants are the second most important park attribute in terms of preference for a local open space (see Figures 9.2(a) and 9.2(b)).

One recurring theme in such research is the importance of the outdoor environment as a social context. Our research with older people suggests benefits to well-being and quality of life may be as likely to arise from social contact in the outdoor environment as from contact with nature or engaging in physical activity (Sugiyama and Ward Thompson, 2007b). As environmental psychologists have pointed out (Canter, 1985; Scott, 1998), while the physical environment has a significant role to play in everyday life, this role is rarely explicit unless a feature of the physical environment obstructs, prevents or otherwise interferes with a person's objectives (Myers and Ward Thompson, 2003). Of course, these objectives may have to do with enjoyment of aspects of the physical environment, as our I'DGO project participants told us when they highlighted the natural environment and wildlife as reasons for getting outdoors. But for some age groups, especially teenagers, the physical environment is often no more than a backdrop to the all-important social aspects of life.

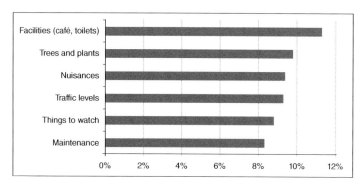

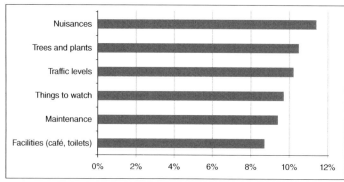

Figure 9.2 Most important attributes of a local park for older participants (aged over 60 years) who (a, above) live with someone else and who have difficulty getting about and (b, below) who live alone and have no difficulty getting about. This illustrates the results of a choice-based conjoint approach, using redundancy analysis to explore how differences in importance are related to individuals' personal characteristics (from Aspinall et al., 2010, in press).

When we were exploring young people's needs and desires in relation to the outdoor environment (Travlou, 2007), we frequently found that, when we asked what they liked about the physical environment, they described the social. The physical environment was often only described when it was considered negative or unpleasant, a detractor to desired social goals. Yet landscape architects and other environmental professionals are focused on planning, designing and managing the physical environment, and it is this aspect that we want to understand better through our research. We often get a sense of the barriers to access and enjoyment of the environment – people seem to find such things easy to describe – but we also need to explore the factors in the physical environment that attract people outdoors. These are not simply the opposite of what constrains access and use, and our work with a range of different social groups reinforces the importance of understanding these too, difficult though it is to elicit the information at times. In recent I'DGO research with older people, the constraints to using parks and outdoor space included graffiti, dog fouling and other signs of incivility, as well as heavy traffic on roads, but the natural environment – trees, natural vegetation and wildlife – was shown to be an important attractor, in some cases overriding negative aspects of the environment (Alves et al., 2008; Aspinall, Chapter 7, this volume; Aspinall et al., 2010, in press). It is just this kind of trade-off that we need to understand better.

Environmental support for physical activity

The above suggests that the physical environment may offer support for, or hinder, dimensions of health and well-being in a number of different ways. One conceptualisation of environment–person interaction is the notion that there may be salutogenic environments: that is, environments that support healthy behaviours and responses, by contrast with, for example, obesogenic environments which support lifestyles that are conducive to people being overweight (Bull et al., Chapter 4, this volume), or stressful environments that affect mental and physical health in other ways (Hartig, 2007). Public health concerns over sedentary lifestyles and imbalance between energy expenditure and energy intake in the populations of the developed world have led to a particular focus on environments that encourage people to walk more, since walking has been called 'the nearest activity to perfect exercise' (Morris and Hardman, 1997: 328), is available to young and old, rich and poor, and requires no specialist skills or equipment. The question for researchers like us is: what qualities in the outdoor environment (where most walking is likely to happen) might have an influence on how much people walk?

Such a simple-sounding challenge is immensely difficult to address, as Chapter 4 by Bull and colleagues attests. OPENspace research has identified some of the salient factors for older people in Britain (Sugiyama and Ward Thompson, 2008) and underlines the fact that, in walking for leisure, people seek different support from the environment compared with walking for transport – where getting from A to B is the primary objective (see Figure 9.3).

In the context of growing international interest in 'walkability' (Cortright, 2009; Bull et al., Chapter 4, this volume), OPENspace researchers have recently been engaged in developing audits to assess the quality of the urban environment in a more precise way, and in particular to assess how well it encourages walking. Our work initially attempted to assess the walkability of an area in Glasgow, as part of a SPARColl (the Scottish Physical Activity Research Collaboration) project researching the effectiveness of methods to modify walking behaviours (Fitzsimons et al., 2008). The focus for OPENspace has been, first, to develop a reliable objective audit tool that is appropriate to the European city, by contrast with North American and Australian instruments developed to date. We have produced a Scottish Walkability Assessment Tool (SWAT: see Millington et al., 2009) which is now being tested in other residential urban areas in England and Wales as part of the I'DGO project (see <www.idgo.ac.uk>). In doing this, we have noted that many British urban contexts are very well connected for pedestrians in terms of street pattern, and almost universally served with footways (pavements or sidewalks), by comparison with North American examples in particular. The challenge, then, is to test the sensitivity of our walkability tool to walking levels by seeing how well audits of the neighbourhood environment predict project participants' step counts using pedometers.

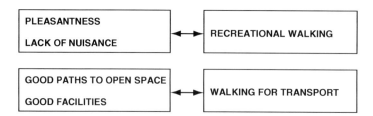

How do perceived quality and accessibility of neighbourhood open spaces affect patterns of activity?

A more pleasant neighbourhood open space is associated with a 40% increase in the likelihood of achieving more than 1 hour of recreational walking per week

(Logistic regression, odds ratio 1.41, (95% confidence intervals 1.01–1.98, p<0.05)

Figure 9.3

Features of local open spaces that make a difference to recreational walking as opposed to walking for transport, for older people. Pleasantness includes an attractive, relaxing open space that is good for chatting and for children to play in; nuisance includes vandalism and dog fouling and 'youngsters hanging around'; good paths are ones that are easy to walk on and enjoyable; facilities include public transport, toilets and shelters, and a range of activities (after Sugiyama and Ward Thompson 2008).

Initial results on baseline walking levels in the Glasgow project suggest that there are comparatively low levels of association between street environment audits and walking activity (Millington et al., under review). It seems likely that the everyday street environment of many urban areas in Britain is good enough to make walking easy if people wish to do so, and that other factors (social as well as physical) are the principal determinants of how much walking people undertake. Further analysis is being undertaken to explore whether the physical environment plays a stronger role in relation to interventions such as pedometer use to increase walking levels. Whatever the outcome of this latter analysis, it will be important to see whether we can identify what makes a 'good enough' environment for walking. Future research can usefully explore where thresholds lie for different groups in terms of environmental support for walking.

Our I'DGO TOO (phase two) project is exploring older people's outdoor activity in urban areas of high multiple deprivation, where a longitudinal study will assess what difference environmental changes to the residential streets make in terms of this activity. We are using sites where Home Zone type environmental modifications are being implemented, to change the residential streets to shared space streets under Sustrans' 'DIY Streets' programme (Department for Transport, 2005; Sustrans, 2009). Comparison with control sites nearby will help in assessing whether this kind of small-scale, local change to the street environment around people's homes makes a difference to the time older people spend outside the home, the kinds of activities they undertake and the level of activity (particularly walking). A modified version of the SWAT walkability audit is being used, along with behaviour observation of street use and accelerometers to measure activity levels of older participants (see Figures 9.4, 9.5, 9.6 and 9.7).

Such research will help address questions of environmental support for walking using objective measures – very useful to environmental designers – but in order to understand the mechanisms behind any relationship between physical environment and walking, we need to compare such measures with local participants' subjective assessments of their environment and their desired activities and needs. In all of the projects just described, subjective assessments of participants' perceptions, activities and use are also being elicited. Comparisons between subjective and objective measures, and assessments of which best predict walking and other activity levels, will help our understanding of what aspects of the physical environment make a place 'walkable' and, of particular interest, where the physical environment is a constraint on walking (where that threshold may lie) or where it is an enticement to walk. We continue to use a Personal Projects approach (Little, 1983; Sugiyama and Ward Thompson, 2007a) as part of the methodology, to elicit what is idiosyncratic in participants' desires and needs for outdoor activities, to help understand how environmental support for walking may vary according to these projects, and what difference that may make to overall levels of activity and quality of life.

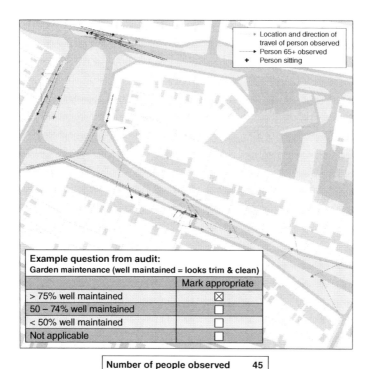

Figure 9.4
Behaviour
observation map
of street use from
the I'DGO TOO
project, showing a
typical case study
street (before
implementation of
any 'DIY Street'
environmental
changes) with
mapped
observations of
use, and (lower
left) an example
question from the
modified SWAT
walkability street
audit undertaken
on all such case
study streets.

Example question from audit:
Garden maintenance (well maintained = looks trim & clean)

	Mark appropriate
> 75% well maintained	☒
50 – 74% well maintained	☐
< 50% well maintained	☐
Not applicable	☐

Number of people observed   45

Gender

Males	25
Females	20

Age group

Child	11
Teenager	6
Young adult (<40)	15
Older adult (40 to <65)	15
65+	7

Mobility

No mobility issues	44
Using a wheelchair	1

Social interaction

Alone, no interaction with anyone	32
Talking to another person	12
Playing	1

Physical activity

Walking/using a wheelchair	32
Cycling	5
Walking a dog/other pet activity	3
Walking a baby/other child activity	2
Standing	1
Sitting	1
Running/other exercise	1

Support for walking in the natural environment

Much emphasis has been placed on the urban environment as salutogenic (or otherwise), since Britain (and the Western world) is such an urbanised society. Yet the tools for measuring walkability that have been developed recently, as part of the push to understand what encourages active lifestyles, have largely focused

Figure 9.5
Attributes
included in the
I'DGO TOO street
audit tool for the
first phase of the
case study surveys
(a modified
version of the
Scottish
Walkability Audit
Tool (SWAT),
Millington et al,
2009).

Types of building or features	On-road features (continued)
Residential buildings	Crossing aids
Types of commercial destinations	Bike parking facilities
Types of public or government services	Driveway crossovers
Transportation facility	Surveillance
Types of recreational facilities	Garden maintenance
Path for walking	Verge maintenance
Type of path	**Cleanliness**
Path location	Graffiti and vandalism
Path material	Litter / discarded items
Usable width of pavement	Dog fouling
Slope	Seating
Path condition and smoothness	Public toilets
Permanent path obstructions	**Trees**
On-road features	Tree height
Slope (only assessed on-road if no path is present)	Percentage of hedge along the segment
	Hedge height
Condition of road (only assessed if no path is present)	**Types of views**
	How alike are the building designs?
Vehicle parking	**Attractiveness**
Traffic control devices	**Continuity of path**
Type of pedestrian crossings	**Signage**

Figure 9.6
London, England:
a typical case
study street from
the I'DGO TOO
project, (before
implementation of
any 'DIY Street'
environmental
changes) 2008.

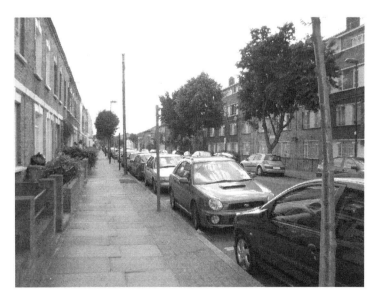

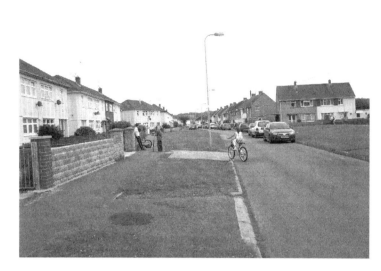

Figure 9.7
Bridgend, Wales: a
typical case study
street from the
I'DGO TOO
project, (before
implementation of
any 'DIY Street'
environmental
changes) 2008.

on walking for transport, and that in turn has meant a focus on street walkability. Important though street walkability is for understanding people's activity levels as part of daily life, it ignores walking within (rather than alongside) more natural environments such as parks, riversides or woodlands. Such environments are likely to play a much larger role in walking for leisure than in walking for transport, but this can be an important part of daily activity too, especially for certain groups within the population, as our I'DGO research with older people (a growing proportion of the population) has shown (Sugiyama and Ward Thompson, 2008). Since we know that natural environments may offer health benefits in addition to those derived from physical activity (de Vries, Chapter 3, this volume), it is a noticeable gap that audit tools have yet to be developed to adequately address this, although a number of contributors to this volume have begun to address some of the issues. The range of variability in topography, vegetation, visual permeability, surface quality and so on that is displayed in natural or green environments, especially as seasons change, is much greater and more complex than in hard, built environments and, for this reason, natural environments are much more difficult to map and audit in meaningful ways. Yet, for landscape designers and managers, this is of crucial interest.

Kaplan and colleagues (1998) have contributed much to our understanding of responses to the visual structure of the landscape as a whole, but the approach has focused more on static views than on the dynamic, spatial experience of moving through the landscape. Giles-Corti's team in Western Australia have developed a Quality of Public Open Space Tool (POST) (Broomhall,

Giles-Corti and Lange, 2004) which has an emphasis on individual elements in the landscape but is less good at recording the whole as a spatial composition and experience. Space Syntax approaches (Conroy Dalton and Hanson, Chapter 8, this volume) take movement through the environment as a key to understanding how places are used, but ultimately pay more attention to connectedness than to the detailed experience of environmental features. Such considerations raise larger questions about how the environment, natural or built, is experienced in real life, highly relevant to walking but poorly served by the range of audit tools currently developed. And it is in the context of green environments, where natural elements may predominate or play a significant role, that these issues come to the fore.

Understanding the dynamic experience of the landscape

In attempting to understand the experience of the landscape and responses to that experience, much has been much written over many years on landscape aesthetics (for instance, Appleton, 1975; Bourassa, 1991) and how this might influence preference and use (for example, Kaplan and Kaplan, 1989). Abstract experiential qualities such as perceptions of 'safety' and 'attractiveness' have been identified as important factors in stated preferences for parks and green spaces (Bedimo-Rung, Mowen and Cohen, 2005; CABE Space, 2007). However, there are few tools to measure the dynamic spatial experience in practice.

At OPENspace we have been working for some time to develop a mapping tool, drawing on the pioneering work of Appleyard, Lynch and Myer (1964) and University of Edinburgh graduate student work (1974), to record the experience of moving along a path in the landscape in relation to the changing pattern of the surrounding vegetation, landform and structures. This 'view from the path' mapping has been used in a number of research projects relating to forest and woodland landscapes (Ward Thompson et al., 2004; Ward Thompson, Roe and Alves, 2007) and we hope to develop it further as a reliable form of data collection which can be compared with other data on attitudes to the landscape and landscape use. Uniquely, it offers a means to research links between the spatial and structural properties of landscape design and human behaviour. It has also provided a basis for understanding aspects of wayfinding that are relevant to countryside users (Southwell and Findlay, 2007) and has informed the production of a wayfinding assessment toolkit for countryside site managers (Southwell, Ward Thompson and Findlay, 2007).

We are conscious that we need to develop audit or mapping tools that can be used reliably by different auditors to record the dynamic experience of

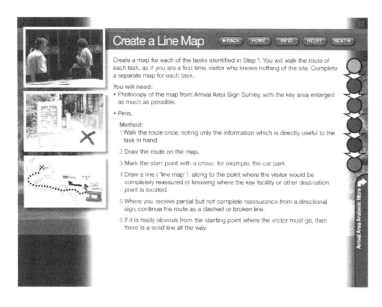

Figure 9.8
A page from Site
Finder, the
wayfinding
assessment toolkit
for countryside
site managers,
based on
researching the
links between the
spatial and
structural
properties of
landscape design
and human
behaviour (from
Southwell, Ward
Thompson and
Findlay, 2007).

landscape but also that we need to record this in a way that speaks the language of landscape designers and articulates the landscape's underlying structure meaningfully to such professionals. It is no easy task. We have been developing a vocabulary of mapping symbols to help capture the experience of walking through a green or wooded landscape (see Figure 9.9), and these, in the hands of someone trained, can quite effectively convey something of the difference between sites and experiences (see Figures 9.10 and 9.11 a and b). The experience can be quite different in summer from in winter, and so such mapping may need to be done at least twice in the course of a year to capture the seasonal change in experience.

There is much work still to be done on testing reliability and, more crucially, testing how well such mapping can predict users' perceptions and levels of use for pathways mapped in this way. Nonetheless, we hope that we are developing a tool that can start to bridge some of the divides between different theoretical perspectives and their manifestations in research practice. It can encompass ecological approaches relating both to natural science and to human ecology; it helps link environment–behaviour relationships with the dynamic experience of the physical and spatial structure of the landscape; it might even offer a way to map affordances (Heft, Chapter 1, this volume).

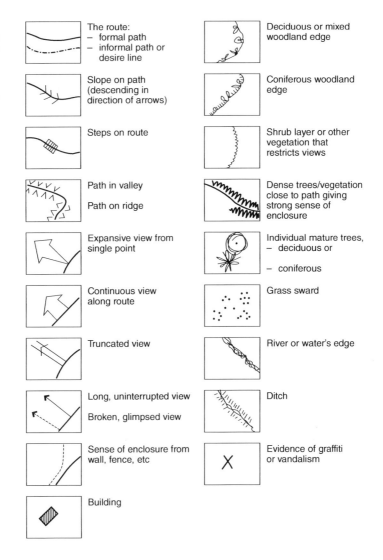

Figure 9.9
Mapping symbols
developed to help
capture the
dynamic
experience of
walking through a
green or wooded
landscape (after
Appleyard et al.,
1964; Edinburgh
University, 1974;
Ward Thompson
et al, 2004;
Southwell et al,
2009).

Where do we go from here?

Overall, within landscape research, there remains a need to better understand what level of availability and/or qualities of the landscape are important or relevant for different people's health and quality of life. More particularly, we need to understand what kinds of interventions in the physical environment (recognising these may need to be accompanied by social interventions) are likely to make a difference to well-being, and for whom.

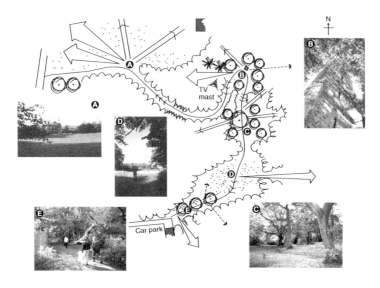

Figure 9.10
Mapping the
experience of
walking through a
wooded landscape
in Corstorphine,
Edinburgh (after
Ward Thompson
et al., 2004).

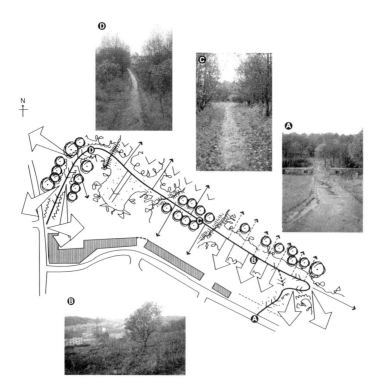

Figure 9.11a
Mapping the
experience of
walking through a
wooded landscape
in Drumchapel,
Glasgow, in winter
(after Ward
Thompson et al.,
2007).

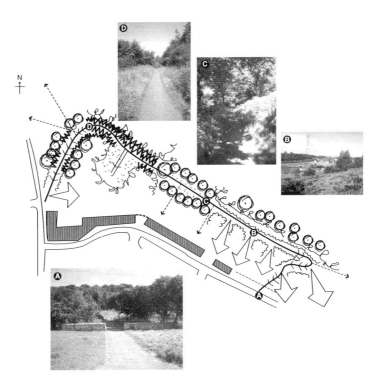

Figure 9.11b
Mapping the
experience of
walking through a
wooded landscape
in Drumchapel,
Glasgow, in
summer (after
Ward Thompson
et al., 2007) .

Heft's approach to affordance (Chapter 1, this volume) places the environment in the spotlight but recognises the vital importance of the person in relationship with that environment. Little's work on personal projects (this volume) places the individual person in the spotlight but recognises the importance of environment as supporting or thwarting projects. Heft talks about affordances as opportunities for action; he makes clear that some environments attract action and others repel, and that such relationships are culturally laden. Observation of behaviour settings is a valuable tool in understanding better what opportunities different kinds of environments offer to different people (Moore and Cosco, Chapter 2, this volume; Goličnik and Ward Thompson, 2010) but, unless we also engage with those people directly, we are unlikely to understand the culturally infused motivations behind affordances. Certainly a personal projects approach can help us unpack some of this, as we have found in OPENspace research. As always, the challenge for landscape designers is to determine what one, common environment can offer that best serves the range of individual needs and desires.

A student of landscape architecture here in Edinburgh has produced a nice diagram to illustrate a way to conceptualise the places of plurality that we need to plan and design, to integrate different users, people from different ages and backgrounds (see Figure 9.12). It recognises that different parts of, say, the neighbourhood environment will offer affordances for individuals, depending on their lifestyles, and that there will be places in common, where the affordances intersect, as well as places that only serve a subset of the population, often a minority, but that may be valuably integrated into the whole.

The park plan is based on a model of spatial use by different characters and their interaction. This is a conceptul diagram of how to lay out the characters' spaces: the larger the circled outline, the greater the character's range; the darker the shade, the more the character interacts with other characters.

Figure 9.12
A conceptual diagram of how to plan a park for different users' needs and range of movement. Diagram: Thomas Clark, Landscape Architecture student, Edinburgh College of Art.

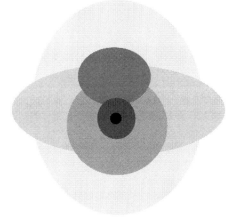

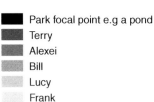

Park focal point e.g a pond
Terry
Alexei
Bill
Lucy
Frank

| Terry squirrel | Alexei child | Bill older person | Lucy teenager | Frank and Alfie dog walker and dog |

What might a landscape design based on affordances, personal projects and encouragement to be healthy and physically active look like? One fundamental question is, what will entice people out of doors? This is especially important for older people and others living in some form of care home, where there is often quite restricted access outdoors (see Zeisel, 2007). Once out of doors, what will encourage people into places that are salutogenic? Despite much research high-lighting people's fears for their safety in green and public spaces (Croucher, Myers and Bretherton, 2007; Greenspace Scotland, nd), there is also evidence that green space and nature can be enticing, that biophilia may be at the heart of what is attractive in many cases, despite these fears (Kaplan and Kaplan, 1989; Kellert and Wilson, 1993; Frumkin, 2001; Hartig, 2007). So green places do seem to be important, and perhaps our 'view from the path' tool can help understand the affordances of such places offer as people enter and move around within them. Certainly, within the broader landscape of the neighbourhood environment, there would need to be opportunities for energetic activity, places for children to scramble and explore; access for people with different physical abilities and requirements; places to be noisy and boisterous and places to be quiet, separate, to 'get away' and feel alone, or protected and calm.

Many of these already exist, of course, so perhaps a neighbourhood mapping is needed to get sense of what is missing. We need to look at a variety of scales and social contexts if we are to address socio-spatial inequalities in planning and designing our communities. Audits by different groups can help us understand some of the diversity of needs and users' perspectives, as has been promoted by CABE Space (2007) for example, and been implemented in different ways in many different contexts, from local parks to neighbourhood woodlands (for example, Ward Thompson et al., 2007; Elders Council of Newcastle, 2008). Such approaches, combined with a mapping of the spatial experience, can offer valuable insights into the kinds of affordances that are available or lacking. In the case of green space such as woodlands, for example, we have started to artic-ulate some of the questions that help pinpoint where design intervention may be necessary. 'Where do I go to get to the woodland? Is this the woodland I'm looking for? Where is the entrance? What can I do here? Is it safe? Will I be able to find my way back? What kinds of views will I get (and will there be a bench where I'd like it when I want to enjoy the view or need a rest)?' (Southwell, Ward Thompson and Roe, 2009). Such simple questions as these may be all that is necessary to elicit a sense of whether a place entices or repels, and what it offers different individuals, but they need to sit within a wider theoretical understanding of the relationship between environment and health, between the quality of the landscape and quality of life, if we are to be truly effective in designing land-scapes to make a difference.

In OPENspace, we continue to undertake research building on the opportunities offered by projective approaches to engagement with place, and the concept of affordance. In addition, the use of personal projects analysis makes it possible to conceptualise and assess environmental supportiveness based on individuals' needs, wants and personally available environments. We believe such approaches can help build the theoretical link for understanding the relationship between the individual, the quality of the landscape (especially the local outdoor environment) and quality of life. And, finally, we believe that the development of 'view from the path' mapping techniques offers the possibility of linking environment–behaviour relationships with the dynamic experience of the physical and spatial structure of the landscape in a manner that can speak directly to landscape designers, planners and managers.

References

Alves, S., Aspinall, P., Ward Thompson, C., Sugiyama, T., Brice, R. and Vickers, A. (2008) 'Preferences of older people for environmental attributes of local parks: the use of choice-based conjoint analysis', *Facilities*, 26 (11/ 12): 433–53.

Appleton, J. (1975) *The Experience of Landscape*, New York: Wiley.

Appleyard, D., Lynch, K. and Myer, J. R. (1964) *The View from the Road*, Cambridge, Mass.: MIT Press.

Aspinall, P., Ward Thompson, C., Alves, S., Sugiyama, T., Vickers, A. and Brice, R. (2010, in press) 'Understanding the relative importance of older people's preferences for different attributes of neighbourhood open space', *Environment and Planning B*.

Bauer, G., Davies, J. K., Pelikan, J., Noack, H., Broesskamp, U. and Hill, C. (2003) 'Advancing a theoretical model for public health and health promotion indicator development. Proposal from the EUHPID consortium', *European Journal of Public Health*, 13: 107–13 (supplement).

Bedimo-Rung, A. L., Mowen, A. J. and Cohen, D. A. (2005) 'The significance of parks to physical activity and public health: A conceptual model', *American Journal of Preventive Medicine*, 28 (2S2): 159–68.

Bell, S., Morris, N., Findlay, C., Travlou, P., Montarzino, A., Gooch, D. et al. (2004) *Nature for People: The Importance of Green Spaces to East Midlands Communities*, Research Report 567, Peterborough: English Nature.

Bourassa, S. C. (1991) *The Aesthetics of Landscape*, New York: Belhaven.

Bronfenbrenner, U. (1979) *The Ecology of Human Development*, Cambridge, Mass.: Harvard University Press.

Bronfenbrenner, U. (ed.) (2005) *Making Human Beings Human: Bioecological Perspectives on Human Development*, Thousand Oaks, Calif.: Sage.

Broomhall, M., Giles-Corti, B. and Lange, A. (2004) Quality of Public Open Space Tool (POST). Perth, Western Australia.

Burton, N. W., Haynes, M., Wilson, L. M., Giles-Corti, B., Oldenburg, B. F., Brown, W. J., Giskes, K. and Turrell, G. (2009) 'HABITAT: A longitudinal multilevel study of physical activity change in mid-aged adults', *BMC Public Health*, 9: 76.

CABE Space (2005a) *Does Money Grow on Trees?* London: Commission for Architecture and the Built Environment (CABE).

CABE Space (2005b) *Start with the Park: Creating Sustainable Urban Green Spaces in Areas of Housing Growth and Renewal*, London: CABE.

CABE Space (2007) *Spaceshaper: A User's Guide*, London: CABE.

CABE Space (2009) *Making the Invisible Visible: The Real Value of Park Assets*, London: CABE.

Canter, D. (1985) 'The Road to Jerusalem', in D. Canter (ed.) *Facet Theory: Approaches to Social Research*, New York: Springer-Verlag.

Convention on Biological Diversity (1993) Convention on Biological Diversity (with annexes). Concluded at Rio de Janeiro on 5 June 1992, registered ex officio on 29 December 1993, available at: <http://www.cbd.int/convention/convention.shtml> (accessed 21 August 2009).

Cortright, J. (2009) Walking the Walk: How Walkability Raises Home Values in U.S. Cities, Cortright, Impresa, for CEOs for Cities, August 2009, available at: <http://blog.walkscore.com/wp-content/uploads/2009/08/WalkingTheWalk_CEOsforCities.pdf> (accessed 23 August 2009).

Croucher, K., Myers, L. and Bretherton, J. (2007) The Links Between Greenspace and Health: A Critical Literature Review, York: University of York.

De Bourdeaudhuij, I., Teixeira, P., Cardon, G. and Deforche, B. (2005) 'Environmental and psycho-social correlates of physical activity in Portuguese and Belgian adults', Public Health Nutrition, 8 (7): 886–95.

Department for Transport (DfT) (2005) Home Zones: Challenging the Future of our Streets, London: DfT.

Dramstad, W. E., Olson, J. D. and Forman, R. T. T. (1996) Landscape Ecology Principles in Landscape Architecture and Land-Use Planning, Washington, D.C.: Harvard University GSD, Island Press and ASLA.

Edinburgh, University of (1974) Applecross Peninsula Study 2, Postgraduate Diploma in Landscape Architecture, Second Year Project, 1973-74, University of Edinburgh.

Elders Council of Newcastle (2008). Older Person Friendly City Parks and Recreation Areas: Report from Working Group, September 2008, Newcastle upon Tyne: Elders Council of Newcastle.

Fitzsimons, C., Baker, G., Wright, A., Nimmo, M., Ward Thompson, C., Lowry, R., Millington, C., Shaw, R., Fenwick, E., Ogilvie, D., Inchley, J. and Mutrie, N. (2008) 'The 'Walking for Well-being in the West' study, a pedometer-based walking programme in combination with a physical activity consultation with 12-month follow-up: rationale and study design', BMC Public Health, 8: 259.

Forman, R. T. T. (1995) Land Mosaics: The Ecology of Landscapes and Regions, Cambridge: Cambridge University Press.

Frumkin, H. (2001) 'Beyond toxicity: human health and the natural environment', American Journal of Preventive Medicine, 20 (3): 234–40.

Gibson, J. (1979) The Ecological Approach to Visual Perception, Boston, Mass.: Houghton-Mifflin.

Goličnik, B. and Ward Thompson, C. (2010) 'Emerging relationships between design and use of urban park spaces', Landscape and Urban Planning, 94: 38–53.

Greenspace Scotland (2008) Greenspace and Quality of Life: A Critical Literature Review, Research Report, Stirling: Greenspace Scotland.

Greenspace Scotland (nd) Greenspace and Community Safety. Making the Links: Technical Briefing Note No. 9. Commissioned jointly by Communities Scotland, NHS Health Scotland, Scottish Natural Heritage and Greenspace Scotland. Stirling: Greenspace Scotland.

Greenspace Scotland (2009) Making the Links: Greenspace for a more Successful and Sustainable Scotland, Stirling: Greenspace Scotland.

Handley, J., Pauleit, S., Slinn, P., Barber, A., Baker, M., Jones, C. et al. (2003). Accessible Natural Green Space Standards in Towns and Cities: A Review and Toolkit for their Implementation, Research Report 526, Peterborough: English Nature.

Hartig, T. (2007). 'Three steps to understanding restorative environments as health resources', in C. Ward Thompson and P. Travlou (eds), Open Space: People Space, Abingdon: Taylor & Francis: 163–79.

Hartig, T., Evans, G. W., Jamner, L. D., Davis, D. S. and Garling, T. (2003) 'Tracking restoration in natural and urban field settings', Journal of Environmental Psychology, 23 (2): 109–23.

I'DGO (Inclusive Design for Getting Outdoors) <http://www.idgo.ac.uk>.

James, P., Tzoulos, K., Adams, M. D., Barber, A., Box, J., Breuste, J., Elmqvist, T., Frith, M., Gordon, C., Greening, K. L., Handley, J., Haworth, S., Kazmierczak, A. E., Johnston, M., Korpela, K., Moretti, M., Niemalä, J., Pauleit, S., Roe, M. H., Sadler, J. P. and Ward Thompson, C. (2009) 'Towards an integrated understanding of green space in the built environment', Urban Forestry and Urban Greening, 8: 65–75.

Kaplan, R. and Kaplan, S. (1989) The Experience of Nature: A Psychological Perspective, New York: Cambridge University Press.

Kaplan, R., Kaplan, S. and Ryan, R. L. (1998) With People in Mind: Design and Management of Everyday Nature, Washington, D.C.: Island Press.

Kellert, R. and Wilson, E. O. (eds.) (1993) *The Biophilia Hypothesis*, Washington, D.C.: Island Press.

Kelly, G. (1955) *The Psychology of Personal Constructs*, New York: Norton.

Little, B. R. (1983) 'Personal projects: A rationale and method for investigation', *Environment and Behavior*, 15 (3): 273–309.

Little, B. R. (2000) 'Persons, contexts, and personal projects: assumptive themes of a methodological transactionalism', in S. Wapner, J. Demick, T. Yamamoto and H. Minami (eds), *Theoretical Perspectives in Environment–Behavior Research: Underlying Assumptions, Research Problems, and Methodologies*, New York: Plenum.

Maas, J., Verheij, R. A., Spreeuwenberg, P. and Groenewegen, P. P. (2008) 'Physical activity as a possible mechanism behind the relationship between green space and health: a multilevel analysis', *BMC Public Health*, 8: e206.

Margulis, L. (2000) *Symbiotic Planet (A New Look at Evolution)*, New York: Basic Books.

Millington, C., Ward Thompson, C., Rowe, D., Aspinall, P., Fitzsimons, C., Nelson, N. and Mutrie, N. (2009) 'Development of the Scottish Walkability Assessment Tool (SWAT)', *Health and Place*, 15: 474–81.

Millington, C., Aspinall, P., Baker, G., Fitzsimons, C., Mutrie, N. and Ward Thompson, C. (under review) *Does the environment around people's homes predict how much they walk?*

Morris, J. N. and Hardman, A. (1997) 'Walking to health', *Sports Medicine*, 23: 306–32.

Myers, M. S. and Ward Thompson, C. (2003) 'Interviews and questionnaires', in S. Bell (ed.), *Crossplan: Integrated, Participatory Landscape Planning as a Tool for Rural Development*, Edinburgh: Forestry Commission: 17–29.

Pikora, T., Bull, F., Jamrozik, K., Knuiman, M., Giles-Corti, B. and Donovan, R. (2002) 'Developing a reliable audit instrument to measure the physical environment for physical activity', *American Journal of Preventive Medicine*, 23: 187–94.

Pikora, T., Giles-Corti, B., Knuiman, M., Bull, F., Jamrozik, K. and Donovan, R. (2006) 'Neighborhood environmental factors correlated with walking near home: Using SPACES', *Medicine and Science in Sports and Exercise*, 38 (4): 708–14.

PPS (2009) *Key Factors in Planning, Designing and Maintaining Safer Parks*, available at: <http://www.pps.org/info/design/toronto_safety_2> (accessed 12 September 2009).

Saelens, B. E., Sallis, J. F., Black, J. B. and Chen, D. (2003) 'Neighborhood-based differences in physical activity: an environment scale evaluation', *American Journal of Public Health*, 93: 1552–8.

Scott, M. J. (1998) *The Environmental Correlates of Creativity and Innovation in Industrial Research Laboratories*, Ph.D. thesis, University of Liverpool.

Southwell, K. and Findlay, C. (2007) '"You just follow the signs": understanding visitor wayfinding problems in the countryside', in C. Ward Thompson and P. Travlou (eds), *Open Space: People Space*, Abingdon: Routledge: 11124.

Southwell, K., Ward Thompson, C. and Findlay, C. (2007) *Site Finder: Assessing the Countryside Visitor's Wayfinding Experience*, Edinburgh: OPENspace research centre, Edinburgh College of Art.

Southwell, K., Ward Thompson, C. and Roe, J. (2009) *Better Woodland Walks* (Unpublished pilot audit tool by OPENspace research centre), Edinburgh College of Art, for Forestry Commission Scotland.

Sugiyama, T., Leslie, E., Giles-Corti, B. and Owen, N. (2008) 'Associations of neighbourhood greenness with physical and mental health: do walking, social coherence and local social interaction explain the relationships?' *Journal of Epidemiology and Community Health*, 62:e9.

Sugiyama, T. and Ward Thompson, C. (2007a) 'Measuring the quality of the outdoor environment relevant to older people's lives', in C. Ward Thompson and P. Travlou (eds.) *Open Space: People Space*, Abingdon: Taylor & Francis: 153–62.

Sugiyama, T. and Ward Thompson, C. (2007b) 'Older people's health, outdoor activity and supportiveness of neighbourhood environments', *Landscape and Urban Planning*, 83: 168–75.

Sugiyama, T. and Ward Thompson, C. (2007c) 'Outdoor environments, activity and the well-being of older people: conceptualising environmental support', *Environment and Planning A*, 39: 1943–60.

Sugiyama, T. and Ward Thompson, C. (2008) 'Associations between characteristics of neighbourhood open space and older people's walking', *Urban Forestry and Urban Greening*, 7 (1): 41–51.

Sustrans (2009) *DIY Streets, Project Review 2009*, Bristol: Sustrans.

Thompson, I. (2000) *Ecology, Community and Delight: Sources of Values in Landscape Architecture*, London: E. & F. N. Spon.

Travlou, P. (2007) 'Mapping youth spaces in the public realm: identity, space and social exclusion', in C. Ward Thompson and P. Travlou (eds), *Open Space: People Space*, London: Taylor & Francis: 71–81.

Ward Thompson, C. (2002) 'Urban open space in the 21st century', *Landscape and Urban Planning*, 60 (2): 59–72.

Ward Thompson, C. (2005) 'Common threads in a changing world: landscape and health.' Keynote paper presented at 'Landscape Change', 17th European Council of Landscape Architecture Schools (ECLAS) Conference, Ankara University, 14-18 September 2005.

Ward Thompson, C., Aspinall, P., Bell, S., Findlay, C., Wherrett, J. and Travlou, P. (2004). *Open Space and Social Inclusion: Local Woodland Use in Central Scotland*, Edinburgh: Forestry Commission.

Ward Thompson, C., Aspinall, P., Bell, S. and Findlay, C. (2005) ''It gets you away from everyday life': local woodlands and community use what makes a difference?', *Landscape Research*, 30 (1): 109–46.

Ward Thompson, C. and Scott Myers, M. (2004) 'Community perceptions of local landscapes', *Landscape*, 21 (1): 7–18.

Ward Thompson, C., Roe, J. and Alves, S. (2007) *Woods in and Around Towns (WIAT), Evaluation: Baseline Survey*, unpublished report for Forestry Commission Scotland, Edinburgh, UK: OPENspace research centre.

World Health Organization (WHO) (1948) Definition of health, available at: <http://www.who.int/about/definition/en/print.html> (accessed 12 September 2009).

Worpole, K. (2007) '"The health of the people is the highest law": Public health, public policy and green space', in C. Ward Thompson and P. Travlou (eds), *Open Space: People Space*, Abingdon: Taylor & Francis: 11–21.

Zeisel, J. (2007) 'Healing gardens for people living with Alzheimer's: challenges to creating an evidence base for treatment outcomes', in C. Ward Thompson and P. Travlou (eds), *Open Space: People Space*, Abingdon: Taylor & Francis: 137–50.

Part V

Conclusions

Chapter 10

Challenges for research in landscape and health

Simon Bell

Introduction

This final chapter of the book aims to take stock of where research and its application have got to, and what kinds of challenges face the research and practice
community over the next few years in advancing this field. It is mainly based on
reflections arising from the preceding chapters, and represents a personal view
of the author. In that respect I hope it will also challenge readers to consider
whether my views are valid and whether they agree with my prognoses.

The book has so far been divided into four sections broadly dealing
with theory, evidence, methodology and application, although some chapters
have spanned several of these themes. It seems logical to consider them in turn,
and also to consider how each is related to the rest. While the book is limited and
cannot consider all possible theories, methods or applications, it does aim to
present a wide range and to focus on especially strong and compelling approaches
relevant to its theme. We recognise the results of relevant research are being
published at an increasing rate, and this reflects not only the general increase in
interest in the field by policy makers and others, but also the strong basis to the
field provided by the authors represented here.

Before discussing the issues raised in the book chapters themselves,
it is worth noting that many of the contributors are part of a wider research
community focusing on the general theme of nature/landscape/green space and
health (the terms vary depending on the context), and have already been involved
in a number of research, meta-research or networking projects on this theme.
This background and some of the results are worth noting because they help to
place the specific issues I shall raise later in the chapter in the wider debate at a
research and policy level.

Simon Bell

The broader research context

Some years ago, in 2004, my colleagues and I at OPENspace completed a wide-ranging research mapping project and compiled a database of high quality literature about green space, which included a number of studies on green space and health, for the UK government (what is now the Department for Communities and Local Government) (Bell, Montarzino and Travlou, 2006; Bell, Montarzino and Travlou, 2007). We updated this compilation of research and also carried out a review for the organisation Greenspace Scotland in 2008 (Bell et al., 2008). For both of these studies we were asked to identify gaps in research and to look at the main trends emerging.

The earlier study, Mapping 'green and public space research', showed imbalances in the volume and coverage of research under different topics, with physical health and environments for physical activity having received considerable recent interest (related to types of green space such as parks and gardens, natural areas, outdoor sport facilities, amenity green spaces, community gardens and urban farms). Children were the age group and play was the activity that had received the lion's share of attention in research at that time. Little research had been undertaken on green and public space in relation to physical activity in other age and social groups, a point I return to later (Bell et al., 2007). Pollution and its effect on health had also received a lot of attention, again related mainly to children. Mental health issues, such as the effect of green areas on stress, were quite limited in research coverage at that time, as was the more general consideration of well-being.

The broad findings suggested that there were several aspects worthy of improvement in future research efforts, these being:

- provision of better baseline data on how people use (or do not use) green spaces and other areas of the landscape, especially in terms of different demographic categories (gender, age, ethnicity, and so on), and longitudinal studies to test the longer-term effects of green areas on health and well-being
- a methodological/analytical need for some standardisation of data collection methods and techniques for improved comparison between datasets compiled by different organisations (and indeed internationally)
- a more refined classification of age and social groups under which research on green space and health was undertaken, such as a subdivision of the category 'children and young people'.

The Greenspace Scotland project included a systematic review of evidence (Bell et al., 2008), and included a lot of new material published since the 2004 study, which demonstrated how the subject had grown. It found clear evidence for a positive relationship between green space and health: on the proximity of green space having an effect on levels of physical activity in all age groups of people; on physical exercise in green space having a positive effect on promoting well-being and recovery from stress; and on exposure to green space helping restoration from stressful situations and behavioural or emotional disorders in children. The weakness of the body of research lies in the understanding of the mechanisms – the studies find associations, correlations or linkages, but by and large, have not established cause and effect relationships (see Chapter 3 by de Vries in this volume). Moreover, the evidence comes from a range of types of data and indicators, some much less objective than others – the preponderance of self-reported data in many studies being a case in point. While, on the one hand, self-reported data may sometimes be a better indicator or predictor of activity than objective data, on the other hand it is subject to error and may be prone to overestimation, especially with regard to levels of physical exercise.

The possibility of obtaining a psychological benefit, such as stress reduction, from viewing green space is identified in the evidence (Kaplan, 2001), but as before, the mechanism is unknown. However, the methods used in the research may create problems for the reliability and interpretation of the evidence, for example, where photographs of nature rather than views of real nature have been used (Verlarde, Fry and Tviet, 2007). We found that the evidence of proximity (the closer an area of green space is to residential areas the more likely people are to use it (Cohen et al., 2006 and Roemmich et al., 2006)) noted above does appear to strengthen the evidence base on the green space–health relationship, as does the walkability of the neighbourhood (the ease with which people can walk through it to reach a green area without encountering too many obstacles or barriers (Li et al., 2005)). There are links between health and social/community benefits when people participate in communal activity in green space but it is unclear to what extent the green space itself is a factor (Coley, Kuo and Sullivan, 1997).

A number of gaps in the evidence and potential areas for further research were identified, some of most relevance to the present discussion being:

- The need to test more widely the issue of proximity, accessibility and type of green space for different age, social, economic and ethnic groups in relation to health and well-being. This suggests there would be value in a large-scale project using mixed methods, including recording activity levels, and a conjoint-type choice experiment to test the trade-offs amongst different factors, similar to work being undertaken in the I'DGO project at OPENspace (as mentioned in several chapters in this volume).
- The impact of views to green space on mental health and general well-being expressed through increased rates of restoration, could be significant, but more work in a range of locations is needed to be able to capture enough data to form a definitive view based on good evidence.

- More work on the role of green spaces in promoting increased health and well-being through community activity is needed, in order to be able to isolate the role of green space from other aspects, such as social contact and integration.

These reviews provide a good overview of the subject area which some of the chapters in this book examine in more depth (Chapters 3–5 in particular as well as Chapter 8).

Finally, before entering a deeper discussion of the themes raised in previous chapters, it is worth mentioning recent work undertaken by a wide group of European researchers, including some of the authors represented in this book, in a project funded by the COST organisation (COoperation in Science and Technology), which looked at trees, woods and human health and well-being (in fact the extent of coverage was not just trees and woods but extended to all types of green space). This project brought together a variety of work, and a book is in preparation. One of the chapters (Van Herzele et al., in preparation) looks at how research evidence is applied in practice, and also contains a useful approach for differentiating between different life stage or social groups, in part to answer some of the issues raised in the 2004 project mentioned earlier, for example, about classifying children and young people into a more refined and meaningful set of categories for research purposes.

Finally, in reviewing the wider context of discussions and research in the field, a COST-sponsored strategic workshop took place in Cyprus in 2007 at which the issues surrounding nature/green space/trees and forests and health were discussed by a multidisciplinary group from around Europe. A number of recommendations were made, among which those of particular relevance to this book are (Nilsson, Baines and Konijnendijk, 2007):

- The salutogenic (that is, positive) effects of nature on human health and well-being need wider recognition. So far, relationships between environment and health have mostly been considered from a 'negative' perspective, for example, in terms of environmental hazards.
- A more persuasive evidence base is needed on the links between natural outdoor environments and human health and well-being. Studies should investigate the mechanisms at work, and look at effects for different target groups. Questions about 'natural health' need to be incorporated into national health surveys.
- New research should be based on a more comprehensive catalogue of existing studies. Substantial research has been carried out, but it is widely dispersed. Findings need to be cross-referenced, for example, against other health care and epidemiological research.

- Future research requires common theoretical frameworks and more robust methodologies. Application of more rigorous methods will lead to greater acceptance in medical and related fields. Common methodologies will enable cross-border comparison.
- Cross-sectoral and multidisciplinary research is needed, following a 'joined-up' approach. Studies should look at health benefits of outdoor environments, as well as issues such as food security and quality, environmental protection and social cohesion.
- Relationships between the natural outdoors and human health need to be considered in public policy. So far, these relations have only very slowly been translated into strategies for development, environmental protection, or into mainstream healthcare policy.

I return to these recommendations and the gaps identified in the concluding section to the chapter.

Theoretical aspects

It will be noted by readers that one of the key aspects of theory that runs through the book is affordances. Not only is the broad theory explained fully and clearly by Heft in Chapter 1, its use or application is also demonstrated in several other chapters, notably the work by Grahn, Ivarsson, Stigsdotter and Bengtsson, described in Chapter 5. Heft's chapter leads to the concept of affordances through the interpretation of the 'ecological' approach to visual perception. Our visual senses are, for most people, the most important ones (while not dismissing the others), so it would seem logical that some aspect of the mechanism linking landscape and health is derived from our perception of our surroundings, whether or not we are participating in any special activity. Thus the arguments leading to the utility of perception as a means of discovering what the landscape affords us, as described in Chapter 1, seem clear. This ecological view of landscape generally applies when we are in it and not just looking at it – the act of movement (which also uses other senses in a more integrated fashion than if we are looking at a scene from a distance) being a necessary aspect of this perception – the so-called 'aesthetic of engagement' (Berleant, 1992).

In other chapters, aspects of affordances are discussed and applied in practice, showing that the theory has considerable utility. I would like to speculate a little that the concept has potentially a very wide application, and that in fact it could offer a key tool in the search for the 'missing link' or the underlying mechanisms leading to the positive relationships between health and nature or landscape: as noted in the earlier section of this chapter and also in Chapter 3 by de Vries, there are linkages and correlations but no causal mechanisms identified as yet. If there is something about a green area that causes us to feel better, then there must be a mechanism linking some quality of the space to our emotions, as well as potentially to our actions. I venture to speculate that when we observe – as Ward Thompson notes in Chapter 9 – that it is common sense that 'the quality of the landscape in which we lead our lives makes a difference to the quality of the lived experience', in fact the quality of one (our lives) is contingent in many (but not all respects) upon the accumulated affordances provided by the landscape.

When discussing 'supportive features' that help older people to get outdoors, this is another way of describing a specific set of affordances; and when Little discusses personal projects in Chapter 6, the aspects that make it possible to pursue a project are clearly linked to a set of affordances unique to an individual or a group undertaking a specific project (also as used in the project on older people described by Ward Thompson). Perhaps the highest degree of direct application is to be found in this volume in the design of play areas for children described by Moore and Cosco in Chapter 2 and in the therapeutic garden at Alnarp as described by Grahn and his colleagues in Chapter 5. The observational techniques used to understand how children at play uncover those aspects of a play area offering more or less play value clearly provide a window into the affordances of that particular landscape type. At Alnarp, the concept of the different landscape rooms with varying built-in features aimed at providing specific affordances provides a glimpse of how affordances can be used in practice by designers.

When affordances are discussed they are mainly about what the environment affords us when we are undertaking some activities; in other words, often a positive set of features, such as a rock which provides an affordance for sitting or a grassy slope which provides an affordance for rolling down. This is somewhat the same concept as supportive features. However, affordances can also be negative, and there is not necessarily any way of clearly separating features that prevent us doing something – a bench that is too low for an old person to sit on is a negative affordance for them while it may be fine for a younger person – from the positive affordances. A wide-open space may offer affordances for playing games or seeing open views, but for a person with agoraphobia it might be a frightening prospect. The observational techniques of children's play areas described in Chapter 2 also allow for the identification of negative affordances.

Part of the reason a natural area contributes to stress reduction or to attention restoration could therefore be that it lacks many of the negative factors presented by stressors found in other settings, such as noise, traffic, concern over personal safety, as well as the affordances for meditation or contemplation provided by quietness, soothing sounds or attractive plants. Clearly this has limitations, and I do not want to stretch the application too far; when stressors are not associated with the physical environment – when they are social factors and problems such as chronic depression suffered by the clients using the healing garden at Alnarp – the factors the people are escaping from which triggered their condition may be hidden or difficult to define as being connected to the environment. However, when it comes to physical activity and using places, it is known that the absence of negative features is as important as the presence of positive features (or affordances).

In economics, it is normal to talk about values of commodities, goods or services in different ways – as use values, option values, existence values, bequest values and so on – and this applies to many environmental goods and services such as the landscape. I raise this idea here because it may be possible to apply it to the concept of affordances, especially to the cases where viewing nature or green spaces is seen to have a therapeutic effect. It is often noted that we value the Amazon rainforest highly even though few of us will ever visit it (and therefore make no use value of it) because it has an existence value – we want to know it is still there – and an option value – it may supply many new drugs not yet discovered, for example. If we can see a landscape from a window there is only a limited immediate use value (the attractive view yields an aesthetic utility) but a big option value ('I can go over there whenever I want to and just knowing this makes me feel less trapped in this flat'), which can itself have positive effects on well-being. These values are potentially another way of describing affordances. The aesthetic value of the view is in itself an affordance –an attractive view (containing the properties described by the Kaplans such as coherence, legibility, complexity and mystery: Kaplan and Kaplan, 1989) affords a positive emotional response – while the latent affordances visible or known from other sources provide the option value. Thus it may be possible to talk about different classes or categories of affordances which affect different people in different ways and which may help account for the benefits provided by green areas. It may also be similar to the idea of the availability and actualisation of affordances used in the literature on the subject (e.g. Chemero, 2003).

While many approaches to understanding the links between green space or landscape and health try to take a population view – much of the work described by de Vries and by Conroy Dalton and Hanson is of this nature – it is clear too that there is also a lot involved in individual differences. Little's approach, for example, focusing on personal projects rather than looking at broader populations, is an example of this, and he notes a number of factors that are often not taken into account in broader studies, for example, whether a person has certain personality traits such as being an extrovert or an introvert. However, if affordances hold one of the keys to understanding the relationship between nature or landscape and health, then the way that affordances are perceived by different individuals, perhaps belonging to or classifiable as being part of specific groups, needs to be understood. One potentially fruitful route is the 'SoftGIS' method of Kahila and Kyttä, using aerial photographs of local districts and asking people to mark on them places that are important to them, as well as to fill in questionnaires which provide a spatially explicit insight into that person's affordances in their neighbourhood. This method uses a broader concept of affordances, including emotional, social, and sociocultural opportunities and restrictions (Kahila and Kyttä, 2008).

Related to the concept of affordances outlined above – though developed originally for different purposes – is the theory of so-called 'hygiene factors' (Herzberg, 1966). Herzberg, in the context of workplace satisfaction, developed a theory based on two aspects, which he referred to as hygiene factors (or dissatisfiers) and motivators (or satisfiers). The theory contends that before a person is motivated to perform well, the hygiene factors have to be taken into account – the negative or dissatisfying aspects have to be removed. By applying this same notion to the motivation for visiting green areas, it is possible to see that negative factors and perceptions (dissatisfiers = deterrents) can act as barriers to people, preventing them from obtaining the benefits (satisfiers = affordances). Research into some of these aspects is quite well known. For women brought up in urban areas, woods, forests and natural areas in general can be seen as fearful. Perceptions include fear of getting lost and fear of being attacked by strangers (Burgess, 1995; Ward Thompson et al., 2004).

Other factors that are known to affect the level of comfort people have include low evidence of management, neglected sites, the presence of litter, and evidence of perceived antisocial behaviour such as alcohol bottles, drug syringes, fires, vandalism and graffiti. According to the principle of hygiene factors, these issues must be dealt with first, in order for people to feel comfortable about visiting a place, and then to be able to take advantage of the motivating factors such as the desire for fresh air, to take exercise, to meet friends or to seek solitude, availing themselves of the positive affordances.

Without stretching the concept of affordances too far, and certainly without making claims that the theory is the answer to everything concerning the links between nature or landscape and health and well-being, it does seem that there remains a good deal of mileage in the whole notion of affordances and in applying it more explicitly in research.

There are many other theories that are mentioned by the authors in this volume and which contribute to our understanding of some aspects of the links between nature/landscape/green space and health and well-being. Grahn and colleagues discuss several, such as attention restoration theory and aesthetic affective theory, as a basis for developing the therapeutic setting in the Alnarp healing garden. The scope of meaning/scope of action theory has been developed by Grahn to explain aspects of the way the environment communicates with a person. Interestingly, he directly connects this with affordances – indeed, it is a kind of interpretation of an application of affordance theory to a specific situation (see Chapter 5).

Ward Thompson identifies several theories as informing the work undertaken at OPENspace, such as personal construct theory, place theory and human ecology theory. These help to understand how people relate to places and local environments and how they identify with them, and in many ways it is possible to see links with affordance theory, even if this was not available or considered at the time by their originators.

All these theories have arisen from a range of different fields within environmental psychology, primarily, and are generally associated with specific bodies of work by key individuals or by research groups who have applied them, reinforced them, and in some cases perhaps jealously guarded them against rival theories (such is the cut and thrust of academia). It would be enormously helpful if these theories could be evaluated and their strengths and weaknesses in application tested (whether in research design, the interpretation of results or the application of results) to see whether the undeniable connections between them can be recognised and their limits described. It might help to refine or develop further theories, which help to explain more about the causal relationships between landscape/environment/green space and health.

Evidence on the relationship between landscape and health

Three chapters cover this in different ways. De Vries looks at four categories of potential mechanisms linking nearby nature to health. The first of these is the most direct as it concerns a physical agent, pollution, causing ill-health by the clear mechanism of triggering allergic responses and asthma in people, and identifies ways of reducing it using trees to filter particulate matter out of the air. However, this is notable for the low degree of effect, and is more or less dismissed as a primary mechanism. The other three are less tangible, in that the mechanism is not the result of a direct cause and effect in the way that pollution is. These sections refer to the evidence, which comes from the literature, and also from the author's own studies. In terms of reducing stress and mental fatigue, for example, the relationship is known to be there from the evidence, but the causal mechanism is not understood – as de Vries notes in his introduction, correlation does not equal causation. The same is true for stimulating physical activity, where there is no apparent causal mechanism in nature that stimulates greater physical activity. When it comes to facilitating social contacts and cohesion, however, there is a surprise since it is the least researched aspect but the evidence for nature being a mediator is the most convincing to date.

The second chapter looking at the evidence is that of Bull, Giles-Corti and Wood. They note the importance of population-based approaches and research focusing on everyday environments. They note that there needs to be a supportive landscape for physical activity, and identify that many aspects of the layout of urban residential areas are not conducive to regular physical activity. They also find that some kinds of activity are related to different environmental properties. They present a number of wide-ranging and very interesting challenges for research in the field.

The third chapter is that of Grahn and his colleagues, looking at the very specific aspects of therapeutic landscapes, where the careful evaluation of the progress of clients using the healing garden shows convincing evidence of the special settings designed for the purpose contributing to the improvement in mental well-being.

One aspect I would like to discuss further here relates to the physical aspects of the landscape or neighbourhood. This is because de Vries proposes that an instrument to assess the restorative potential of a (green) environment based solely on its physical characteristics should be developed. Bull and colleagues also identify a need to develop measures of the urban environment, among other things, noting the potential offered by GIS to do this, and making use of different audit tools. It seems that the potential is there to do so but we need to know more about what we can measure in so-called objective ways. Since the environment, as noted by Ward Thompson in Chapter 9, offers different barriers or supportive features to different people, surely it is important to look at what features are important to whom and then to measure them, and to seek correlations between aspects of the landscape and the behaviour of the residents. It seems that the SoftGIS of Kahila and Kyttä mentioned earlier neatly bridges this gap by capturing the values and affordances in an area. If this could be linked with audits and walkability indices, for example, a much more comprehensive way of uncovering the mechanisms might be found. It would undoubtedly be more complicated but also more likely to discover something new.

De Vries puts forward some suggestions for how green areas in a neighbourhood might be organised, taking him into the territory of landscape design, which I shall come on to when considering Ward Thompson's chapter in particular. The ideas appear to run into some problems when attempting to design places that meet many different needs. This relates to something Harry Heft noted in his chapter:

> that an action-based approach highlights the properties of environments that are engaged by users, pointing to properties that are 'where the action is'. Environments offer an abundance of relational affordance properties, some of which might be realised by particular users at a given time.
>
> (Heft, Chapter 1, this volume, p.31

As a result, tools such as SoftGIS can help to uncover what the residents of a particular neighbourhood use places for, what negative features there are, and how new supportive features that meet the needs of the residents can be incorporated into the design and layout of places. Understanding the behaviour patterns is also possible using either a personal project and/or a conjoint approach (see Little in Chapter 6, Aspinall in Chapter 7 and Ward Thompson in Chapter 9).

Both de Vries and Bull and colleagues discuss the role of the social environment – de Vries exploring the role of green space in facilitating or supporting social contacts and cohesion, and Bull and colleagues raising the issue of how to incorporate measures of both the urban and social environments, along with physical and psychological health outcomes, so as to be able to understand better the relationship and the role of the one affecting the other, with obvious implications for planning and design. There are methodological challenges here. Ward Thompson also notes the complexities of describing and classifying the landscape with its multiple scales and dynamic nature, and relating this to measures of the social environment. This issue reflects the division among researchers to date – those who focus on the people and those who look at the landscape. Clearly, if we wish to understand more fully the mechanisms and causes behind the relationships between landscape and health, a more joined-up approach would help, as would the use of mixed methods in research. A good example is the space syntax method described by Conroy Dalton and Hanson, which currently only looks at the physical layout of a city or green area, and makes good predictions about which places will be used the most. These authors themselves point out that the way forward for space syntax is to include an element of environmental psychology input which attempts to elicit the affordances of the landscape. This might include a range of methods of data collection, including self-reporting and observation. Thus it seems that most people are in agreement about this need, as Ward Thompson puts it, to shine the spotlight on both environment and people together.

In conclusion to this section, it seems that while the evidence of a positive relationship between environment/green space/landscape and health increases, we are really no nearer to knowing how any cause–effect mechanism works. A promising area is to explore the two constituent parts of people and environment together, focusing on the affordances which, as Heft notes, are something that somehow forms a combination of the person and the environment, and then looking at the characteristics of the people on the one hand and the environment or landscape on the other. It may be that also focusing on the supportiveness of the landscape for social contacts and cohesion will show that this is the necessary precondition (a hygiene factor?) for making a place more likely to be used for physical exercise, for example.

Another promising approach to testing out the difference between associational and causal influences is through the use of a statistical technique known as Structural Equation Modelling (Pearl, 2000). This allows us to build a series of hypothetical models that we think might explain a dataset. We can then test the models to find which comes closest to fitting the available data through one-way (causal) or two-way (associational) relationships between variables. Peter Aspinall at OPENspace has begun to explore this avenue of research.

Methodology

The section in this volume on methodology contains chapters discussing personal projects, by Little, and conjoint analysis, by Aspinall. In addition, there is discussion on the use of observation and behaviour mapping (Moore and Cosco, Chapter 2), approaches based on statistical analysis of population data in relation to spatial analysis of green areas (de Vries, Chapter 3), the use of walkability and other scales (Bull et al., Chapter 4), space syntax (Conroy Dalton and Moore, Chapter 8) and a range of examples including many of these plus aspects of design research by Ward Thompson (Chapter 9). Design research can also be considered part of the approach in the healing garden work discussed by Grahn and colleagues in Chapter 5. What these examples all show is the methodological complexity of work in this area and the inadequacy of any single method in isolation. The methodological challenges are significant. Some were identified in the reviews and gap analyses mentioned in the earlier section of this chapter, where the wider research context was summarised.

A starting point is the level of evidence needed to convince the people that matter – primarily the people who demand a high level of evidence and who, for example, are used to large-scale randomised controlled trial experiments, especially those from the medical professions. While this demand is not ubiquitous – there are examples where randomised control trials are not needed and where the evidence using different methods is acceptable – it remains a major challenge for the field under discussion here, noted by Ward Thompson in Chapter 9, and has been highlighted in, for example, the results from the COST strategic workshop (Nilsson et al., 2007). Some approaches, such as the use of randomised control trials, may be more difficult to conduct in the field under discussion here (although work by University of Strathclyde and OPENspace has shown that they can be successful: Scottish Physical Activity Research Collaboration, 2009), so that more work is needed not only on the development of robust methods but also on persuading more of the medical world to accept different kinds or standards of evidence from those they are used to.

In any studies looking at the salutogenic effects of the outdoors on people at the population level, as opposed to the individual, it is always necessary to obtain baseline data against which to measure the effects of exposure to different conditions. This has been underlined by Bull and colleagues in Chapter

4. The challenges include obtaining data on potential sample populations and all the issues of privacy and ethics, especially when dealing with children. The practicalities of measuring against baselines over a long time period and the control of a range of demographic and environmental variables are extremely difficult, as noted by de Vries in Chapter 3.

Controlling for a range of variables is also complex in several ways (as noted by Ward Thompson in Chapter 9) because the relationship between environment and health works differently for different people. This may relate to their life-stage, to different lifestyle parameters or to their social context. De Vries notes that the more control is made for these independent variables within the sample, the less easy it may be to isolate the significance of the dependent variable under exploration, suggesting the need for larger sample sizes so as to obtain larger subsets in which any differences between the various life-stage groups are likely to be statistically significant.

Bull and colleagues also raise the issue of maintaining response rates. This is a major challenge when behavioural changes such as increasing amounts of exercise are under investigation, as well as aspects connected with psychological health (where time spent in nature or a healing garden is part of the 'dose') or where social contacts and cohesion are also being explored. There are a number of methods that have been tried – incentives of various kinds – to maintain response rates for the duration of a particular study and perhaps beyond, but more work will be needed, especially if very long-term studies are to be undertaken which are more likely to provide the evidence of sustained impacts on health of various interventions, for example, and where long-term commitment by participants is needed. When approaches such as action research are more likely to be adopted, as being practical and cost-effective, this aspect becomes even more important (as does the issue of baseline data). It is possible that the personal projects method described by Little in Chapter 6, although not so easily adapted to larger populations (yet still applicable for groups such as demonstrated by Ward Thompson for the I'DGO project), may help to improve the maintenance of response rates, especially when accompanied by supportive measures to encourage participants. There may be more of a problem in providing effective supporting measures when there are larger numbers of people in the samples.

In many of the studies mentioned by de Vries and also reviewed in the work described at the beginning of this chapter, the measurement of the dependent variable, be it physical activity levels, changes to mental health or increases in social integration, can be more problematic than for conventional medical trials. This is in part because of measurement instruments, especially of the self-report variety, which have been common in the past and remain popular. Objective measures are often seen as being much more reliable and trusted, as well as being more tractable to quantitative analysis, than qualitative data. Physical activity may be easier in this respect because, as noted by Bull and colleagues in

Chapter 4, pedometers or accelerometers are quite acceptable measurement instruments. However, self-report methods are still needed in many projects, in part because they are the only way of obtaining some data (on how people feel, for example), so that improvements in how these data are collected, using better questionnaire instruments to try to overcome problems of overestimation, for example, are likely to help the evidence obtained from them to be more acceptable. When working with children, this problem of measurement becomes more serious – small children can be fitted with pedometers but cannot fill out questionnaires, nor do they respond well to interviews. The observation and behaviour mapping method described by Moore and Cosco is a very useful alternative, and can be used in other circumstances as long as the sample sizes are not too big and the territorial limits for the study are not too extensive – a whole neighbourhood raises practical problems for observation and behaviour mapping which are not an issue in a smaller children's playground, for example. The SoftGIS method may be a good compromise here because it combines behaviour mapping with self-reporting and some quantitative data collection.

Methods of research that attempt to predict behaviour in the context of changing environments or other factors have also been of interest. The conjoint approach described by Aspinall and used in several projects undertaken by OPENspace and partner organisations offers many benefits. While this method was developed initially for marketing purposes (but probably because of this), it is very good at discriminating between a number of different factors that people have to choose amongst and make trade-offs between when making decisions, whether it is about buying a house, choosing where to live or deciding which of two parks is a better one to visit. By mimicking the real-life decisions, such approaches demonstrate both the complexity of decision making and how real-life decisions are contingent upon other factors not necessarily apparently connected to the issue under consideration.

The discussion of methodology has so far concentrated on the people part of the equation linking health and landscape. The other main dimension is that of the landscape or environment or green space itself, in relation to the way people perceive it, use it and obtain benefits from it. Several of the chapters are concerned with this. De Vries discusses research where green areas were evaluated using GIS, and spends the last part of his chapter discussing what landscapes might need to be like to provide benefits that fall into the four categories he reviewed, showing that, at a relatively basic level, it might be the case that different environmental layouts offer some but not all benefits.

Grahn and colleagues spend considerable time describing the design of the sections of the healing garden at Alnarp, which have received careful design so that they present specific affordances as part of the therapeutic process offered there. In this respect, the landscape design is of key importance as part of the methodology. In the case of children's play areas, Moore and Cosco also show how the spatial layout and content of the play areas have a direct relationship with children's play and the use children make of different elements for different types of play. Behaviour mapping correlated to the landscape seems to be another good way of combining the people and the landscape. Ward Thompson also shows how landscape characteristics can be seen as important factors for older people visiting parks, for example, thus influencing the way a future park is designed. All these methods involve some sort of design intervention, and mean that there is some control of the variability in the setting where different behaviours take place.

When it comes to evaluating environments or landscapes that are not specifically designed as spaces for recreation or play but happen to be the broader living environment, including streets and unplanned natural or semi-natural areas, then the landscape variables are less easy to describe and evaluate. The method that is most developed in this regard but – perhaps ironically – does not necessarily involve people in its application (although it was developed from observing patterns of people's use of spaces correlated to measurable features of those spaces) is space syntax, described by Conroy Dalton and Hanson in Chapter 8. Thus there are a number of tried and tested ways of describing landscapes but there remain some methodological issues yet to be resolved.

The use of GIS is mentioned frequently, and there are some challenges in how to use it most effectively. Bull and colleagues raise some issues such as the validity of the datasets and their stability over time – in longitudinal studies the environment may change quite considerably over the time duration of the research project, and have a marked effect on the results. The GIS dataset needs to be kept up to date with these changes. Scale issues, resolution of data and the way the data is described and classified also need further work. Datasets may originate from sources where the data was not collected for the purpose of the research and may not describe the environment in the most suitable way. For example, data on green areas may have been collected by ecologists and classified by habitat type, whereas for a designer a different classification such as height, species or spacing of trees may be more useful. The street network (for vehicular traffic) may be the available dataset for studying how people move throughout urban areas, but research may be more interested in the pedestrian network, which may be quite different. The scale issue is also reflected in the resolution of the data, such as the level of detail at which polygons are drawn to show different details that people would see on the ground. For example, if the data is from a large area, clumps of trees may be defined as simple polygons whereas, at the level of evaluation in the field, more complex and detailed shapes may be needed in order to relate behaviour to settings. SoftGIS (Kahila and Kyttä, 2008) and the use of aerial photographs may help to overcome this.

Conroy Dalton and Hanson summarise their chapter with the observation that:

the way forward should include a synthesis of three types of expertise: an ability to objectively quantify natural spaces (the contribution of space syntax), environmental/cognitive psychology methods of, for example, verbal protocols and other forms of self reporting in order to elicit the types of affordances provided by the natural landscape and knowledge of the landscape itself, providing structured methods of classification and evaluation.

(Conroy Dalton and Hanson, this volume, p.228).

I think that this neatly sums up the general direction in which methodological development should proceed, combining many disciplines and both qualitative and quantitative methods, selecting sampling methods, survey methods and analysis methods which can be combined and compared, delivering a synergy not available by limiting the research to a single approach. This may present challenges in how the results are presented to those who need it, and may also provide challenges for finding academic publication outlets. It also suggests multidisciplinary teams of researchers who need to be creative, open minded and who can learn enough about each other's disciplines to communicate and make the theoretical, methodological and analytical connections needed to harness such a synergy.

Applications in practice: spatial structure, landscape design and landscape use

The final section of the book moves into the landscape, and looks at aspects of the structure and quality of the environment where people undertake activities, which may be improving their health and well-being. While establishing the causal mechanisms between landscape and health is challenging enough, converting the findings of research into guidance on landscapes most likely to have the greatest effect is in some ways even more of a challenge. Designers are frequently not very interested in research that seems to tell them nothing new or merely restates the obvious. Designers work very pragmatically and empirically, learning from experience of what does and does not 'work' in particular cases (according to their own, their clients' and their peers' design criteria), and applying the knowledge thus gained in their next projects. Design criticism is used to evaluate their work in the same way that peer review is used for scientific work. Landscapes – as opposed to buildings – develop over time and can easily be modified, especially in terms of planted area, grass-mowing regimes and the introduction, repositioning or removal of elements such as benches or paths. Thus it should be possible for robust research that produces surprising results (and therefore not the obvious, which will be ignored) to be implemented in many circumstances relatively quickly. Retrofitting buildings is much more complicated by comparison.

Designers also have to be sensitive to many different factors in their work – as Ward Thompson noted, a design may have to fulfil nonsocial requirements such as providing habitats for wildlife or dealing with storm water, so that an optimum design solution for all aspects may be difficult. The same is true of the client or user groups for a park, for example. People of different life stages, ethnic backgrounds, ranges of ability and behaviours may need to be considered, which may add challenges over the layout of spaces and the arrangement of component elements. This is especially difficult in a small area.

Conroy Dalton and Hanson, in Chapter 8, describe and illustrate the application of space syntax. This is a good example of a method for evaluating spaces, and with further development, should be better at describing natural areas or places with less well-defined boundaries or edges such as parks, as opposed to purely built environments. This is a tool of real value for designers who wish to evaluate and optimise their design by telling them how likely it is to promote social integration, for example, before the design is implemented. Communication between researchers and designers is therefore vital. A good example of researchers in a particular field communicating research to designers or managers is that of the Kaplans who, together with a landscape architect colleague, wrote a very effective book communicating how to apply their theory of landscape perception into designs which people were more likely to find attractive (Kaplan, Kaplan and Ryan, 1998). The combination of designers, researchers and practitioners at the healing garden in Alnarp also enables best practice in design to be communicated to the design profession. Likewise, the use of behaviour mapping and the conclusions drawn about the effectiveness of different elements and layouts for children's play areas can have a direct benefit on future designs if the findings are communicated effectively.

Ward Thompson, in Chapter 9, points out the need to understand the dynamic experience of the landscape and the way it is experienced spatially and temporally. Being able to model landscapes, to make changes to key variables and to evaluate the likely responses of users to those changes can now be achieved to increasingly sophisticated degrees using technology such as a Virtual Landscape Theatre (Macaulay Institute, 2009). This makes use of GIS data and modelling software to create a landscape that can be surprisingly realistic, and enables people to 'enter' and experience it. There are ways of capturing perceptions about the landscape – different aspect of the layout and composition, for example – and for evaluating different design options (Macaulay Institute, 2009). Seasonal changes can also be simulated to see what differences may arise as a result of these. This is likely to be a very fruitful route for helping to improve the understanding of how the 'ecological' model of perception, tied as it is to affordances and the dynamic nature of landscape experience, can be linked to the landscape structure, composition and quality, for improving design. It should also help to overcome some of the limitations of the static viewing of landscapes.

Space syntax analysis of the same layout used in the virtual model should also be possible, and enable further analysis of the landscape structure.

Engagement with users of a landscape or neighbourhood is another important route by which to improve designs, helping to find out who uses an area for what, who does not, why they do not and what might make them use it more. Participatory design, while valuable in its own right, can also be used as a mode of action research. The initial step would be to measure a baseline of community perceptions and use before any planning or design is carried out, after which the subsequent effects of the interventions are measured. This could not only improve the lives of the clients for the particular project, but also contribute to the body of knowledge of what design interventions work best and have the most cost-effective results.

Summary and conclusions

In this chapter I have reflected on the content of the earlier chapters and have tried to place their contents in the wider context of the fast-developing field of research into landscape (or environment or green space, depending on the terms used) and health (as defined by the WHO, 1948). The book, subtitled 'Innovative approaches to researching landscape and health', focuses on a selective number of key areas, particular methodological approaches and opportunities for innovation. Clearly there are innovative aspects in all of the work presented, and there are many identifiable challenges ahead for the research community. I suggest the following main challenges arise which, if addressed by researchers as well as practitioners (therapists, planners, designers), will help the research field to advance:

- Develop and refine the theoretical basis upon which the work rests. Without continual development of theory the empirical work will run the risk of lacking a grounding and the elusive causal mechanisms will remain beyond our grasp. The utility of affordance theory has been established but it, together with related theories, could be developed further.
- Strengthening the evidence base requires establishing the causal mechanisms, and this in turn needs some fresh thinking and some larger-scale, well-designed research, using more multidisciplinary methods.
- Since the issue of distinguishing between association and causal mechanisms still seems to plague the area it is worth considering how to apply structural equation modelling in order to test models arising from data.
- The methodological basis for the research is strong but there are many challenges and a number of improvements to be made by using multidisciplinary methods, improving baseline data, and solving problems of incorporating spatial and aspatial, qualitative and quantitative forms of data.

- Ways of understanding the key characteristics of the landscape that best promote better health and well-being also need improvement. Moving from static to dynamic modes of experiencing environments is increasingly possible using new technology, and enables theoretical aspects such as affordance theory to be linked more strongly to the planning and design process for landscapes.

In conclusion, it can be seen that these points are in turn reflected in the identified gaps, methodological challenges and recommendations which emerged from the mapping exercise for the UK Department for Communities and Local Government (Bell et al., 2006, 2007), the Greenspace Scotland review (Bell et al., 2008, and the COST strategic workshop (Nilsson et al., 2007) summarised in the opening section. A book such as this enables some of these themes to be explored in greater depth than a broad review, and it also allows us to focus on the areas that may be most promising for helping to improve research and to set high standards for new research excellence.

References

Bell, S., Montarzino, A. and Travlou, P. (2006) *Green and Public Space Research: Mapping and Priorities*, London: Department for Communities and Local Government.

Bell, S., Montarzino, A. and Travlou, P. (2007) 'Mapping research priorities for green and public urban space in the UK', *Urban Forestry and Urban Greening*, 6: 103–15.

Bell, S., Hamilton, V., Montarzino, A., Rothnie, H., Travlou, P. and Alves, S. (2008) *Greenspace and Quality of Life: A Critical Literature Review*, Stirling: Greenspace Scotland.

Berleant, A. (1992) *The aesthetics of Environment*, Philadelphia, Pa.: Temple.

Burgess, J. (1995) *Growing in Confidence: Understanding People's Perceptions of Urban Fringe Woodlands*, Publication CCP 457, Cheltenham: Countryside Commission.

Chemero, A. (2003) 'An outline theory of affordances', *Ecological Psychology*, 15(2): 181–95.

Cohen, D. A., Ashwood, J. S., Scott, M. M., Overton, A., Evenson, K. R., Staten, L. K., Porter, D., McKenzie, T. L. and Catellier, D. (2006) 'Public parks and physical activity among adolescent girls', *Pediatrics*, 118: E1381–E1389.

Coley, R. L., Kuo, F. E. and Sullivan, W. (1997) 'Where does community grow? The social context created by nature in urban public housing', *Environment and Behavior* 29 (4): 468–94.

Herzberg, F. (1966) *Work and the Nature of Man*, Cleveland: World Publishing.

Kahila, M. and Kytta, M. (2008) 'Web-based SoftGIS method in research and urban planning practices', in U. Bucher and M. Finka (eds), *The Electronic City*, Berlin: BWV.

Kaplan, R. and Kaplan, S. (1989) *The Experience of Nature: A Psychological Perspective*, Cambridge: Cambridge University Press.

Kaplan, R., Kaplan, S. and Ryan, R. (1998) *With People in Mind: Design and Management of Everyday Nature*, Washington, D.C.: Island Press.

Kaplan, R. (2001) 'The nature of the view from home: psychological benefits', *Environment and Behavior*, 33: 507–42.

Li, F. Z., Fisher, K. J., Brownson, R. C. and Bosworth, M. (2005) 'Multilevel modelling of built environment characteristics related to neighbourhood walking activity in older adults', *Journal of Epidemiology and Community Health*, 59: 558–64.

Macaulay Institute (2009) The virtual landscape theatre <http://www.macaulay.ac.uk/landscapes/> (accessed 2 September 2009).

Simon Bell

Nilsson, K., Baines, C. and Konijnendijk, C. C. (2007) 'Health and the natural outdoors', final report, COST Strategic Workshop, Larnaca, Cyprus, 19–21 April 2007.

Pearl, J. (2000) *Causality: Models, Reasoning, and Inference,* Cambridge: Cambridge University Press.

Roemmich, J. N., Epstein, L. H., Raja, S., Yin, L., Robinson, J. and Winiewicz, D. (2006) 'Association of access to parks and recreational facilities with the physical activity of young children', *Preventive Medicine,* 43: 437–41.

Scottish Physical Activity Research Collaboration (2009) <http://www.sparcoll.org.uk/> (accessed 2 September 2009).

Van Herzele, A., Bell, S., Hartig, T., Camilleri Podesta, M.-T. and van Zon, R. (in preparation) 'Health benefits of nature experience in practice and research', in Nillson et al. (eds), *Trees, Woods and Human Health and Well-Being.*

Velarde, M. D., Fry, G. and Tveit, M. (2007) 'Health effects of viewing landscapes: landscape types in environmental psychology', *Urban Forestry and Urban Greening,* 6: 199–212.

Ward Thompson, C., Aspinall, P., Bell, S., Findlay, C., Wherrett, J. and Travlou, P. (2004) *Open Space and Social Inclusion: Local Woodland Use in Central Scotland,* Edinburgh: Forestry Commission.

World Health Organization (WHO) (1948) Definition of health <http://www.who.int/about/definition/en/print.html> (accessed 2 September 2009).

Index

Page numbers in *italics* denotes an illustration/diagram

23909652R00173

Printed in Great Britain
by Amazon